ORGANIZATIONAL SKILLS TRAINING FOR CHILDREN WITH ADHD

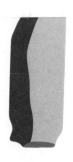

Organizational Skills Training for
Children with ADHD

AN EMPIRICALLY SUPPORTED TREATMENT

Richard Gallagher
Howard B. Abikoff
Elana G. Spira

THE GUILFORD PRESS
New York   London

© 2014 The Guilford Press
A Division of Guilford Publications, Inc.
370 Seventh Avenue, Suite 1200, New York, NY 10001
www.guilford.com

Printed in the United States of America

This book is printed on acid-free paper.

Last digit is print number: 9   8   7   6   5   4   3

The authors have checked with sources believed to be reliable in their efforts to provide
information that is complete and generally in accord with the standards of practice that are
accepted at the time of publication. However, in view of the possibility of human error or
changes in behavioral, mental health, or medical sciences, neither the authors, nor the editor and
publisher, nor any other party who has been involved in the preparation or publication of this
work warrants that the information contained herein is in every respect accurate or complete, and
they are not responsible for any errors or omissions or the results obtained from the use of such
information. Readers are encouraged to confirm the information contained in this book with other
sources.

Library of Congress Cataloging-in-Publication Data

Gallagher, Richard, (Psychiatrist)
  Organizational skills training for children with ADHD : an empirically supported treatment /
by Richard Gallagher, Howard B. Abikoff, Elana G. Spira.
      pages cm
  Includes bibliographical references and index.
  ISBN 978-1-4625-1368-0 (paperback)
  1. Attention-deficit-disordered children—Education.   2. Attention-deficit-disordered
children—Behavior modification.   3. Study skills.   4. Time management.   I. Title.
  LC4713.2.G36 2014
    371.94—dc23
                                                    2014003700

About the Authors

Richard Gallagher, PhD, is Associate Professor of Child and Adolescent Psychiatry and of Psychiatry at New York University (NYU) and Director of Special Projects at the Institute for Attention Deficit Hyperactivity and Behavior Disorders at the Child Study Center at NYU Langone Medical Center. Dr. Gallagher is a clinical psychologist and neuropsychologist. He has been treating and evaluating children for over 30 years, has played roles in developing training programs for child and adolescent psychologists and psychiatrists, and has numerous presentations and publications on clinical research to his credit. With Howard B. Abikoff, Dr. Gallagher coauthored the research manual on which this book is based, as well as the Children's Organizational Skills Scales.

Howard B. Abikoff, PhD, is Professor Emeritus of Child and Adolescent Psychiatry at the NYU School of Medicine. Previously, he was the Pevaroff Cohn Professor of Child and Adolescent Psychiatry and Professor of Psychiatry at NYU and Director of the Institute for Attention Deficit Hyperactivity and Behavior Disorders at the Child Study Center at NYU Langone Medical Center. For more than 40 years, his work has centered on the development and evaluation of assessment measures and treatments for children with attention-deficit/hyperactivity disorder (ADHD). Dr. Abikoff has published over 165 papers, chapters, and reviews, and serves on the editorial boards of numerous psychology and psychiatry journals. With Richard Gallagher, Dr. Abikoff coauthored the research manual on which this book is based, as well as the Children's Organizational Skills Scales.

Elana G. Spira, PhD, is Clinical Assistant Professor of Child and Adolescent Psychiatry at the Child Study Center at NYU Langone Medical Center. As a child behavior therapist at the NYU Child Study Center, she provided Organizational Skills Training to children and parents in all five years of the research study on which this manual is based. Dr. Spira is an Adjunct Lecturer at the NYU Silver School of Social Work, where she teaches courses in research methods and program evaluation. She has published papers in prominent journals on emergent literacy and behavior problems in early childhood and has presented workshops on the development of executive functions and organizational skills, behavior management techniques, ADHD, and emergent literacy for teachers, parents, and mental health professionals. Dr. Spira is Director of Research and Evaluation at Westchester Jewish Community Services, a leading social service agency in Westchester County, New York.

Preface

This book presents the rationale and treatment manual for organizational skills training (OST), an evidence-based intervention addressing a significant problem in children with attention-deficit/hyperactivity disorder (ADHD): difficulties with organization, time management, and planning (referred to as OTMP). The content reflects an intensive process that has taken more than a decade—a time period needed to develop, refine, and evaluate the treatment in a randomized clinical trial. Although OST is a novel treatment, it is grounded in principles derived from a wealth of research and clinical experience.

The need for effective treatments for childhood ADHD has motivated numerous research investigations. Findings from these studies have clarified the benefits and limitations of medication, intensive psychosocial treatment, and their combination. Research has supported the utility of behavioral treatments for ADHD, focusing mainly on the ways that contingency management implemented by parents and teachers can help children with ADHD carry out behaviors that are challenging for them. However, prior to the research efforts described in this book, there were no systematically evaluated assessments or interventions targeting organizational skills in elementary school children with ADHD, despite the fact that deficits in these skills can have a strong detrimental impact on functioning in home and at school. Furthermore, there was no evidence for the effectiveness of a skills-based intervention in producing generalizable improvements in children's organizational behaviors that could be transferred to and maintained in real-life settings.

Dr. Howard Abikoff's extensive participation in clinical research on ADHD assessment and treatment highlighted several overarching concerns regarding treatment goals and outcomes. These issues, which informed many of the decisions regarding the intervention and assessment procedures described in this book, include the following: (1) the short-lived effects of treatment, which tend to dissipate once treatment ends; (2) the minimal effects of treatment on important functional domains, including interpersonal and social competence and academic achievement; (3) the extent to which treatment targets are directly relevant to and reflect children's dysfunctions; (4) children's ongoing difficulties with managing school responsibilities and demands in school and at home, despite symptomatic improvements on medication; and (5) a dearth of measures and interventions specifically focusing on children's organizational impairments.

In his clinical work, Dr. Abikoff was struck by the observation that many children with ADHD did not seem to know how to get and stay organized. He and other practitioners found that these children often did not know what assignments they had for homework, did not always get home or back to school with needed papers and books, had difficulty with time management, and could not create or follow a plan for even simple projects. The children often misplaced items and had rooms and schoolwork areas that were in constant disarray. Parents reported that family arguments and meltdowns often accompanied the morning routine and homework time. Teachers also reported a notable pattern of forgetfulness in their students with ADHD. In light of these OTMP difficulties and their adverse effects on school and home functioning in many children with ADHD, Dr. Abikoff embarked on a clinical research program to assess how these problems were manifested in children's daily lives at school and home, and to determine whether these difficulties could be remediated by using established behavior therapy principles and procedures. Cognizant of the treatment issues and concerns noted previously, the researchers carried out this work with the proviso that clear evidence of usefulness and impact had to be demonstrated in a rigorous controlled study before the assessment procedures and treatment components made their way into a final manual.

To start the process, Dr. Abikoff partnered with Dr. Richard Gallagher, who had experience in creating treatment manuals, including collaborating with Dr. Abikoff on the development of a social skills intervention for the New York–Montreal Multimodal Treatment Study. From the outset, Drs. Abikoff and Gallagher had extensive discussions about the day-to-day organizational challenges that many children with ADHD face in responding to school and home demands. Important input from teachers and other clinicians helped further identify and clarify the skill sets that children needed for effective organizational functioning, and contributed to the selection of treatment targets for the treatment research manual that was adapted for the present book. However, in developing the treatment program, we recognized the importance of the "generalization problem," which is common in ADHD psychosocial clinical research. As found in numerous investigations, ranging from studies of social skills training to those of interpersonal problem solving, children with ADHD can demonstrate new skills when guided in sessions, but they generally do not show those skills in real-world situations. To address the problem of transfer of training, Dr. Gallagher drew upon his clinical and research experience in the treatment and assessment of ADHD. It was determined that OST should focus on building skills that can be linked to easily recognizable situations and are directly relevant to children's daily functioning at school and home; that skills should be practiced extensively; and that skills should be prompted and praised in order to assure their use in appropriate situations.

The initial development of assessment measures and the creation of OST were supported by a grant from the Leon Lowenstein Foundation and a National Institute of Mental Health (NIMH) R21 Treatment Development grant (No. MH62950). The successful pilot test of OST was followed by a large-scale randomized clinical trial supported by an NIMH grant to Dr. Abikoff (No. MHR01074013). These studies, which are detailed in Chapter 1 of this book, indicated that OST had a strong effect in improving the home and school lives of children and their families right after treatment was provided—and, notably, into the next school year. This was an exciting development that provided support for a new evidence-based tool in the treatment of children with ADHD. Refereed presentations at national conferences, peer-reviewed publications, and responses by colleagues in the field encouraged us to make the OST intervention widely available.

Once the results of the randomized clinical trial were known, we began preliminary discussions with Kitty Moore of The Guilford Press to see whether we could make the manual available to a wider audience. She was very receptive and helped us on the path of making the work as accessible as possible. To help "translate" the research protocol into a user-friendly treatment manual, Dr. Elana Spira joined the team. Throughout the randomized clinical trial, Dr. Spira was one of the primary study therapists at our New York site. Her experience in implementing the intervention with a variety of cases contributed significantly to this treatment manual. Her translation of session content, helpful hints, and suggestions for variations in treatment are well informed by her practical experience in implementing OST and other behavioral treatments.

As this brief history illustrates, our intention is to offer an intervention guide that we hope can meaningfully alter the lives of children with a significantly impairing chronic condition. If clinicians find that the guide contained in this book can be practically and successfully implemented, our goal in disseminating this material will have been achieved. We hope that this book enables therapists, parents, and teachers to help children who struggle with organizational demands.

A few words on our use of pronouns in the text are in order. To avoid awkwardness, we try to alternate between "he" and "she" whenever gendered pronouns are necessary. After our broad overview of the OST program in Chapters 1 and 2, we also switch to addressing our therapist readers as "you" in Chapter 3, where we begin our detailed descriptions of procedures.

We must acknowledge multiple people whose support and collaboration were invaluable in the process of developing, evaluating, and disseminating OST. We are indebted to the Leon Lowenstein Foundation and the NIMH for providing funding for measurement development, assessment, treatment development, and evaluation efforts, and for allowing us the opportunity to create highly talented research and treatment teams. The Lemberg Foundation supplied crucial funding to facilitate implementation of OST in real-world outpatient clinical settings. This support contributed to the development of helpful hints and adaptations to the treatment manual, which are presented in the session guidelines. For providing us with the setting, resources, and practical and emotional support for conducting the research, we owe great thanks to the New York University (NYU) School of Medicine and the NYU Child Study Center and their faculty and staffs. The former chair of the Department of Child and Adolescent Psychiatry and Director of the NYU Child Study Center, Harold Koplewicz, MD, and the current chair and Director, Glenn Saxe, MD, provided us with continued, unwavering assistance in using the Center as the incubator for this originally fledgling project.

We are immensely grateful to the dedicated, skilled research and clinical teams that made the development and evaluation of OST possible. Three research coordinators—Sasha Collins-Blackwell, for the pilot study; Robin Stotter, for the entire randomized clinical trial; and Christina DiBartolo, for coordinating efforts to evaluate the implementation of OST in clinical settings—proved doggedly determined in recruitment and daily operation of the research activities. Their time was given generously, well beyond their appointed hours. Dr. Karen Wells and Dr. Desiree Murray spearheaded the expansion of the research to a second study site at Duke University Medical Center. They created an alternative version of the intervention, made certain that we had excellent recruitment success, and established a top-notch clinical and research team for the randomized clinical trial. They were and are excellent colleagues whom we regard with great respect and affection. We enjoyed our stimulating and constructive twice-weekly conference calls with them and their team. A cadre of experienced therapists, both at NYU and at Duke, helped ensure that the treatment was delivered in a clinically sensitive and skillful manner. A large number of research assistants had a tremendous impact as they sensitively and effectively interacted with research participants, their parents, their teachers, and us.

Kitty Moore, our senior editor at Guilford, was encouraging from the start. She provided invaluable guidance in formulating the structure of the book and was consistently pleasant, patient, and thoughtful. Barbara Watkins, the developmental editor, was exceptional in altering our presentation and language, always improving what we presented to her in raw form. She truly understands clinicians and their need for clarity and constructive guidance. Marie Sprayberry served as copyeditor.

Finally, for all of our research and clinical efforts, we have to thank the children, families, and dedicated teachers who allowed us to test out our ideas for assessment and treatment with good faith, great patience, and exceptional honesty. We are grateful to them for their willingness to place their trust in the potential benefit of our unproven intervention. They went well beyond self-interest, knowing that by participating in our research study, they could possibly be providing help to other children in the future. We are humbled by their cooperation and commitment.

For all of us, our families deserve special notice. Conducting this work has required many hours pulled away from our relationships and home lives. We fully appreciate our family members' patience, their support, and their open ears in listening to our frustrations and successes throughout this long process. Without their backing and affection, this project would have been much less fun and rewarding. We dedicate this book to our families, with immense gratitude.

Contents

List of OST Forms and Handouts

TEACHER FORMS

PART I

AN INTRODUCTION TO THE ORGANIZATIONAL SKILLS TRAINING PROGRAM

CHAPTER 1

The Need for Organizational Skills Training for Children with ADHD

This book provides an evidence-based intervention designed to improve key organizational skills in elementary school children with attention-deficit/hyperactivity disorder (ADHD). Organization, time management, and planning skills are needed to meet school demands and associated tasks that must be completed at home. Without these skills, children in general, but especially children with ADHD, are at risk for school disengagement, school failure, and subsequent negative outcomes (Barkley, Fisher, Smallish, & Fletcher, 2006; Bernardi et al., 2012). Reviews of the literature; case analyses; and consultations with parents, teachers, and professionals all indicate that significantly impairing organizational problems emerge around third grade, persist into later grades, and are major contributors to poor outcome.

In childhood, organizational difficulties, such as misplacing, forgetting or losing materials, failing to record homework assignments and due dates, and not completing or handing in assignments on time not only hinder academic performance and scholastic attainment, but lead to diminished confidence and engagement in school (Power, Werba, Watkins, Angelucci, & Eiraldi, 2006). Teachers report reduced achievement in children who misplace assignments or take too long getting materials ready for in-class assignments (Diamantopoulou, Rydell, Thorell, & Bohlin, 2007; Langberg, Molina, Arnold, Epstein, & Altaye, 2011). Indeed, teachers indicate that failing to execute organizational behaviors can even hinder the academic performance of intellectually talented students (Baker, Bridger, & Evans, 1998; Clemons, 2008), as well as gifted students with ADHD (Assouline & Whiteman, 2011; Leroux & Levitt-Perlman, 2000). At home, many parents of children with ADHD affirm that organizational difficulties contribute to intense and frequent family conflict (Abikoff & Gallagher, 2009), especially at homework time (DuPaul, 2006; Power et al., 2006). Notably, organizational difficulties tend to persist into adulthood (Barkley & Fischer, 2011) and adversely affect the work productivity of adults with ADHD (Doshi et al., 2012). Marital relationships are also negatively affected by organizational difficulties, as exemplified by spouses who report significant conflicts when a partner with ADHD forgets to pay bills on time or loses important papers (Minde et al., 2003; Solanto et al., 2010). In light of the adverse consequences and chronic nature of organizational difficulties, it is critical to intervene early with children with ADHD and address their organizational impairments before they enter middle school, when organizational challenges increase and adult supervision decreases.

The cardinal symptoms of ADHD (inattention, hyperactivity, and impulsivity), in conjunction with the associated features of poor frustration tolerance and delay aversion (Thorell, 2007), ineffective social skills (Ronk, Hund, & Landau, 2011), motivational difficulties (Volkow et al., 2009), and executive functioning (EF) deficits (Barkley, 2012), contribute to problems in key aspects of functioning. Among the most prominent and well-documented functional difficulties during childhood are impaired peer relationships (Mikami, 2010), conflicts with parents and teachers (Kos, Richdale, & Hay, 2006; Woodward, Taylor, & Dowdney, 1998), disruptive classroom behaviors (Abikoff et al., 2002), and poor academic performance and achievement (Eisenberg & Schneider, 2007; Hinshaw, 1992; Sexton, Gelhorn, Bell, & Classi, 2012). Many different behavioral interventions have been used to treat these problems. Treatment approaches that primarily involve working directly with the children have included social skills training, self-instructional training, and training in interpersonal problem solving. In contrast, other treatment approaches have targeted parents and/or teachers as change agents, and include parent management training, parent friendship coaching, classroom behavior management, and contingent reinforcement of on-task and academic performance. Reviews of the treatment literature indicate considerable differences in the efficacy of these approaches, with minimal support for child-based treatments and broader evidence for contingency management procedures and parent behavior management training (Hinshaw, Klein, & Abikoff, 2007).

Until recently, few systematic treatments have directly targeted organizational functioning in children with ADHD. Rather, most efforts have focused on improving children's academic performance, productivity, and homework functioning. For example, Power and colleagues have created a homework solutions program for children with ADHD (Power, Karustis, & Habboushe, 2001; Power, Mautone, Soffer, Clarke, Marshall, et al., 2012). Implemented by parents, the intervention rewards children for staying on task, completing homework in a timely fashion, and determining what rules should be followed while completing work. DuPaul and Stoner (2003) describe a variety of school-based approaches, including the use of peer buddies and peer tutors to help students with ADHD write down assignments and pack up needed materials, and the use of daily behavior report cards to reinforce on-task behavior and turning in work. A number of reports utilizing multiple-baseline designs for single or a small number of participants have also emphasized work completion; on-task behavior in school and at home; and (at times) minimal aspects of organization, time management, and planning, with noted improvements in work completed and quality of work (Axelrod, Zhe, Haugen, & Klein, 2009; Currie, Lee, & Scheeler, 2005; Dorminy, Luscre, & Gast, 2009; Gureasko-Moore, DuPaul, & White, 2006, 2007; Raggi & Chronis, 2006).

Although many of these interventions have demonstrated positive effects, they also have empirical and practical limitations. Reports of success are often based on a small number of children, and efficacy has not been established in randomized controlled trials. Furthermore, many of the interventions cannot be easily implemented by clinicians unless they are working in a school setting. But, most importantly, the utility of some of these approaches is limited for children with organizational difficulties. For example, the success of a homework improvement plan will be suboptimal if a child does not know what homework has been assigned or has lost important materials needed for the work. In addition, even though adverse effects resulting from organizational difficulties often begin in elementary school, most interventions that have directly addressed such difficulties have focused on children in middle school (Langberg, Epstein, Becker, Girio-Herrera, & Vaughn, 2012) and on adults with ADHD (Solanto et al., 2010). These programs with older children and adults are of significant value; however, the lack of established, effective interventions for organizational difficulties in elementary school-age children with ADHD is noteworthy. The organizational skills training (OST) program described in this book addresses these issues.

OST is based on a programmatic body of clinical research that spanned more than a decade, including a randomized controlled trial (summarized later in this chapter). Designed for elementary school children in grades 3–5, OST uses behavioral skills training procedures to improve children's organizational skills. It also includes a prompt–monitor–praise–reward component for teachers and parents, as well as home-based contingency management procedures. The program is time-limited and consists of 20 sessions lasting 1 hour each and held twice weekly over 10–12 weeks. In addition to two orientation sessions for the child and parent and a concluding session, four key skills modules are taught: Tracking Assignments, Managing Materials, Time Management, and Task Planning. Chapter 2 presents an overview of the treatment program and offers guidelines for assessment. Detailed session-by-session guidelines are presented in Part II of this book. Two initial contacts are held with the child's teacher to determine the child's level of functioning in school and to determine the teacher's ability to provide direct assistance in implementing the program. If the teacher agrees to participate, five subsequent structured contacts between the therapist and the teacher are built into the program. These are described in detail in Chapter 3. Copies of all handouts and forms provided to each teacher, parent, and child, as well as forms used by the therapist, can be found in Part III of this book. In the rest of this chapter, we first review specific organizational deficits found in many children with ADHD. We then describe the development of OST, the rationale for its components, and the treatment's evidence base.

ORGANIZATIONAL DEFICITS IN CHILDREN WITH ADHD

Clinical observations, as well as functional and factor analyses, reveal that many (but not all) children with ADHD experience difficulties in four broad domains of organizational behavior: tracking assignments, managing materials, time management, and task planning (Abikoff & Gallagher, 2009). OST was designed to address weaknesses in these four key organizational skill domains, especially as they relate to school performance. The abbreviation OTMP is used throughout this book to represent organization (O), time management (TM), and planning (P) functions.

Tracking Assignments

Children with ADHD often do not systematically keep track of short-term and long-term assignments. They also do not consistently use tools for tracking assignments, such as planners for writing down homework assignments or calendars for noting the due dates of long-term assignments. Without these critical tools, children are unable to complete their assignments appropriately, and receive negative feedback from disappointed teachers and frustrated parents.

Inefficient tracking of assignments can have long-lasting detrimental consequences, especially in academic settings. In clinical interviews with clients ranging in age from 8 to 19, weaknesses in tracking assignments were highlighted as key factors limiting school success. One male client, Jack,[1] a 19-year-old college student who had been accepted to a college ranked within the top 50 universities in the United States, was asked to take a leave of absence due to multiple course failures. When asked why he had failed so many courses, he indicated that he consistently missed deadlines for handing in papers and other major assignments, because he did not note due dates on a calendar. Jack's multiple course failures cost his parents tens of thousands of dollars, as he was unable to obtain credit for more than 25% of the courses for which he had registered. Another male client, Andrew, a high school junior with ADHD, reported that he used random scraps of paper to record homework assignments instead of using the school-supplied planner. He often lost these scraps of paper and had to call his increasingly annoyed classmates to ask about the homework assignments each evening. Anne, a sixth-grade student, reported that she was overwhelmed by efforts to keep track of assignments for the five classes she had each day. She was often successful at recording the assignments for two or three of those classes, but made errors or forgot to record the assignments for the other classes. For all of these students, failure to use organizational tools effectively for tracking assignments contributed to significant academic, social, and (in Jack's case) financial consequences.

Managing Materials

Children with ADHD also have difficulty managing the materials that are necessary for completion of school assignments. They may write down the homework assignments for a given day, but forget to pack the requisite textbooks or notebooks in their backpacks, making it impossible for them to complete those assignments. They find it especially challenging to manage the multiple papers that are distributed in school. These children often arrive home with crumpled papers at the bottom of their backpacks, or return to school without their completed homework, which has been forgotten on a desk at home. They do not take the time to consider the materials they will need to complete various tasks, and find themselves unprepared for class or for completing their homework.

In clinical interviews with parents and children, problems with managing materials are frequently reported as causing significant conflicts related to schoolwork. Hugh, a fifth-grade boy, and Pam, a fourth-grade girl, told similar stories of their struggles with managing materials for schoolwork. Both children often forgot books or papers at school, forcing their parents or other caregivers to travel back to the building or call friends to get copies of missing papers. In Pam's case, devastating fights ensued when she forgot items at school. In the intake interview, she cried for 10 minutes as she recounted how much she hated those fights. She said she did not want her mother to think that she did not care about school or that she was a bad girl. Her mother stated that she hated the fighting, too, but had trouble controlling her frustration when Pam did not respond to frequent reminders to be "better organized." Hugh and his parents had similar experiences, reporting that Hugh often lost significant time going back to school or getting copies of papers from friends, forcing him to stay up late or miss beloved sport practices or games to complete his homework. His parents were not as harsh in their criticism, but were very concerned that untimely completion of assignments could cause Hugh to lose the necessary credit and grades to take advanced classes, for which he possessed the requisite intellectual abilities.

If problems with managing materials are not addressed early in elementary school, they can cause long-lasting difficulties in middle school and beyond, when the demands for

---

[1]Case presentations have been modified to protect confidentiality.

juggling materials for multiple classes increase. Benjamin, a seventh grader, struggled with the demands of managing his class materials throughout the school day. He would often arrive at a class without the appropriate books or other materials, and would have to request permission to go to his locker to retrieve the necessary items. Benjamin reported that some teachers would not grant this permission, and would penalize him for not handing in homework that he had actually completed but left in his locker. Edward, a sixth-grade student, experienced similar problems with being prepared for class; he decided that using his locker was too risky, given his tendency to forget essential items there. Instead, he carried all of his materials with him throughout the day, so he would never be without a needed item. To avoid using his locker, he carried two fully packed bags with him. His parents reported that he was experiencing significant back problems—probably because the combined weight of the bags was over 25 pounds, and he was a slight boy, weighing just 90 pounds.

Time Management

Children with ADHD also have difficulty managing time effectively, and this negatively affects their ability to complete schoolwork and other important tasks. These children typically cannot accurately predict how much time will be required to complete tasks; thus they do not plan their schedules appropriately, and are unable to complete required tasks in a timely manner. Difficulties with time estimation can cause daily problems, as children may not leave enough time for homework completion, throwing the entire evening routine into turmoil. Time estimation problems also pose significant issues in relation to long-term assignments, which must be completed over the course of several days or weeks. Children who underestimate how long it will take to complete an extended assignment often find themselves stressed as they attempt to complete complicated tasks at the last minute. In addition to problems with understanding time and schedules, children with ADHD also tend to "lose time"—by getting off task. Multiple internal and external distracters cause them to lose focus on tasks, which slows them down; parents and teachers often complain that these children "waste time" or take an inordinate amount of time to complete simple tasks.

Pam, the fourth-grade student described above, reported that homework often took her 2–3 hours to complete, even though her teacher insisted that homework should take only 45 minutes daily. Pam reported that it was difficult for her to focus on her homework for extended stretches of time; things like her brother's watching TV in the next room or her own doodling on her papers distracted her from her work, slowing her down. Hugh's parents described their frustration with Hugh's inability, even as a fifth grader, to manage the evening schedule appropriately. A babysitter watched Hugh after school and was supposed to monitor his homework completion. However, Hugh often told her that his homework would take only 15 minutes to complete, and then watched TV or played outside for an hour or more before starting his work. When his parents came home at 6:00, Hugh would often just be starting his homework, which would inevitably take close to an hour to complete. This delay in the evening routine caused significant stress and conflict in the home.

Problems with time management cause functional impairment not only in academic situations, but in daily routines. Julie, a third grader, fought with her mother every morning because Julie was never on time for the bus. Her mother complained that even though Julie's alarm clock went off an hour before the bus arrived, Julie was not dressed and ready in time. Furthermore, Julie was slow to complete her bedtime routines; her mother reported that Julie often daydreamed in the shower, which took her 20–30 minutes to complete, and then she had to be repeatedly reminded to get her pajamas on and brush her teeth. Julie's mother reported that the morning and evening hours felt like a never-ending series of arguments; both she and Julie were exhausted and frustrated by the end of the day.

Task Planning

A final organizational area that poses difficulty for children with ADHD is task planning. Children who are poor planners often do not know how to start projects, and they tend to get stuck in the middle of their work because they do not know how to complete projects appropriately. They do not exercise good planning skills, which include breaking goals down into smaller steps, obtaining the needed materials for completion of those steps, fitting steps into their schedule so that they are completed in a timely fashion, and checking work for neatness and completeness. Thus they often rush to complete projects at the last minute and hand in assignments that are missing important components. Furthermore, because they do not plan appropriately for other activities or events (such as family occasions or extracurricular activities), they often find themselves unprepared for these situations, because they have failed to consider items that might be needed or steps that should have been taken.

Both Hugh and Pam received multiple long-term assignments that required extended work over a period of several days or weeks, such as book reports, biographies, and science projects. Their parents reported that Hugh and Pam were often paralyzed by fear of these assignments, not knowing how to get started or what steps were required to complete these assignments. They would become more anxious as deadlines approached, and their parents would end up putting in hours, sometimes the night before a project was due, helping the children put together a subpar product. Hugh's teachers were especially disappointed in the poor-quality work he handed in, as they knew he was intellectually capable of doing better work. However, Hugh simply did not know how to plan appropriately to complete assignments that required sustained effort over an extended period of time.

Jack, the college student who failed multiple courses, reported that poor planning significantly impaired his ability to work productively in a university environment. He was unable to spread out the steps for studying for exams or completing papers and projects. Without his parents there to organize him, as they had done throughout elementary and high school, Jack was unable to plan a schedule that would allow him to complete all of the steps necessary for his course assignments.

Tom, an eighth grader on a traveling swim team, reported that poor planning caused problems for him in the team's activities. He was responsible for packing his swim bag before each practice, and he often forgot to include all of the equipment he needed. He often had to borrow items for practice or call his mother to bring him needed items. His inability to plan ahead and consider what might be needed caused stress for him, the members of his swim team, and his parents.

POSSIBLE CAUSES OF CHILDREN'S OTMP PROBLEMS

The causes of children's OTMP difficulties have not been fully established. It is likely that the cardinal symptoms of ADHD contribute to these problems. For example, daydreaming while the teacher describes the homework assignment can result in a child's not writing down the homework, and attending to a conversation with a peer while packing up can lead to materials' being misplaced or overlooked. Inattention can even interfere with the learning of OTMP routines, so that, for instance, teacher instructions on how to write down assignments or how to use a planner may be missed if a child is attending to something else in the classroom. Impulsivity, manifested by rushing, can also lead to OTMP problems. Examples include making errors while writing down instructions in a planner, skipping important steps when working on a long-term assignment, or leaving important materials at school or at home while rushing to catch the bus.

The potential impact of ADHD symptoms on OTMP functioning suggests that a treatment targeting the former, such as stimulant medication, might improve functioning in both areas. To address this issue, a small, placebo-controlled, crossover study evaluated whether the use of stimulant medication in medication-naïve children with ADHD and OTMP difficulties would improve ADHD symptoms and OTMP functioning (Abikoff et al., 2009). Significant medication effects were found for parent and teacher ratings of ADHD and OTMP behaviors. However, OTMP scores were not normalized for 61% of the children, who continued to show impairments in OTMP functioning while on medication. The study findings, which suggest that medication may be helpful in ameliorating OTMP difficulties in some but not all children with ADHD, are in accord with clinical observations that some stimulant-treated children with ADHD continue to present with significant OTMP problems (Abikoff & Gallagher, 2003).

It is also conceivable that OTMP difficulties are behavioral manifestations of EF deficits in children with ADHD, and stem from impairments in inhibitory control, delay tolerance, working memory, time perception, and self-monitoring (Barkley, 2006; Pennington & Ozonoff, 1996). For example, deficits in working memory in general, and visual–spatial working memory in particular (Martinussen, Hayden, Hogg-Johnson, & Tannock, 2005), could affect children's storage and recall of verbal information and instructions and could impede their recall of where essential supplies and materials have been placed (Reck, Hund, & Landau, 2010). In addition, poor time estimation (Sonuga-Barke, Bitsakou, & Thompson, 2010) could interfere with children's ability to determine how long it takes to complete tasks, resulting in problems with setting schedules to meet deadlines. It has been suggested that these EF deficits hinder self-regulatory behaviors, and interfere with organizing actions and planning (Willcutt, Doyle, Nigg, Faraone, & Pennington, 2005).

EF is addressed in more detail later in this chapter. However, it is important to point out here that, notwithstanding the presumed neuropsychological underpinnings of OTMP dysfunction, the relationship between performance on neuropsychological measures of EF and measures of daily life activities is quite low, with correlations typically ranging from 0 to .30 (Barkley & Murphy, 2011). These findings call into question the ecological validity of these EF measures and suggest that they assess functional constructs with little relationship to real-world behavior (Barkley & Murphy, 2011). These findings are also reflected in the goals and intentions of OST. Namely, the OST intervention is not intended to target and change putative aspects of EF underlying ADHD. Rather, to the extent that these EF deficits are present, our position is that through OST, children can be taught to minimize their functional consequences.

OST TREATMENT MODEL: RATIONALE AND THEORETICAL ASSUMPTIONS

The OST intervention primarily relies on the use of behavioral skills training procedures to improve children's organizational skills and enhance their OTMP functioning. The initial impetus for OST derived from our clinical work with children with ADHD who had organizational difficulties. We were struck by two observations. First, it became clear that OTMP difficulties had adverse effects on children's academic functioning, as well as their confidence and their engagement in school, homework behaviors, and family relations. Second, we observed that many youngsters with OTMP difficulties appeared to lack the relevant knowledge and specific skills to organize their materials, manage their time, and plan their work effectively. Their organizational abilities were compromised because they did not know what behaviors to use in specific situations, and/or they lacked the proficiency to use the behaviors effectively and efficiently. Moreover, many of the children could not state what they would do in response to organizational demands or demonstrate effective OTMP behaviors, even when told what to do.

We considered that these difficulties were primarily a result and reflection of OTMP skills deficits. As such, we deemed that an appropriate intervention had to emphasize behavioral skills training procedures to facilitate the development and use of effective OTMP behaviors. In addition, to increase children's motivation to participate in treatment and to facilitate training, skill usage, skill acquisition, and learning, several basic behavior modification elements and principles are incorporated into the OST program. These include a prompt–monitor–praise–reward component for teachers (see Chapter 3) and parents (see Session 2), and home-based contingency management procedures as described in the Part II treatment sessions.

INTERVENTION DEVELOPMENT

Developing a Measure of OTMP Functioning

Because there was a lack of validated, normed measures that assessed children's functioning on a wide range of ecologically valid behaviors reflecting OTMP demands at home and school at the time OST was being developed,[2] we focused on developing such a measure. Our intention was that the availability of this kind of measure would (1) assist in treatment development by providing information on the various domains and their associated behaviors that characterize children's OTMP functioning; (2) yield age- and gender-based normative scores indicating typical levels of OTMP functioning; (3) establish cutoff scores signifying problematic functioning in the clinical range, which could be used to identify children in need of treatment; and (4) enable evaluation of change in children's OTMP functioning by assessing their skill levels before and after treatment.

To this end, we developed the Children's Organizational Skills Scales (COSS), with versions for parents and teachers, and a self-report version for children. The questionnaires assess a child's functioning on a 4-point rating scale, ranging from 1 = "Hardly ever or never" to 4 = "Just about all of the time." They contain items describing a wide range of situations at home and school that call for OTMP behaviors, as well as items assessing how much interference in functioning and conflict result from the child's OTMP difficulties. The initial COSS dataset consisted of teacher ratings of a representative sample of over 900 third- to eighth-grade general education students attending schools in the New York metropolitan

---

[2]Other measures that assess aspects of OTMP functioning include the Behavior Rating Inventory of Executive Function (BRIEF; Gioia, Isquith, Guy, & Kenworthy, 2000) and the Comprehensive Executive Function Inventory (Naglieri & Goldstein, 2012).

area (Abikoff, Gallagher, & Alvir, 2003). In addition, parent ratings of 138 students in this sample were obtained, as were self-ratings provided by these 138 children.

To broaden the normative database, COSS ratings from teachers, parents, and children were subsequently obtained on a larger national sample. Confirmatory factor analyses yielded the same primary factor structure obtained on the initial 2003 COSS dataset (Abikoff & Gallagher, 2009). Specifically, three factors were identified, with item content considered to reflect Memory and Materials Management, Task Planning, and Organized Actions. Memory and Materials Management contained items that indicated problems in recalling assignments, forgetting needed materials, losing needed materials, and losing track of due dates. Task Planning items reflected problems in timely completion of tasks, not knowing how to start on tasks, not being able to follow a schedule even when one had been created, and rushing to complete tasks, which often results in messy work. A set of proactive behaviors, such as using calendars, making outlines, and using folders for needed papers, constituted the Organized Action factor.

The psychometric properties of the COSS (Abikoff & Gallagher, 2009) include important validity data, which confirm earlier findings (Gallagher, Fleary, & Abikoff, 2007) that the scales differentiate children with ADHD from typically developing children. Notably, although these group differences are marked (OTMP problems are significantly greater in the group with ADHD), a *majority* (slightly more than 50%), but *not all* children with ADHD have impairing OTMP problems. This finding has important clinical implications, and speaks to the target population that OST is intended for—namely, children with ADHD who have demonstrable OTMP difficulties.

Rationale for the Treatment Components

OST was developed and pilot-tested in a treatment development grant provided by the National Institute of Mental Health (NIMH). In addition to the organizational domains identified by the COSS, a functional analysis of school demands for elementary school children indicated that tracking assignments was another key aspect of organizational functioning that could be problematic for children with ADHD and negatively affect their productivity and performance. Thus treatment modules were developed to address four broad organizational areas: Tracking Assignments, Managing Materials, Time Management, and Task Planning. Specific skills associated with Tracking Assignments and considered critical were recording homework in written form and using a calendar to keep track of test dates and other due dates. Managing Materials incorporated tools and routines to organize and transfer papers; develop methods for packing and transferring needed books, writing instruments, and other supplies; create reminder checklists for school backpacks and other bags (e.g., for sports, for lessons, or for going from one parent's house to another if a child had separated or divorced parents); and organize work areas and desktops. Time Management focused on improving children's awareness of time by estimating and tracking how long tasks and activities took to complete; determining when specific assignments and work on projects should be scheduled through parent–child and teacher–child discussions; and developing a personal calendar of after-school and weekend activities. Task Planning emphasized the process of systematically considering all of the steps needed to complete a task, determining how long each step should take, gathering the needed materials for each step, and reviewing each step to make certain the project was done neatly and completely by the deadline.

During treatment development, an iterative process was utilized for clinical evaluation of each treatment session. Child, parent, and teacher feedback was used to alter session content and materials that were hard for children to understand, and to determine whether the actions that were taught to children made sense and could be carried out without undue difficulty. The feedback was also used to ascertain whether using the actions targeted in treatment was effective in improving the children's OTMP functioning.

Several crucial lessons were learned in the iterative development of the intervention components. Most critically, it became apparent that treatment required working directly with the children, while incorporating extensive involvement of parents and teachers to facilitate children's skill acquisition and implementation. Developing methods for parents and teachers to support children's use of the recommended tools and routines was vital in several ways. It was observed that even the most cooperative children found the process of changing their actions and implementing new strategies a challenge; children were more likely to meet this challenge when parents utilized behavior management methods that incorporated prompting, recording, praising, and rewarding their children's efforts. It was also essential to inform teachers about the specific tools and routines children were learning to use for tracking assignments, managing materials, using time well, and task planning. Teachers had to be engaged so that they understood the sequence of treatment and knew what actions children should be prompted and praised for using each school day. Teachers were instrumental in providing parents with reports on a daily record about whether or not a child used the target actions, so that parents could incorporate school behaviors into the home-based positive behavior management program. Engaging parents necessitated providing them with instructions in behavior management prior to skills training for children, and guiding the parents in the effective implementation of behavior management throughout the remainder of the program. A separate set of procedures engaging teachers was also developed.

During initial work with the children in skills building, two further lessons were learned. First, it became clear that many of the children were highly sensitive about their organizational problems. They had often received many requests simply to "remember" to engage in tasks (e.g., writing down assignments or storing papers in backpacks) from parents and teachers, who could not understand why these actions were so difficult. In many cases, arguments, reprimands, and punishments resulted when children showed persistent problems. Parents and teachers sometimes wondered whether the children were doing poorly on purpose, in order to avoid work. The children often believed that there was something terribly wrong with them; they could not understand why they could not engage in simple routines that other children seemed to manage easily. Thus parents, teachers, and children were all frustrated by the children's seeming inability to exercise basic organizational skills.

In order to engage the children in a cooperative and collaborative process, it became necessary to remove blame from the equation. To do so, the children, their parents, and their teachers were asked to consider that poor OTMP skills were the result of factors that were not completely in the children's control. Rather than blaming the children for doing poorly, participants were presented with an explanatory model suggesting that "Glitches" in their brains were at fault, and that all persons are susceptible to these glitches. Lapses in OTMP skills were presented as the work of the Glitches (described later in this book), personified as mischievous creatures that "live" in people's brains and send messages designed to trip them up. For example, the Go-Ahead-Forget-It Glitch tells children that they do not need to write down assignments, because they will remember the assignments when they get home. However, this Glitch knows that children are prone to forgetting and actually wants the children to fail. When a child is reprimanded, the Glitch dances and laughs, knowing that its trick worked. In the first phase of treatment, children, their parents, and teachers were asked to work together to beat the Glitches. Thus an orientation component that explained this belief system was added to facilitate a good start to treatment. This form of reframing the problems that children encountered proved very successful, as children, parents, and teachers all found themselves less tense and more willing to meet the challenge of beating the Glitches. In particular, children seemed to be comfortable with this model, especially when they were told that all people succumb to the tricks of the Glitches. Use of the model clearly helped in establishing a therapeutic alliance with the children.

The second major lesson we learned pertained to scheduling of the treatment sessions. It became clear that sessions had to be held during the school year and more than once a week. Initial efforts that provided sessions during the summer months just before school indicated that children did not find simulated practice very useful. The few children with whom this schedule was tried were cooperative, but the skills did not seem to "stick" with just in-session practice. Trying to adapt summer situations for the children to practice the skills between sessions did not make the intervention relevant enough for the children, who then had to apply the skills during the school year. Moreover, even during the school year, it became evident that at least two sessions a week were needed. A schedule of once-weekly meetings did not enable the children to recall the session content sufficiently. In addition, children fell back upon ineffective routines if they were not exposed more frequently to the new skills they were learning and were unable to practice the skills between sessions that were relatively close in time. Twice-weekly sessions addressed these concerns and allowed the children sufficient guided practice to overcome ingrained patterns. In addition, more frequent contact with a therapist provided the children with needed encouragement and feedback as they took on challenges and ensured continued follow-through from parents in implementing behavior management principles at home.

Completion of this iterative phase resulted in a 20-session OST intervention that has been subsequently evaluated in a pilot study and a randomized controlled trial (described below), and that forms the basis of this book. The 20 hour-long sessions include an initial orientation session; one session devoted to training parents in the use of behavior management procedures to prompt, praise, and reward their child for skill use; two sessions on Tracking Assignments; five sessions on Managing Materials; five sessions on Time Management; five sessions on Task Planning; and a final wrap-up session to provide guidance on continuing use of skills.

Pilot Study

An initial pilot test of OST was conducted with 20 third- to fifth-grade children who met the following inclusion criteria: a *Diagnostic and Statistical Manual of Mental Disorders*, fourth edition (DSM-IV; American Psychiatric Association, 1994) diagnosis of ADHD; OTMP problems at home and/or school that were in the clinical range and were causing a high level of interference in functioning, based on Parent and Teacher COSS scores; in a general education classroom, with a teacher willing to participate in the child's treatment; IQ score of at least 85; a standard score of 85 or better on a language comprehension screen; and no other serious psychiatric conditions that would interfere with their participation or required other treatment. Children's OTMP functioning was evaluated immediately before and after treatment with the COSS, and their homework functioning was assessed with the Homework Problems Checklist (Power et al., 2006). In addition, OTMP functioning was assessed weekly by parents on a shortened version of the COSS, and teachers completed a shortened version of the COSS at midtreatment.

Results from the pilot study were encouraging and indicated that OST had important positive effects (Abikoff & Gallagher, 2008). Parent and teacher ratings of children's OTMP behaviors improved significantly from pretreatment to posttreatment, and parents reported significant reductions in homework problems. Notably, a sequential analysis of change, based on weekly COSS ratings, indicated that the timing of change in the OTMP targeted areas (i.e., tracking assignments, managing materials, time management, and task planning) almost perfectly matched the provision of skills building for the associated area. Finally, there was evidence of OST's feasibility and acceptability. All children and their parents attended at least 17 of the 20 sessions (90% attended all 20), and there were no dropouts. Parent and teacher ratings indicated satisfaction with the program, with both groups reporting that their roles and the actions required of them were reasonable.

Randomized Clinical Trial

The positive outcomes related to OST's clinical utility in the pilot study led to a large-scale, dual-site (New York University Langone Medical Center and Duke University Medical Center), randomized clinical trial of OST's efficacy in comparison to an active comparator treatment and a wait-list control group. The study was supported by the NIMH, and results were obtained on 158 children with ADHD and OTMP problems who met the same inclusion criteria used in the pilot study, with the exception that performance on a language comprehension task was not measured.

Children were randomly assigned to either OST; a second intervention, which emphasized instructing parents and teachers in the use of systematic contingency management procedures to reward the child for attaining target endpoints indicative of effective organization; or a wait-list control group. The contingency management program was entitled Parents and Teachers Helping Kids Organize (PATHKO; Wells, Murray, Gallagher, & Abikoff, 2007). In PATHKO, a social learning theory model was used to train parents in the use of positive and negative consequences to increase the frequency of their children's organized behaviors. Children were not provided with skills instruction or informed about how they should reach the targeted organizational endpoints. The active ingredients in PATHKO included the use of a home token economy; a daily behavior report card implemented by teachers; and appropriate use of negative consequences and response cost procedures. Children were rewarded for knowing what homework had been assigned; arriving home with all needed materials; turning in assignments on time; demonstrating actions that reflected planning; and other end results that were selected by parents, therapists, and teachers.

Substantial support was found for OST's efficacy (Abikoff et al., 2013). Children treated with OST improved more than controls in organizational functioning at home and school ($p < .001$). The magnitude of these effects was very high, with effect sizes of $d = 1.18$ on the Teacher COSS and 2.77 on the Parent COSS. Notably, OST's efficacy extended beyond OTMP functioning: It resulted in significant improvements in key aspects of school, homework, and family functioning. Teachers reported positive changes in children's academic performance and productivity ($p < .001, d = 0.76$) and in their academic proficiency relative to expected standards ($p < .01, d = 0.42$). Parents reported significant reductions in homework problems among children receiving OST relative to controls ($p < .001, d = 1.37$), as well as significant improvements in family relationships ($p < .001, d = 0.47$) and significant decreases in family conflict resulting from the children's organizational functioning ($p <$ .001, $d = 1.26$). Of special clinical relevance was the finding that at the end of treatment, 60% of the OST-treated children, compared to 3% of controls, no longer had COSS scores in the clinical range; that is, they no longer met the criteria for organizational difficulties required for admission to the study.

All of these improvements persisted at a short-term follow-up, 1 month after treatment ended during the same school year. More importantly, the gains achieved with OST in family relations, in OTMP-related conflicts, in children's academic performance and productivity, and in organizational functioning in school were sustained without any fall-off into the next school year. The school findings at follow-up are especially notable, given that ratings were obtained from teachers who had no involvement in and were unaware of the children's treatment status. There was some drop-off in homework behaviors and organizational functioning at home, although the level of functioning in both areas remained significantly better than pretreatment levels. Academic standing was the only outcome measure that did not show evidence of maintenance effects. Overall, the follow-up findings regarding the sustainability of gains with OST are very encouraging, given the well-documented difficulties in achieving maintenance effects in ADHD behavioral treatment studies (Hinshaw et al., 2007).

The PATHKO intervention, which focused on training parents and teachers to reward children for achieving OTMP endpoints, also had a significant impact on children's functioning. Children who received PATHKO showed similar significant improvements, relative to controls, in most of the study outcomes, with the exception of no group differences in academic proficiency scores. Furthermore, the PATHKO group was statistically equivalent to the OST group on all outcomes except for parent ratings on the COSS, which indicated significantly more improvement in OTMP functioning at home for children treated with OST ($p < .005$, $d = 0.69$).

There were several other important results from the study. First, wait-list children demonstrated no significant change in OTMP behaviors during the 10- to 12-week waiting period, which is in accord with anecdotal reports that OTMP deficits are persistent and do not change over time. Second, children's outcomes were similar, regardless of their medication status. That is, the beneficial effects of OST did not differ in youngsters who began the study on medication, compared to those not treated with medication. Third, OST was similarly effective when applied by clinicians in two geographically distinct clinical settings, providing additional support for OST's generalizability.

Although both OST and PATHKO resulted in significant improvements immediately after treatment and during the next school year, there were some advantages associated with the skills training intervention. First, parent reports indicated that children's overall OTMP functioning at home, especially their use of Organized Actions, improved significantly more with OST and continued to be significantly better than with PATHKO during follow-up. Second, children treated with OST maintained their gains in homework functioning in the next school year, whereas PATHKO-treated youngsters showed a slight, but steady increase in homework problems once treatment had ended. Third, OST-treated children improved significantly more than controls in their academic proficiency scores and in self-ratings of their organizational functioning on the Child version of the COSS, whereas PATHKO-treated children did not differ from controls on these outcomes. Finally, after the waiting period was over, the wait-list parents were able to choose which treatment they wanted for their children. They had no knowledge (nor did the investigators) of the study results and were provided only with full, unbiased descriptions of each treatment's principles, focus, and procedures. Of

30 wait-list cases, 28 (93%) of the parents selected OST for their children. These results have important clinical implications: They speak to OST's acceptability and appeal, and suggest that a treatment format emphasizing direct skill development for the children is and will be more attractive to parents in clinical settings.

OST versus EF Training

OST is a treatment that is intended to improve children's organizational abilities so that they can effectively manage essential tasks, especially those related to school functioning. As described above, there is also empirical support for the expectation that improving children's organizational functioning will be associated with concomitant benefits in other key functional domains, including academic performance, homework management, and family relations (Abikoff et al., 2013). However, in discussing OST, it is also important to reiterate what it is not. Specifically, OST is not designed or considered to be a treatment that improves overall EF in children. To help clarify this point, we emphasize several fundamental differences between OST and general EF treatment (or what has come to be called "cognitive training").[3]

First, OST primarily focuses on teaching children skill sets to meet the demands of relatively specific, recurring situations, many of which are school-related and call for organization. In contrast, EF training is more general in its approach and objectives. Specifically, as noted in a recent article on training cognition in ADHD, EF training attempts to target underlying cognitive "processes that are putatively expected to automatically govern behaviors across multiple situations, making this particular type of intervention a hypothetically broad-reaching treatment" (Rutledge, van den Bos, McClure, & Schweitzer, 2012, p. 543). Second, whereas OST focuses on enhancing skills related to organizational functioning in real-world situations, EF training primarily relies on the use of computerized laboratory tasks as a means of enhancing the development of cognitive control processes (e.g., attention, working memory, response inhibition). General EF training assumes that enhancements in underlying cognitive processes will result in "top-down" behavioral effects, which ostensibly include not only effective application of specific behavioral skills, but also the recognition of when to use the skills. Thus the implicit, if not explicit, expectation is that effective EF training will by its very nature lead to generalization, and result in wide-ranging cognitive and behavioral improvements. Unfortunately, with few exceptions, there is a dearth of empirical support for this hypothesis from randomized, well-controlled trials (Rutledge et al., 2012). More importantly, from a clinical perspective, the current general absence of evidence for behavioral improvements (especially regarding children's organizational behaviors) on ecologically valid outcome measures that assess functioning in real-world settings is especially noteworthy; it speaks to the clinical utility, or the lack thereof, in this approach.

There are likely multiple reasons why generalized behavioral improvements have not been achieved with EF training. Prominent among these is the lack of correspondence

---

[3]The term "cognitive training" as used here is to be distinguished from the cognitive training approaches used with children with ADHD in the 1970s and 1980s, which attempted, unsuccessfully, to enhance children's reflective problem-solving skills and reduce impulsive behaviors through the use of self-instructional and self-reinforcement techniques (Abikoff, 1985).

between the skills and associated tasks targeted in training and the behavioral outcomes expected to change with treatment. Another related possibility is the failure of EF training to clearly tie the use of the cognitive skills focused on in training to exact situations or situational cues outside of training, leaving a significant gap between the training context and the environment in which the skills should be used. This gap is in marked contrast to OST, which emphasizes and clearly identifies for children the connection between the settings (antecedent conditions) and the specific skills to be used in these settings; provides a rationale for and practice in how to use each skill; and teaches parents and teachers to prompt and cue the children to use each skill when needed. A third factor that may contribute to the lack of behavioral improvements with EF treatments is that reinforcement procedures are typically not used to reward the children for showing generalized behavior change outside the training sessions. In comparison, to increase children's motivation to use the skills targeted in training, OST works with the parents to provide the children with contingent rewards for implementing the skills outside the treatment setting.

In considering the relationship between EF and the clinical treatment of organizational difficulties, it is important to emphasize that there is still no consensus regarding which processes fall under the rubric of EF (Castellanos, Sonuga-Barke, Milham, & Tannock, 2006). Numerous aspects of EF deemed to be crucial have been described in theoretical writings, including attention control, resistance to distraction, behavior sequencing, response inhibition, set shifting, working memory, goal-directed behavior, problem solving, planning, delay tolerance, and temporal processing. Moreover, various theoretical models have been proposed, which differ in the aspects of EF considered to be core in individuals with ADHD (e.g., Barkley, 2012; Sonuga-Barke et al., 2010).

A more practical concern pertains to the relevance of the measures and procedures used to assess EF, and their questionable clinical utility in case identification and treatment planning in children with ADHD. A few clinical research findings illustrate these concerns. First, it is worth repeating that the ecological validity of EF measures is dubious. As noted previously, the association between test scores and daily life activities in adults with ADHD is quite low (Barkley & Murphy, 2011), and there is evidence that although some adults with ADHD have neuropsychological EF test scores in the normal range, they perform badly on real-life analogue tasks with high organizational demands (Torralva, Gleichgerrcht, Lischinsky, Roca, & Manes, 2013). A poor relationship between test scores and organizational behaviors has also been found in children with ADHD. Youngsters in the initial pilot study of OST (Abikoff & Gallagher, 2008) had COSS scores in the clinical range, reflecting organizational difficulties in daily life. However, their scores on EF tests of attention, inhibitory control, planning, and working memory were in the normal range. Moreover, although the children showed significant improvements in OTMP behaviors after treatment, the improvements were not correlated with improvements on EF tasks, and changes in EF tasks were minimal following intervention.

In summary, at this stage of development, many of the readily available tests of EF for children are not useful in assisting in treatment planning, in identifying children with OTMP deficits, or in tracking change in OTMP functioning. These objectives are better served by functional assessments of specific organizational behaviors needed for daily life activities. Additional detailed comments regarding the role, assessment, and treatment of EF in individuals with ADHD are beyond the purview of this book, and are addressed elsewhere (Barkley, 2012).

CONCLUSION

As described in this chapter, the content of the OST program was developed in the context of a comprehensive program of research. The intervention relies on basic principles of behavioral skills training, which are incorporated into the format of each session. These principles include detailed descriptions of each skill; a rationale for using the skill and for its effectiveness; modeling the specific actions and substeps that encompass implementing the skill; guided practice of the actions by the child in simulated situations that reflect those the child encounters at home and at school; and reinforced *in vivo* practice. To maximize cooperation and skills usage, OST also incorporates behavior management approaches, including the use of prompting, monitoring, praising, and rewarding skills usage. In addition, OST emphasizes an engagement strategy involving the use of a "Glitch" metaphor, which objectifies the problems that children face, facilitates collaborative participation, and helps to avoid resistance and discouragement. In Part II of this book, there are "Helpful Hints" and "Troubleshooting Note" boxes, which are based on our clinical and supervisory experience with the program. These boxes address and provide information about a variety of situations that may arise during the course of treatment, including how to maximize children's participation and how to manage barriers to treatment resulting from problematic or insufficient parental and/or teacher involvement.

Our hope and expectation is that this treatment manual will prove to be a very useful clinical tool for improving the lives of children with ADHD whose functioning is compromised by their organizational difficulties.

CHAPTER 2

The OST Program and Guidelines for Assessment

RATIONALE FOR THE SEQUENCE OF SKILL MODULES AND SESSIONS

The sequence of OST sessions has been based upon a careful review of school demands and the problems that children encounter as they attempt to meet those demands. Table 2.1 outlines the sequence of sessions. Skills training follows a logical sequence of what must be done to complete school tasks and demands. The Tracking Assignments module comes first, so that the child knows what to do each evening. Then, once a child is certain of the assignments, working on them requires that the needed papers, books, and other materials are available. Thus a module that presents skills for Managing Materials follows the module on Tracking Assignments. Knowing the details of assignments and having the required materials are essential prerequisites for Time Management; after these skills are addressed, the child can then focus on the other skills related to Time Management, including fitting tasks into a schedule and avoiding time-wasting distractions. All of the preceding skills are required for effective planning to occur. Thus, once the child has learned how to track assignments, manage materials, and manage time, the final module on Task Planning is introduced, so that the child knows how to complete tasks and projects successfully.

The sequence of skills training also reflects the increasing complexity of the skills utilized. Initially, the child is concerned with the concrete tasks of writing down information and of selecting and packing needed materials. Next, actions related to the abstract concept of time are addressed. Finally, the child develops and follows a plan by identifying and anticipating what needs to be done in the future, and, after completing steps, reviews the actions taken, to make sure that the task has been completed appropriately. Thus the number and complexity of cognitive functions increase as treatment progresses. The training sequence allows a child to be successful in acquiring more concrete skills before being presented with skills training in routines that make more abstract demands. The following sections describe the sessions and modules in more detail.

TABLE 2.1. Overview of the OST Treatment Program

Two Preliminary Contacts: Assessment of School OTMP Problems and Brief Treatment Overview

Introduction
- Session 1. Introduction: Parent and Child Orientation
- Session 2. Introduction: Using Social Learning Strategies to Motivate Skills Building (for Parents Only)

Teacher Contact #1: Teacher Orientation and Introduction to Tracking Assignments

Module 1: Tracking Assignments
- Session 3. Tracking Assignments: Implementing Behavior Management Procedures and Getting It All Down
- Session 4. Tracking Assignments: The Daily Assignment Record and the Assignment and Test Calendar

Module 2: Materials Management

Teacher Contact #2: Prompting and Praising Paper and Backpack Materials Management
- Session 5. Managing Materials: Managing Papers for School
- Session 6. Managing Materials: Review of Routines for Tracking Assignments and Managing Papers
- Session 7. Managing Materials: Introducing Backpack Checklist
- Session 8. Managing Materials: "Other Stuff" and Other Bags
- Session 9. Managing Materials: Getting Work Areas Ready to Go

Teacher Contact #3: Prompting and Praising Getting Work Areas Ready to Go

Module 3: Time Management
- Session 10. Time Management: Understanding Time and Calendars

Teacher Contact #4: Guiding Time Management with Time-Planning Conferences
- Session 11. Time Management: Time Tracking for Homework
- Session 11a (Optional). Time Management: Instruction in Telling Time and Calculating the Passage of Time
- Session 12. Time Management: Time-Planning Conferences at Home and School
- Session 13. Time Management: Time-Planning for Longer-Term Assignments and Avoiding Distractions
- Session 14. Time Management: Time Planning for Regular Routines

Module 4: Task Planning
- Session 15. Task Planning: Introduction to Task Planning

Teacher Contact #5: Guiding Task Planning with Task Planning Conferences
- Session 16. Task Planning: Next Steps—Managing Materials and Time
- Session 17. Task Planning: Fitting the Steps into the Schedule
- Session 18. Task Planning: Planning for Long-Term Projects
- Session 19. Task Planning: Checking It Out and Planning for Graduation

Program Summary
- Session 20. Program Summary: Personalized Commercial and Graduation

Teacher Contacts

A full guide with recommendations for engaging teachers in the school-based component of treatment is provided in Chapter 3.

Orientation to Treatment

The first two sessions provide parents and children with an orientation to treatment, which lays the groundwork for the positive approach used to address OTMP deficits. The first session is intended to help parents and children understand that skill development will be used to help the children improve their organizational performance in school and at home. They will understand that a proactive approach will be used to overcome OTMP difficulties, through a forthright discussion of specific OTMP skills that could be improved. The therapist introduces and reviews the Guide to the Glitches (see Handout 3), which helps parents and children frame OTMP problems in a way that is free of blame and criticism. The therapist also conducts a functional assessment of a child's OTMP problems. Session 2 provides one-on-one training to parents in the application of behavior management methods for prompting and motivating their child to consistently use the new skills taught. Parents are shown how to use the Home Behavior Record (for example, see Handout 7) to record their prompting, monitoring, praising, and rewarding of the child's specific skill use. Also during this session, a parent and therapist review possible rewards that can be used to motivate the child. This is preparation for a system in which the child earns points that can be used to obtain rewards.

During this introductory period, the therapist will hold the first of five scheduled teacher contacts, and will orient the teacher to the goals and objectives of OST and the teacher's role in treatment. Suggested content for the five teacher contacts is included in Chapter 3.

Module 1: Tracking Assignments

Sessions 3 and 4 teach the child skills related to tracking assignments. At the end of this module, children should be consistently using a simple but effective tool for recording daily assignments and noting materials that they need for those assignments. In addition, they should have a routine for keeping track of due dates and test dates on a calendar. Parents will be using behavior management methods for prompting the use of a Daily Assignment Record (see Handout 10) and an Assignment and Test Calendar (see Handout 11), and will be providing rewards for consistent use of those tools at home and in school. Teachers will be prompting and praising children for use of the Daily Assignment Record at school and noting children's use of this tool, so that parents can provide appropriate rewards at home.

Module 2: Materials Management

Sessions 5–9 focus on methods for organizing papers, books, and work areas. In these sessions, children learn and practice a new way to organize and transfer their papers, and will develop and use a simple checklist for effectively packing their backpacks. They will also learn a routine for getting work areas ready to go, so that all required materials are present and distracting items are put away. At the end of this module, children should arrive at school and home with the materials they need, and should be efficient in setting up work areas. Parents should be consistently prompting their children to use tools that help them manage papers, to pack up their items, and to manage their work areas, and should be providing praise and rewards for these actions. Similarly, teachers should be supporting children's use of these tools in school through prompting and praise.

Module 3: Time Management

Sessions 10–14 focus on teaching critical time management skills. In this module, children learn to estimate how long it takes to complete tasks and to determine when to fit tasks into their personal schedules. In addition, they will learn strategies for controlling the "Time Bandit," by identifying things that distract them and taking steps to manage those distractions. By the end of these sessions, children should be better able to estimate how much time should be dedicated to specific tasks, and should be able to set up an after-school schedule that allows for appropriate work and fun time. Parents support children's use of time-planning skills by engaging in a daily Time-Planning Conference with their children, and will provide rewards for good time management skills. In addition, teachers will prompt and record children's use of time management routines in class.

A review of a child's time-telling ability is conducted in Session 1, and the therapist will also get a sense of the child's competence with telling time by reviewing activities conducted in Sessions 10 and 11. If it is determined that a child requires some direct instruction in time telling, a supplemental session for instruction in time telling may be included after Session 11.

Module 4: Task Planning

In Sessions 15–19, children learn the components of good planning: breaking a task down into its main steps, ordering the steps, getting needed materials, fitting the steps into their schedules so that the entire task is completed on time, and checking work for neatness and completeness. Parents will prompt children to use these planning steps through the use of a daily Task-Planning Conference, and will reward use of these steps. Teachers will prompt children to use selected planning skills as appropriate, and will continue to prompt, monitor, and praise the use of time management skills in school.

Program Summary

Session 20 provides a review of all skills learned throughout treatment, and helps children think of ways to maintain use of these skills after treatment ends. Children and parents will receive an Owner's Manual for Organizational Skills (see Handout 55), which provides helpful hints for integrating organizational tools into the daily routine. Finally, children will record a personalized "commercial," which helps them to reflect upon the lessons learned from treatment (see Handout 52).

SESSION FORMAT

Each session runs approximately 60 minutes and is presented in a standard format in Part II. First, a list of the session goals for the therapist, child, and parents is provided, followed by a list of supplies and handouts needed, so that the therapist can prepare for the session. A "Session Summary Checklist" outlines the main tasks to be completed in session. The therapist can use the checklist as a general orienting tool, or can keep track of treatment implementation by using the "Yes/No" option provided for each session component. After this outline, there is a brief overview of the session content and, in many sessions, a note regarding steps that the therapist should take to prepare for the session.

The "Detailed Session Content" provides a guide to the session activities in narrative form, accompanied by suggestions on how to discuss the topic and the practice procedures with the child and parent. Narrative content in all sessions is provided to suggest ways of discussing the points with parents and children. It is not expected that the suggested statements be followed verbatim. Therapists should use their own words to make the points so that treatment fits their personal style.

After the initial orientation sessions, each session begins with the therapist's meeting the parent and child to review progress, address questions from the prior session, and briefly review implementation of the behavior monitoring and point program. Then the child is seen alone for skills building in a specific area, which incorporates instruction and practice. Instruction starts with a verbal review of the area of concern, and the therapist then leads the child through a review of current difficulties and practices in that area. Next, an explanation of the tools and routines that can be used to address the area is provided. The therapist demonstrates the use of the tools, and then the child engages in guided practice of the procedures. After several rounds of practice, the parent returns for a session wrap-up. The child is guided through the process of explaining to the parent how the tools and routines will be used between sessions. The therapist provides instructions for the parent on how the child's use of the methods should be added to the Home Behavior Record (again, see Handout 7 and similar later handouts). The therapist also provides the parent and child with needed items for completing the session homework. Finally, to close the meeting, the child is awarded points for specific positive actions that were demonstrated in the session, and the child can select a prize for the points.

In addition to the main content outlined in each session, "Helpful Hints" are highlighted in gray boxes, based upon clinical experience in providing OST. These tips for therapists address possible concerns that might arise and methods for making treatment run smoothly. At the end of some sessions, a section on "Alternative Procedures" is provided for those situations when the suggested methods do not match the child's needs or circumstances. Finally, in Sessions 5 and 11, we offer separate "Troubleshooting Note" boxes that address frequently encountered problems.

We advise that therapists become familiar with the treatment sequence and session content before starting work with new cases. Sessions are full of specific procedures that have to be completed, so a thorough review of each session before starting a meeting is also recommended. Occasionally, the activities in a session may not use the full session time. In Session 6, for example, there is a review of skills already taught (tracking assignments and managing papers). If a child is doing well with the methods for tracking assignments and managing papers, the review of these tools should not take very long. If there is time left over, the therapist may move on to the material for the next session—in this case, introducing the idea of a backpack checklist.

THERAPIST EXPERIENCE

To provide OST most effectively, therapists should have an understanding of ADHD and prior experience with parent training and behavior modification techniques. Experience in working with children who have ADHD will help the therapist understand the challenges that ADHD presents to children, parents, and teachers, and the techniques that motivate children to overcome those challenges. Furthermore, therapists will be best able to implement OST when they have a strong background in applying behavior therapy with children, in conjunction with parents and teachers. In addition, clinical observations suggest that the delivery of OST is enhanced when therapists know how to use praise and other forms of positive reinforcement in a natural way when interacting with children, and how to guide parents and teachers in using those methods. In implementations in two community clinics, experienced clinicians have been able to carry out OST after a thorough reading of the manual, followed by some practice of the in-session procedures.

CHILDREN APPROPRIATE FOR OST

The OST intervention was developed for and evaluated in children with an ADHD diagnosis who had quantified OTMP difficulties. Data from the regional and national samples of children used in the development of the COSS (see Chapter 1) indicated that children with ADHD not only had more problems with OTMP behaviors than typically developing children; they also had more problems than samples of children with other psychiatric conditions or with learning disorders (Abikoff & Gallagher, 2009). Thus, among children with adjustment and achievement difficulties, those with ADHD are most likely to show OTMP problems.

It should be noted that the utility and effectiveness of OST for children who have OTMP difficulties but do not have a diagnosis of ADHD are unknown. With this caveat in mind, it seems reasonable to expect that OST may also be beneficial to this population without ADHD. Thus, while clinicians may offer OST to children without ADHD who show OTMP deficits, they should be aware that there is no empirical support for the effectiveness of OST in this population. If OST is applied to children without ADHD, small modifications in some materials (e.g., the Guide to the Glitches, the teacher material, and the Owner's Manual for Organizational Skills) will be necessary, to remove references to ADHD. Additional alterations will be needed in how the treatment is explained to the parent and child in the orientation and second sessions. When and where the modifications will be necessary will become clear as therapists review the material.

ASSESSING THE CHILD

Assessing for ADHD

The assessment of ADHD should follow acceptable standards for determining whether high levels of inattention and/or hyperactivity–impulsivity are present and occur in at least two settings. To this end, we typically obtain information not only from parents, but also directly from teachers, regarding children's functioning in school. Although parents may be able to provide some of this information, we have found that teacher feedback provides a more complete and accurate picture of children's behavior. As described below, we also obtain information from teachers regarding the children's OTMP functioning.

Of course, a thorough psychosocial history and general medical clearance should be incorporated, befitting the standards of practice (see Pliszka & Workgroup on Quality Issues, 2007; Subcommittee on Attention-Deficit/Hyperactivity Disorder, Steering Committee on Quality Improvement and Management, 2011). This must be done in order to avoid misdiagnosis of ADHD, and to ensure that attention and behavior concerns are not the result of an acute or chronic illness or injury, or of another psychiatric condition. Rating scales that assess ADHD in particular—for example, the Conners 3rd Edition (Conners, 2008) and the Swanson, Nolan, and Pelham–IV (Swanson, 1992)—and emotional and behavioral disorders in general can provide relevant norms and be useful components of the evaluation process with parents and teachers. Structured or semistructured interviews that assess childhood mental health conditions according to formal diagnostic criteria, such as the Diagnostic Interview Schedule for Children (Shaffer, Fisher, Lucas, Dulcan, & Schwab-Stone, 2000) or the Schedule for Affective Disorders and Schizophrenia for School-Age Children (Kaufman et al., 1997), can be used to facilitate a systematic and comprehensive clinical evaluation. Given that children with ADHD are often comorbid for other disorders, evaluation for other conditions is important, because OST may not be the most appropriate treatment or may require significant adaptations under certain conditions. This issue is discussed in more detail later in this chapter.

Assessing Functioning

Once a child has been diagnosed with ADHD, it should not be assumed that the child also has OTMP difficulties. Children with ADHD are indeed at significantly greater risk for having OTMP problems; however, as noted previously, not all children with ADHD have interfering OTMP difficulties. Therefore, it is important to assess whether OTMP difficulties are present and of concern for a particular child. Although there are no established procedures for making this determination, there is a general approach that we find useful.

The first step is an initial screen to ascertain whether there are any problems or concerns regarding the child's organizational functioning at home and/or at school. In our randomized controlled trial and in clinical settings, children who have participated in OST fall into one of three categories: children who experience OTMP difficulties at home and school (the majority), at home only, or at school only (just a handful). To determine the appropriateness of OST for a given child, a brief functional assessment with parents and teachers will include a review of difficulties with (1) keeping track of and remembering assignments; (2) managing materials; (3) time management, including a discussion of the child's use of time and timeliness in completing assignments and turning them in; and (4) planning, including effectiveness in developing plans for projects, studying for tests, and handing in work that is neat and complete. Figure 2.1 provides a set of questions that can be used in initial screening interviews with the parent and teacher. The therapist can rely on the functional screening interviews with the parent and teacher to determine whether treatment with OST appears warranted for a particular child.

An alternative approach to deciding whether treatment is needed is to use rating scales to obtain specific information about the nature and severity of any organizational problems, and their impact on the child's functioning. Two rating scales that specifically assess children's organizational functioning are the COSS and the Behavior Rating Inventory of Executive Function (BRIEF). As noted in Chapter 1, the COSS, which includes Teacher, Parent, and Child versions, was used during the development and evaluation of OST. This measure allows for comparisons of children to national norms on a total score reflecting broad problems in deploying OTMP behaviors and on three factors indicating problems in Memory and Materials Management; problems in Task Planning, which include poor planning and problems with time management; and limited use of proactive Organized Actions, such as using a calendar and using separate folders for class materials.

In our research and subsequent clinical applications of OST, the following COSS criteria were helpful in identifying children with impairing OTMP difficulties. First, does the child have a total score or a single factor score that is one standard deviation above the mean on the Parent or Teacher COSS? Second, do Parent or Teacher COSS ratings indicate that lapses in memory, poor materials management, ineffective time management and planning, or low use of proactive strategies interfere with the child's functioning? In addition, parent ratings of the level of conflict experienced at home due to problems in these same four areas provide useful clinical information regarding the impact of the child's organizational difficulties, which can inform on treatment planning. Thus the COSS is directly linked to the targets for OTMP, which facilitates its usefulness in selecting cases and tracking progress.[1]

---

[1]Two of us (Drs. Howard B. Abikoff and Richard Gallagher) receive royalties from Multi-Health Systems, the publisher of the COSS.

Child's Name: _____   Date: _____

General area	Step 1. Conduct a screen. Suggested questions to guide an interview with parents and/or teachers	Step 2. Find out how much of a problem the child has in reaching these specific goals (see ratings on the right).	Not a problem—1 Moderate problem—3 Severe problem—5
Tracking Assignments	Does the child use a certain method for recording assignments other than simply trying to remember them?	Recording assignment information	1 2 3 4 5
	Does the child consistently use this particular method for recording assignments?	Consistency in recording assignments	1 2 3 4 5
	Does the child know what has been assigned for homework and when the assignments are due?	Knowledge of assignment information	1 2 3 4 5
Managing Materials	Does the child arrive home with papers, books, and other items needed to do school work?* *Parent interview only	Arriving home with books and papers	1 2 3 4 5
	Does the child turn in homework that has been completed?	Handing in assignments	1 2 3 4 5
	Does the child remember to bring back important items to school (e.g., books, notebooks)?	Returning needed items to school	1 2 3 4 5
Time Management	Does the child spend more time on assignments than seems necessary?	Completing work in a timely fashion	1 2 3 4 5
	Does the child spend more time on other tasks (e.g., daily routines, chores) than seems necessary?	Completing other tasks in a timely fashion	1 2 3 4 5
	Does the child have to rush just before things are due or just before having to leave one place to go to another?	Turning in work and getting ready on time	1 2 3 4 5
Task Planning	Does the child develop a clear plan for completing tasks at school or at home?	Developing a plan	1 2 3 4 5
	Even if a child has a good plan, does the child have trouble following through?	Executing a plan	1 2 3 4 5
	Does the child fail to check work to determine if it is complete, has mistakes, or is messy?	Checking work	1 2 3 4 5

FIGURE 2.1. Interview questions for reviewing organization time management, and planning (OTMP) behaviors.

Another OTMP assessment measure is the BRIEF (Gioia et al., 2000). The BRIEF has versions that can be completed by parents, teachers, and children, and yields scores that compare children to norms developed on a nationally representative sample. Based on its item content, the BRIEF generates scores on factors labeled Plan/Organize and Organization of Materials, which are directly relevant to OTMP functioning. Elevated scores on these factors, or ratings reflecting problems on critical behaviors when an item-based review is conducted, would indicate that a child is a good candidate for OST.

In the first OST session, an extensive functional analysis is conducted to obtain a clear picture of the organizational challenges that a child faces. It is important to point out that this functional review serves a different purpose from that of the screening interviews. The screening helps to establish whether OTMP difficulties are present and whether OST is appropriate for a child, while the detailed review in Session 1 is designed to help parents and children understand the targets for treatment and to establish that an open approach to problems will be used throughout treatment. Furthermore, an initial meeting with the teacher (Teacher Contact 1, described in Chapter 3) is used to determine the specific ways in which OTMP difficulties affect the child's functioning in the classroom.

Assessing for Common Comorbidities and Determining Their Impact on Providing OST

Because it is well known that additional diagnoses in cases of ADHD are the rule rather than the exception (Connor, Steeber, & McBurnett, 2010), assessing for potential comorbid psychiatric disorders during the initial evaluation is advised, and can help determine whether the provision of OST would be affected by co-occurring conditions. If significant emotional issues, such as anxiety or depression, are having an impact on the child's functioning, it may be more appropriate to address those concerns before initiating OST. Alternatively, the therapist can consider making appropriate adjustments to the delivery of treatment if a child has other conditions. For example, children with significant obsessive–compulsive patterns may find OST anxiety-provoking, as they will be asked to follow specific routines. In some cases, the routines could become compulsive in nature, resulting in heightened anxiety rather than improved functioning. When a child has generalized anxiety disorder or a form of social anxiety disorder that involves significant worries about school performance and meeting goals, the child may react to the monitoring of behaviors and the point program incorporated in OST with increased worries that are counterproductive. A review with parents of the child's prior reactions to tracking behavior or setting specific goals for school and home actions should indicate whether this component of OST may be problematic. The presentation and pace of OST could be influenced when a child has a significant learning disorder, language disorder, or borderline or lower intellectual functioning. Broad suggestions for adaptations to OST that may be required for such children are discussed below.

Receptive language disorders are often present in children with ADHD (Barkley, 2006), and they may affect a child's ability to comprehend verbal explanations and discussions in sessions. For a child with receptive language difficulties, the suggested dialogues in session materials can be distilled down to their main points, in words that match the child's capacity for understanding. As most children with receptive disorders are likely to process language at a slow rate (Tallal, 2000; Tannock, Martinussen, & Frijters, 2000), while often being able to understand the content, a therapist may need to use a slower pace of speech and provide pauses in delivery to allow such a child time to process the content effectively. Questioning parents about any speech and language services or supplemental school support that the child is receiving or has had in the past is recommended.

Learning disorders, particularly reading disorders and writing disorders, are prevalent in children with ADHD. Conservative estimates place the rate of overlap near 20%, whereas some studies report up to 45% overlap (Germano, Gagliano, & Curatolo, 2010). The presence of a learning disorder can be reviewed by asking about the child's use of special services, such as special education, a resource room, or private tutoring. If the child is diagnosed with a reading disorder, the reading materials that are provided in OST may have to be read to the child by the therapist in session, and by the parents at home. A child with a learning disorder in math may require the special supplemental session for instruction in time telling, and is also likely to require support from the therapist, teacher, and parent in completing the handouts and routines in the Time Management module of treatment.

When there is a general problem in learning related to below-average intellectual functioning, a number of challenges in the provision of treatment are to be expected. In one case in our pilot study, a child had low-average intelligence and very significant problems in processing speed and memory. Although the child was cooperative during treatment, he had problems managing the session content because of his slow, labored processing of verbal presentations and his forgetfulness while practicing a skill. To achieve functional competence, he required more than the usual time to understand the verbal review of skills and to complete each practice run. As it was not possible to extend the number of sessions in the research protocol, the goal of treatment was modified and focused on helping him become competent in the skill areas that could be covered in 20 sessions. In clinical practice, such a child could be provided with more than 20 sessions to cover all skills, as long as the need for extended treatment is acceptable to parents.

Oppositional defiant disorder is very common in children with ADHD (approximately 50–60% of cases), and serious conduct disorder is present in a significant minority (20%) (Biederman, 2005). Severe problems with conduct should be addressed before OST is implemented. In our randomized controlled trial, parents of children with conduct disorder generally did not seek out OST. Phone screenings suggested that these parents were primarily interested in finding help for the conduct difficulties. However, children with oppositional defiant disorder were treated as research and clinical cases. The decision regarding when to implement OST for children with concomitant behavioral problems should be made after careful consideration of the frequency, severity, and context of oppositional behaviors. For example, a fourth-grade boy evaluated for clinical treatment with OST demonstrated major oppositionality at home in reaction to parental requests, especially those concerning homework. Tension in the family was extremely high, making OTMP concerns only one of many issues. It was decided to place OST on hold until his parents could be provided with extensive behavioral parent training. This approach was effective, and after he and his parents had established a more cooperative relationship, the child completed OST with good results.

Anxiety disorders, found in up to 25% of children with ADHD (MTA Cooperative Group, 1999), can also complicate the delivery of OST. In a few clinical research cases, anxiety symptoms caused children to worry about reaching point goals for between-session skill use. To address these concerns, we found it helpful to ensure that points earned in the behavior management system earned bonus activities and prizes, rather than a child's typical privileges. For children with obsessive–compulsive disorder, it may be important to determine to what extent the child's obsessions and compulsions may account for OTMP deficits, especially in time management. A child may be very slow in meeting time goals and deadlines because of the need to perform compulsive actions in response to obsessive worries. Improving the child's time management strategies through instruction in OTMP skills may not be possible, as the child might experience too much distress in changing compulsive behaviors; instead, the underlying obsessive–compulsive cycle will probably need to be addressed. Despite these concerns, however, the few children with symptoms of obsessive–compulsive disorder that affected their functioning in situations unrelated to school demands were successfully treated in the research study.

Symptoms of autism spectrum disorder (ASD) should also be considered in implementing OST. Two common patterns in ASD can hinder treatment: rigidity in routines, and disinterest in accepting social conventions. A child with ASD who has rigid organizational routines may be unwilling to change responses to organizational situations, even if the current routines are not successful. Furthermore, a child with ASD who does not agree with social conventions, such as the importance of school success, may not be invested in learning more effective ways to handle school demands. In both situations, motivating the child to alter actions or become invested in school success may not be possible without prior extensive work. In the pilot study and randomized controlled trial, there were a few children with ASD symptoms who were treated successfully with OST, most likely because they were not overly rigid and they valued the importance of school success.

ASSESSING AND ENGAGING
PARENT AND TEACHER PARTICIPATION

Assessing Parent Participation

OST was designed and tested with extensive parent and teacher participation. Thus the initial assessment requires an evaluation of parents' and teachers' ability to participate fully in treatment. Parents are involved at the beginning and end of each twice-weekly session. Less direct parental involvement was tried in pilot work, with limited positive outcomes. When we worked only with the children, and other caregivers brought children for "drop-off" individual therapy, the treatment was not effective. Nor is it effective, for the reasons described in Chapter 1, to hold just one session per week. Thus it is recommended that therapists determine, in the initial assessment, whether parents are able to attend sessions with their children two times a week for the time-limited course of 10–12 weeks. Certainly it is easier to obtain adherence to such a requirement in a research study, when treatment is free of charge. Nonetheless, in our clinical experience with OST, once the reasons for the twice-weekly treatment schedule and parental participation were explained to parents, parents were receptive to these treatment requirements.

Attending two sessions per week can be challenging for many parents, given scheduling concerns. Some parents may suggest that they share responsibility for attendance, with one parent attending each weekly session. This arrangement can work, but it requires the therapist to facilitate adaptations that increase communication between parents. Adaptations that have been successful include making certain that the parents share information about the skills learned in each session and the between-session plans for skill use; providing the parent who is not present with a brief, written description of the target skill that should be practiced between sessions; arranging to phone or e-mail the nonparticipating parent with information, especially when a child lives part-time in separated parents' households.

Another factor that can influence a parent's participation in treatment is the presence of ADHD symptoms in the parent. The likelihood that a parent of a child with ADHD has ADHD is high (25–35%; Faraone & Doyle, 2001), and the presence of parental ADHD can influence how well treatment progresses. Parental ADHD symptoms were reviewed in the research study prior to the initiation of treatment. Knowing parental ADHD status before treatment starts will prepare therapists in several ways. First, the therapists will be ready to continually evaluate how effectively parents with ADHD are following through on prompting, monitoring, praising, and rewarding their children. Second, it will alert the therapists to the possibility that additional efforts may be needed to keep such parents motivated to carry out their role in treatment, as parents with ADHD may become discouraged by any difficulties they have in follow-through. Finally, it will sensitize therapists to the possible impact of parental ADHD on treatment implementation at home, and structure the problem-solving discussions at the start of each session accordingly. If a therapist knows ahead of time that a parent is likely to have difficulties with organizational skills, open discussion can help the therapist and parent find practical solutions for developing self-reminders, establishing a daily time at which the parent will guide and check the child's skill use, and organizing a feasible reward schedule. Although parents with ADHD in the research study did find it challenging to implement the steps needed to support their children's skill use between sessions, anecdotal reports from several such parents indicated that participating in OST helped them improve their own organizational skills.

Assessing Teacher Participation

In addition to at least one parent, a child's teacher is another important member of the OST treatment team. Before contacting a teacher, a therapist should obtain a signed parental release giving the teacher permission to discuss the child with the therapist. The teacher is asked to prompt, monitor, praise, and record the use of skills at school on a daily basis. Optimal participation requires that a child's teacher be contacted at least five times by the therapist once treatment begins, in order to discuss the goals of treatment, the behaviors to prompt and praise, and the recording system that will be used.

As described in more detail in Chapter 3, the therapist typically has two preliminary contacts with the teacher before initiating OST with the child. In the first preliminary contact, which can occur by mail or phone, the therapist will obtain screening information from the teacher regarding the child's ADHD symptomatology and OTMP difficulties in school, using a screening interview and/or rating scales (as discussed above). In a second preliminary contact, typically made by phone, the therapist briefly describes the responsibilities involved in treatment participation and determines whether the teacher is willing to participate in the treatment. In some cases, school guidelines may also require that the principal provide permission for the teacher's involvement in an outside treatment. If a teacher is not able to participate, some suggestions for ways to proceed are discussed below. In the few research cases in which teachers originally agreed to participate but did not follow through, adaptations were made that allowed treatment to continue.

If a teacher indicates initial interest during the second preliminary contact, special strategies can facilitate further teacher engagement. It has been found that a face-to-face contact with the teacher, once treatment begins, enhances participation. In fact, in our years of clinical practice, we have found that teachers find a visit from a child's therapist a refreshingly unusual step that gains a lot of good will and assistance in child treatment. This first contact can be used to establish rapport, to provide an accurate and clear indication of the relatively limited time commitment required, and to discuss any barriers to full participation. The first teacher contact held during the course of treatment, which entails an assessment of the child's OTMP difficulties and the ways in which the teacher handles OTMP requirements, takes approximately 30 minutes. The four follow-up contacts (described in Chapter 3), which are likely to occur by phone, usually take 10–15 minutes; daily teacher activities involve 3–5 minutes with the student.

As noted in Chapter 1, teachers in the pilot study indicated that OST participation was not too demanding, and the vast majority of teachers in the pilot study and randomized controlled trial were satisfied with the impact of OST. We have found that once OST's goals are explained, most teachers are very interested in providing extra assistance to their struggling students with ADHD. For some cases, it may be appropriate to use a Section 504 plan to facilitate teacher involvement in OST. Many children with ADHD have a special Section 504 plan that recognizes their status as children with an impairing condition; ADHD is usually designated in the category of Other Health Impairment. Such a plan provides for teaching accommodations, usually including extended time on tests, preferential seating, and the use of daily behavior report cards (see DuPaul & Stoner, 2003). A therapist could work with a parent and teacher either to add another accommodation to a child's established plan, or to suggest the development of a new plan for a child that does not have one in place. The additional accommodation could provide for "daily teacher supervision of the use of organizational tools and routines, to include a few minutes' time to prompt, monitor, and praise the child's use of such tools and routines." With such an official plan in place, the teacher might feel more comfortable providing the needed assistance.

Even with a strong effort to establish rapport and engage teachers in OST, teachers are likely to vary in their level of participation. At just less than full participation, teachers may be willing to prompt, monitor, praise, and record use of skills throughout the majority of the program, but may not be able to engage in the time-planning and task-planning discussions that are advised in the second half of the program. For this situation, detailed adaptations are provided in the Part II session descriptions. They basically involve requests that, at a minimum, the teacher record that work has been turned in on time and that assignments are correctly, neatly, and completely done. In other circumstances, a teacher may indicate willingness to implement the intervention fully, but may not follow through after the initial sessions. If this occurs, the therapist is advised to discuss the situation with the teacher, to determine whether any practical steps can be taken to reduce barriers to full involvement. If a solution cannot be found, it is then advised that OST continue, with modifications made to the in-school recording of skill use. It may be possible for a teacher to provide a weekly report on the child's use of skills, rather than daily reports. Or, if the teacher cannot be relied upon to record behavior, it may be necessary instead for the parent to evaluate the child's in-school performance by asking the child to show evidence that the skill has been used. A child could complete a checklist of OST skills used at school and then demonstrate positive results upon arrival at home. For example, the use of the backpack checklist in school would be documented by the child's arriving home with all needed papers, books, and items. Or the child could complete a checklist of skills used, and a back-up report from the teacher could provide evidence that the child used the skills. For example, having a report from the teacher that all work has been turned in on time would suggest that time management skills are being used well.

Although the positive results of OST in the clinical trial are based on cases where the majority of teachers participated extensively, the therapists' clinical impressions suggested that the few children whose teachers did not follow through still improved. Therapist creativity was used to work around limited teacher involvement. It is expected that resourcefulness and flexibility will be useful when therapists encounter limited teacher engagement in their clinical practice with OST. Experience in completing school consultations and prior work with teachers should help therapists negotiate these situations.

TRACKING PROGRESS

As children progress through treatment, it is helpful for therapists to monitor the children's understanding of and success in using the various organizational tools and routines taught. In addition, therapists must assess how well parents are implementing behavior management procedures at home, as well as how teachers are following through with prompting and praising organizational behaviors in school. A therapist elicits informal feedback from a parent at the beginning of each session on the child's use of the OTMP skills that were learned in previous sessions, and should have a sense from the continuing teacher contacts about how the child is implementing those skills in the classroom. When a child is not progressing appropriately, Part II of this manual provides "Helpful Hints" and "Troubleshooting Notes" regarding ways to enhance the child's ability to apply the lessons learned in session to the home and school environments (additional practice in session, modifications to procedures, etc.).

Toward the end of the Time Management module, the teacher is asked to complete a brief Skills Check-Up (see Teacher Form 9), providing feedback on the child's progress with the skills learned to that point. If the therapist has decided to use a rating scale (such as the COSS or BRIEF) in the assessment process for determining whether a child needs OST, the same rating scale may be readministered to the parent and teacher at different points throughout treatment (e.g., at the midpoint and end of treatment) to obtain a concrete assessment of the child's progress.

FORMS, HANDOUTS, AND OTHER SESSION MATERIALS

OST is different in many ways from other forms of treatment. Because a great deal of instruction and practice is provided, several handouts and forms are required in many sessions. Each session in Part II begins with a list of the materials needed for that session. Specific forms for the therapist, handouts for the parent and child, and forms for the teacher can be found in Part III of this book. Getting materials together before each session is essential. We have found that having files of materials organized by session is useful. We have also found that having materials in a bin facilitates quick access and reduces the need to rush before a session to get the necessary supplies.

Therapists should obtain supplies for themselves before beginning treatment, and should also consider providing supplies to children to reduce demands on parents. Several items are critical to OST: (1) an accordion binder (introduced in Session 5); (2) a portable file box with hanging folders; (3) a badge holder (introduced in Session 6); (4) cardboard luggage tags (introduced in Session 7); (5) a pencil holder; and (6) a stopwatch. The approximate cost for these materials is $25 to $30. For teacher contacts, we recommend providing a thank-you gift (e.g., gift cards) at the end of treatment, if a teacher is allowed to accept gifts. Handouts and therapist forms can be photocopied by purchasers of this book; copies should be available when sessions begin.

TREATMENT MODIFICATIONS

As with any manualized treatment implemented in clinical practice, modifications to OST may be indicated for different cases (e.g., truncating or extending specific portions of treatment, modifying material presented in sessions, or ordering sessions differently). However, it is important to note that there are no empirical data regarding the effects of different treatment modifications. Modifications occurred very infrequently in the randomized controlled trial: Participants attended 19.8 of 20 sessions, on average, with a range of 17–20 sessions attended; fidelity checklists indicated that on average, 96% of the material in the manual was covered in sessions; and sessions were presented in the order laid out in the manual. Thus the positive results obtained with OST were based upon the implementation of treatment according to the guidelines presented in this book. Individual therapists may decide to alter aspects of the program, such as providing only sections of the treatment that seem most relevant to a child, and these decisions may be clinically appropriate; however, therapists should be aware that there is no empirical evidence for the effectiveness of a modified version of this treatment.

With this caveat in mind, the comments below and in the session guidelines regarding potential variations in the treatment protocol are based primarily on observations regarding how OST has been modified by therapists in clinical settings. The three main variations that have occurred in these settings are (1) skipping part of the protocol, usually the module on Tracking Assignments; (2) breaking up the protocol, so that it is started in one school year and completed in the following school year; and (3) extending the protocol by repeating the content of some sessions when a child is showing slow progress. Other variations that have been used with individual clinical cases have included presenting booster sessions in the next school year, as well as returning to previously completed session content before presenting the full 20 sessions when a child stops using tools and routines that have been previously taught.

Skipping part of the protocol is not generally recommended, because the content and order of sessions were devised to meet the deficits demonstrated by most of the children evaluated during program development. Key portions of the protocol that should not be omitted include the initial orientation session, the parent training in behavior management, and the wrap-up session that involves planning for continued use of tools and routines taught during treatment. However, some of the skills-building sessions may not be relevant for certain children. In particular, some children may be very effective at recording their assignments and marking due dates and test dates in a calendar. If this is the case, the module on Tracking Assignments may be shortened. However, planners that children may use for tracking school assignments usually do not include a space for recording the items that are needed for assignments—an element that is critical for disorganized children. Therefore, a modified version of the module on Tracking Assignments should include a plan for and practice of steps for creating a checklist of materials that have to be brought home for each daily assignment, as well as use of a monthly calendar.

A therapist may also find that some children do not have significant difficulties managing materials needed for school, and thus may not need extensive practice in the Managing Materials treatment module. Some children who are generally disorganized may nonetheless be effective in packing papers and books for transport between school and home. In such cases, a therapist could reduce the amount of time spent on developing a method for storing and transferring papers, creating a backpack checklist, or getting work areas Ready to Go.

However, before accepting a child's seeming organization in the areas of Tracking Assignments and Managing Materials at face value, the therapist must consider the amount of involvement that parents have in keeping their child organized. At times, a child may appear to be organized, but only because parents are completing the tasks for the child. For example, many parents in the clinical trial were packing their children's bags or keeping their children's calendars up to date. In cases such as these, use of the full Tracking Assignments and Managing Materials modules is recommended, so that children become more independently capable of using the OTMP skill sets.

Generally, modifications to the Time Management and Task Planning modules are not recommended, because children with poor OTMP skills are rarely effective in these areas. In fact, one modification—using Session 11a, which provides instruction in telling time—adds a session to the program.

As indicated in Chapter 1, scheduling sessions for less than twice a week is not recommended. Treatment is structured to be implemented with a schedule of two sessions per week, conducted over 10–12 weeks, for a total of 20 sessions. Overall, the use of OST methods requires concerted effort by children, parents, and teachers, and frequent contact with therapists helps maintain motivation. Therapists must provide frequent support to parents in their efforts to prompt, monitor, and reinforce children's behaviors, and give children positive feedback and corrective guidance as they attempt to overcome long-standing problems. This problem-solving support and positive feedback seem to be most effective when provided continually.

TROUBLESHOOTING:
ISSUES THAT MAY REQUIRE SPECIAL ATTENTION

From our clinical experience in using OST, it is clear that the attainment of treatment goals is facilitated by several key factors, including (1) the parent's consistent implementation of the home behavior program; (2) the child's ability to maintain improvement in several organizational skill areas as treatment progresses; and (3) the teacher's consistent use of prompts and praise in school.

As treatment progresses, a therapist may find that a parent is not following through on important aspects of the home behavior program; a "Troubleshooting Note" box in Session 5 provides guidance to the therapist on ways to work with the parent to determine appropriate modifications to the system. In addition, if the child shows drop-off in previously learned skills as new organizational skills are introduced, the therapist will need to adapt the session content flexibly and/or adjust the home or school behavior programs to address the child's needs. A "Troubleshooting Note" box in Session 11 suggests steps that the therapist may take to facilitate the child's maintenance of previously targeted skills. It should be emphasized that although these troubleshooting suggestions are detailed in Sessions 5 and 11, the therapist should feel free to use them as needed later in treatment. Furthermore, the therapist may also find that a teacher is not providing the needed level of support for the program in school; if this is the case, a "Troubleshooting . . ." section in Chapter 3 provides suggestions for ways to increase teacher participation.

ADDRESSING ISSUES OTHER THAN OTMP CONCERNS

If significant concerns arise during the course of treatment regarding other problems that affect the child's functioning, OST can and should be "put on hold" to address those other concerns. During the randomized controlled trial, four adjunctive sessions were allowed to supplement OST. These sessions were intended to address issues that posed a danger to a child, that constituted a major challenge to family or child functioning, or that would interfere with the child's participation,. If a child required a full suspension of OST, or if a greater number of sessions were required to address more pressing concerns, the child was dropped from OST so that the other form of care could continue; however, this situation was encountered very infrequently. We found that it was possible to apply OST flexibly enough to allow for other issues (e.g., significant aggression, family discord) to be addressed, while keeping the main focus on OTMP skills.

We also found that children were able to participate in other forms of treatment while they were enrolled in OST. However, when other treatments are required, the impact on a child's schedule should be considered, and priorities may need to be set. If participation in a second treatment makes twice-weekly OST sessions impossible, the effectiveness of OST will be limited, as discussed above.

CHAPTER 3

A Guide to Teacher Contacts

In order for OST to be optimally successful in promoting improved organizational functioning, you, the therapist, should work together with the parent, teacher, and child as part of a cohesive team. The teacher's role in the program is important, as the teacher is uniquely able to prompt, monitor, and praise positive organizational behaviors in school. As new organizational skills are introduced in treatment sessions, the child is instructed to practice those skills at home and in school. The teacher is responsible for prompting the child to use target skills in school, praising the child when those skills are used appropriately, and monitoring and recording the child's use of those skills so that the parent can provide an appropriate reward at home.

This chapter outlines the suggested content for the two preliminary teacher contacts and five teacher contacts held during the course of treatment. The guidelines for the five primary teacher contacts refer to concepts and procedures that will be reviewed in detail in Part II. As you progress through the treatment manual, you may refer back to the guidelines in this chapter to prepare for each of the teacher contacts.

PRELIMINARY TEACHER CONTACTS

As discussed in Chapter 2, before you initiate OST with a child, two brief contacts with the teacher will facilitate a determination of whether OST is a good match for the child's needs.

Preliminary Teacher Contact 1

After obtaining consent from the parent to discuss the child with the teacher, contact the teacher to obtain brief screening information regarding the child's ADHD symptomatology and OTMP functioning at school. Let the teacher know that the child's parents have spoken with you about initiating OST to help their child with organizational skills problems. Ask the teacher whether she would be willing to provide some preliminary information about the child's behavior in the classroom in general, and the child's OTMP functioning in particular. As discussed in Chapter 2, you may conduct a brief screening interview by phone (see Figure 2.1) or send selected rating scales (e.g., the Conners 3rd Edition Teacher Rating Scale, the Teacher version of the COSS, or the BRIEF) to the teacher, with a return envelope or instructions for faxing the completed scales back to you. After reviewing the screening information, you will be able to determine whether the child is experiencing significant problems with OTMP functioning in school, and should be able to make an informed decision regarding the appropriateness of OST for the child. As noted in Chapter 2, children who do not have significant OTMP difficulties in school may still benefit from OST if they are experiencing significant OTMP difficulties at home. However, the majority of children with OTMP problems in one setting will experience similar or related problems in a second setting.

Preliminary Teacher Contact 2

Briefly summarize the information that the teacher has provided regarding the child's behavior and OTMP functioning in the classroom (e.g., "Based on the ratings you provided on the Teacher COSS, it appears as if [child's name] is having difficulty with some key organizational areas in school, including managing materials and completing tasks on time"). Indicate that you believe OST will help the child improve organizational functioning in school and at home, and that the child will benefit most from the treatment if the teacher is involved. Provide a brief description of the treatment (summarized in Teacher Form 1, Teacher's Guide to Organizational Skills Training, which you should e-mail or fax to the teacher) and ask whether the teacher is willing and able to participate in treatment. If the teacher indicates willingness to participate, schedule a time to meet to discuss the child's needs further and to provide a fuller description and outline of the teacher's role in treatment (Teacher Contact 1).

TEACHER CONTACTS DURING THE COURSE OF TREATMENT

There are five recommended teacher contacts to be held over the course of the program. These are scheduled at the following key points during treatment:

1. *Beginning of Week 1:* Orient teacher to OST and Tracking Assignments.
2. *End of Week 2:* Orient teacher to accordion binder use and backpack checklist.
3. *End of Week 4:* Orient teacher to getting work areas Ready to Go in school.
4. *End of Week 5:* Orient teacher to Time Management and the Time Tracker.
5. *Beginning of Week 8:* Orient teacher to Task Planning, and plan for end of treatment.

These contacts are intended to provide the teacher with essential information about what the child is doing in treatment, how the child is expected to practice specific skills in school, and how the teacher can support the child in the use of these skills. Furthermore, these contacts can help you refine treatment efforts; the teacher's feedback about how the child is able to implement OST skills in the classroom can help you modify organizational routines so that they can be used more effectively, and/or can help you determine which skills require additional practice in session. You should also encourage the teacher to reach out at any point during treatment, with questions or concerns about the OST skills and routines. Building a collaborative relationship with the teacher will ensure greater transfer of training from the treatment sessions to the school setting. The following guidelines provide suggested content for the five recommended teacher contacts over the course of treatment, either by phone or in person.

Teacher Contact 1 (Beginning of Week 1)

In Preparation for This Contact

Contact the teacher to set up a 20- to 30-minute first meeting, either in person or on the phone. Send the teacher (via e-mail or fax) the following forms, and indicate that you will review and discuss the forms during your first meeting. (These and other teacher forms are provided in a separate section of Part III.)

- Teacher Form 2, Detailed OST Schedule
- Teacher Form 3, Guide to the Daily Assignment Record
- Teacher Form 4, Sample Daily Assignment Record

In addition, you should review the information provided by the teacher regarding the child's OTMP functioning, which should have been obtained prior to the start of OST, to determine which areas of functioning the teacher views as most problematic. You will review these areas with the teacher during your first meeting.

Orient the Teacher to the Program

Provide a brief summary of the OST treatment model, which combines one-on-one skills training with children and behavior modification procedures used by parents and teachers to encourage skill acquisition. Briefly discuss the explanatory model that is presented to children and parents, which attributes lapses in OTMP functioning to meddlesome "Glitches," and encourages the child to train the "Mastermind" to be in control by using specific organizational tools and routines. Let the teacher know that the intervention was specifically designed for children who have problems with getting and staying organized. *Do not mention the child's diagnosis of ADHD if that diagnosis has been made, unless you have specific permission from the parent to do so.* You can let the teacher know that the OST intervention has been shown to be effective in research studies. This is important, as other therapists and tutors in your area may be offering a form of organizational intervention that has not undergone any empirical testing. You may obtain more investment from the child's teacher if the teacher knows that the program has been empirically validated.

Explain that the child will attend twice-weekly sessions for 10–12 weeks, for a total of 20 treatment sessions. In each session, the child is taught a new organizational skill, practices the use of that skill in session, and is given homework to use that skill at home. OST modules address functioning in the areas of Tracking Assignments, Managing Materials, Time Management, and Task Planning. The parent is responsible for maintaining a home behavior modification system, which involves prompting the child to perform specific organizational skills at home, monitoring the child's performance, and praising and rewarding the child for performing those skills. Refer the teacher to Teacher Form 2 (Detailed OST Schedule) for a breakdown of the specific skills covered in each session.

Explain that the child is expected to use the organizational skills learned in sessions at school, integrating these new skills into a regular routine. Refer the teacher to the last column in Teacher Form 2, and indicate that the teacher will be asked to support the child's use of these skills in school. The teacher will be asked to (1) *prompt* the child to perform specific target behaviors (these will be noted on the Daily Assignment Record, to be discussed below, and will change as treatment progresses); (2) *monitor* the child's use of these behaviors; (3) *praise* the child for performing the target behaviors; and (4) provide the child with a *point* for performing the target behaviors on a copy of the Daily Assignment Record. The parent will then provide home points and rewards to the child, based in part on the teacher's record of whether or not the child performed the target behaviors.

Indicate that the teacher should not have to spend more than a few minutes each day prompting, monitoring, and praising the child's performance of target behaviors. However, this small investment of time will provide invaluable support to the child, as the child learns and practices new organizational skills.

Finally, note that while the Detailed OST Schedule refers to prespecified target behaviors that the child will practice in school each week, flexibility and individualization are built into the program. For example, later in the program, when the child works on task planning in sessions, the teacher may address planning with the child in school or continue to work on time management or other important skills areas with the child, depending on what makes the most sense in the classroom context and what the child's needs are.

Review the Child's OTMP Problems

Using the assessment information gathered from the teacher and parent prior to the start of treatment, initiate a brief discussion with the teacher about the problem behaviors that are observed in the classroom with regard to the OTMP skills. For each behavior, ask the teacher to indicate how problems with the specific OTMP skill interfere with the child's performance in school. For example, if the teacher indicated in the initial assessment that the child often forgets to bring needed things to school, ask the teacher to describe what sorts of things the child forgets, how often this happens, and how it affects the child's functioning in the classroom. This review will give you a better understanding of the child's OTMP functioning in school, and will facilitate your ability to help the child change problematic routines by using new skills. You can also refer back to the teacher's comments in later contacts, when you introduce a new skill that is intended to help the child improve in an area that the teacher highlighted as problematic.

Review Existing Organizational Routines in the Classroom

Ask the teacher whether the children use any specific organizational routines or tools in the classroom (planners to record assignments, specific folders or binders to organize papers, etc.). Determine whether any of these methods would be incompatible with the methods taught in OST, and ask the teacher for input on the feasibility of using different methods for the child. For example, if the teacher instructs the children to use separate two-pocket folders for management of papers from different subjects, ask whether it would be acceptable for the child to try using an accordion binder for managing papers. If the teacher is hesitant to replace an existing approach with a new method, attempt to reach a compromise (e.g., storing the separate two-pocket folders in the accordion binder).

Introduce the Daily Assignment Record

Tell the teacher that in the initial treatment sessions, the child will learn how to use a Daily Assignment Record (often abreviated as DAR) to keep track of assignments and materials that are needed to complete those assignments. Indicate that use of the DAR is intended to help the child control the Go-Ahead-Forget-It Glitch, which tricks the child into forgetting important assignments and materials.

Ask the teacher to look at Teacher Form 4, the Sample Daily Assignment Record, and review the features of the DAR. Ask the teacher to prompt the child to fill in the DAR each day, and to correct any errors that the child makes in the first week of use. Direct the teacher's attention to the final column, where the teacher will provide a point if the child completes the DAR. Note that in the first week, the teacher should provide a point for any effort to use the DAR; after the first week, the teacher should only provide a point if the child completes the DAR accurately. Also explain that as treatment proceeds, the teacher will see that the target behaviors in the final column of the DAR will change (usually on a weekly basis), according to the schedule outlined on Teacher Form 2. Assure the teacher that you will contact him before any new behaviors are introduced, to discuss how to prompt the child to perform each behavior and how to judge whether the child has earned a point.

If the teacher is not comfortable with the idea of the child's using the DAR to record assignments, and would prefer that the child use the same method of recording assignments as the rest of the class, please see the "Alternative Procedures" section at the end of Session 3 for some modifications that might be suggested.

Schedule the Next Contact

Ask for the best method of contacting the teacher in the future (e.g., e-mail, cell phone, school phone), and indicate that reminders and guidelines will be faxed or e-mailed (ask for the teacher's preference) before a new OST behavior must be prompted in the classroom. Tell the teacher that you will confer again in approximately 1 week (at the end of Week 2), and set a tentative date and time for that contact (which will most likely occur by phone).

Teacher Contact 2 (End of Week 2)

In Preparation for This Contact

Send the teacher, via e-mail or fax, Teacher Form 5 (Guide to the Accordion Binder).

Review Use of the DAR

Ask the teacher whether the child is using the DAR to record homework assignments, and confirm that the teacher is prompting, monitoring, praising, and providing a point for using the DAR. Also ask whether the child is having any problem completing the DAR accurately, so that you can work with the child on this skill in session if necessary. Indicate that beginning next week, the teacher will only give the child a school point for *accurate* completion of the DAR.

Discuss Paper Management

Ask the teacher whether the child has problems with turning in homework. You may already have this information from Teacher Contact 1; if so, do not repeat the question, but note that the teacher reported this as an issue. Indicate that storing papers and transferring them between school and home are often difficult for children with organizational problems. Ask what method children currently use in the class for storing and transferring papers, and determine whether use of an alternative method—specifically, an accordion binder—would be acceptable to the teacher. Explain why the accordion binder is a helpful tool for children with organizational problems, and indicate that use of a binder to manage papers can help the child control the Go-Ahead-Lose-It Glitch, which "tricks" the child into misplacing and losing materials. If the teacher insists upon using a different method for paper storage, see the "Alternative Procedures" section at the end of Session 5, and decide upon a method that meets the child's needs and is acceptable to the teacher.

Explain Use of the Accordion Binder in School

Refer to Teacher Form 5 (Guide to the Accordion Binder), and review how the child should use the binder (or alternative procedure, as discussed above) to file, store, and transfer school papers. Ask the teacher to prompt the child to use the binder for storing papers (e.g., "Please put this math worksheet in the 'Math' section of your binder"). After 1 week of giving the child a point for putting papers in the binder, the teacher will then give a point for putting papers in the binder *and* returning all homework papers to school in the binder. Remind the teacher to praise the child (e.g., "Great job putting that worksheet into your binder!") for using the binder and returning homework papers to school.

Look Ahead: The Backpack Checklist

Tell the teacher that in Week 4, the child will work on creating a backpack checklist, which will list the things that should be packed in the backpack each day. When the target behavior related to using the backpack checklist appears on the DAR, the teacher should prompt the child to use the steps on the backpack checklist when packing up at the end of each day, and should provide praise and a point if the child uses this tool appropriately.

Schedule the Next Contact

Tell the teacher that you will confer again in approximately 2 weeks (at the end of Week 4), and set a tentative date and time for that contact (which will most likely occur by phone).

Troubleshooting Issues Regarding Teacher Implementation of the School Point Program

It is important that the teacher consistently provide prompts, monitoring, praise, and points for the child's use of specific organizational behaviors at school. Therefore, you should review the child's DAR folder during each session, noting whether the teacher has filled in the final column on the DAR appropriately. If teacher points are missing on multiple days, ask the child about how the teacher manages the use of the DAR and other organizational routines in school. If the child indicates that the teacher does not provide reminders for the organizational routines, or that the teacher expects the child to remember to ask for the teacher's initials and points, you should follow up immediately with the teacher. In a separate phone or e-mail contact, remind the teacher that the child will probably forget to use the DAR and other organizational routines in school if an adult does not prompt use of these skills, especially when those routines are first being learned. Reiterate the importance of these prompts, and of the reinforcement that the teacher can provide through praise, and ask the teacher for cooperation in helping the child to learn these new skills successfully. You may need to problem-solve with the teacher to determine how to fit prompts for these new organizational routines into the daily schedule. For example, the teacher may decide that checking the DAR at the end of the day is not feasible, and may want to check the DAR after lunch instead, when the schedule is less hectic. Work with the teacher to develop a routine for prompting, monitoring, and praising the child for use of organizational behaviors, taking into account multiple demands on the teacher's time.

Teacher Contact 3 (End of Week 4)

In Preparation for This Contact

Send the teacher, via e-mail or fax, Teacher Form 6 (Getting Ready to Go: Teacher Guidelines).

Review Use of the DAR, Binder, and Backpack Checklist

Ask the teacher whether the child has been using the DAR and binder regularly in school, and check on whether the child is turning in homework each day. The child has probably just started using the backpack checklist in school; ask the teacher whether the child is responding to prompts to refer to the checklist while packing up. Request that the teacher continue to prompt and praise the use of the backpack checklist, as the child is just learning to follow this routine in packing up. Let the teacher know that the child will be creating checklists for other bags (e.g., bags for extracurricular activities or trips) at home.

Ask the teacher for feedback on how the child is doing in terms of keeping track of assignments and managing materials at school. Determine whether the child needs additional practice with specific routines or skills in session to prepare for challenging situations that arise in school. For example, if the teacher reports that the child is finding it difficult to get all of the papers into the correct sections of the binder at the end of the day, and is cramming the papers into the backpack for fear of missing the bus, you should address this issue with the child in session. Help the child come up with an alternative procedure that does not add stress to the daily routine; for example, the child can put all the papers into one section of the binder in class, and sort them into sections at home (see Session 6). The teacher's feedback can be a valuable tool in helping you to maximize the child's benefit from each of the OST tools and routines.

Explain Use of Ready to Go in School

Indicate that the child will be learning how to be "Ready to Go" for any task, by preparing the work area with items that are needed to complete the task and clearing away any unnecessary items. Refer to the Ready to Go steps listed on Teacher Form 6; tell the teacher that the child will practice these steps extensively in session and at home, and should be prepared to practice them at school as well. Tell the teacher that "Got the desk Ready to Go" will be the next new target behavior on the DAR. Ask the teacher to prompt the child to use the Ready to Go steps once a day, to prepare the desk or other work area for an in-class assignment of the teacher's choosing, and to monitor the child's use of these steps. The teacher should then praise the child and provide a school point for using these steps.

Schedule the Next Contact

Tell the teacher that you will confer again in approximately 1 week (at the end of Week 5), and set a tentative date and time for that contact (which will most likely occur by phone).

Teacher Contact 4 (End of Week 5)

In Preparation for This Contact

Send the teacher, via e-mail or fax, the following forms:

- Teacher Form 7, Introduction to Time Management
- Teacher Form 8, Time Tracker for In-Class Work
- Teacher Form 9, Skills Chheck-Up

Review Use of Skills for Tracking Assignments and Managing Materials

Ask how well the child is doing in tracking assignments with the DAR, managing materials and workspace (with the binder, backpack checklist, and Ready to Go), and turning in assignments. Make note of any difficulties the child is having, and ask the teacher for feedback on how any of these routines can be modified or practiced further to improve their use and effectiveness in the classroom. Let the teacher know that she will be asked to complete a brief Skills Check-Up form (Teacher Form 9) in the next week or so, to check on the child's continued use of organizational routines in the classroom.

Introduce New Module: Time Management

Indicate that as outlined in Teacher Form 7, the next several sessions will focus on time management, in an effort to control the "Time Bandit." Briefly review the Time Bandit's "tricks," which include making the child lose track of time, forget when things are due, encourages procrastination, and distracts during a task so time isn't used well. Review the behaviors that will be covered in this module, as outlined on Teacher Form 7, and describe how the teacher can help the child use the Time Tracker for In-Class Work (Teacher Form 8) to improve time estimation and use in the classroom. Ask the teacher to prompt, monitor, praise, and provide a School Point for use of the Time Tracker in class.

Schedule the Next Contact

Tell the teacher that you will confer again in approximately 2 weeks (at the beginning of week 8), and set a tentative date and time for that contact (which will most likely occur by phone).

Teacher Contact 5 (Beginning of Week 8)

In Preparation for This Contact

Send the teacher, via e-mail or fax, the following forms:

- Teacher Form 10, Introduction to Task Planning
- Teacher Form 11, Sample Task-Planning Conference

Review Use of Skills for Time Management

Ask the teacher how well the child is doing with estimating how long in-class assignments will take and handing in assignments on time. Also review the teacher's feedback on the Skills Check-Up (Teacher Form 9), addressing any issues the teacher has noted regarding the child's use of skills related to tracking assignments, managing materials or time management.

Introduce New Module: Task Planning

Indicate that for the final few sessions of OST, the child will be learning skills that will help control the Go-Ahead-Don't-Plan Glitch. This Glitch sometimes tells the child to engage in tasks willy-nilly, without much planning, which results in problems for the child. Explain that the child is learning to use a Task-Planning Conference to plan for important tasks and/or projects, and will practice the steps in task planning (listed on Teacher Form 10), in sessions and at home.

Ask the teacher whether there are opportunities in the classroom to use task-planning skills—for example, planning independent work time or working on a long-term, independent research project. If the teacher assigns in-class work that requires independent effort over an extended period of time, use of the task-planning steps could be useful for the child. If that is the case, guide the teacher through the planning steps, explaining how the child can use the Task-Planning Conference (a sample copy is provided as Teacher Form 11) to organize a reasonable plan for completing an in-class assignment or project. Ask the teacher to prompt the child to use the Task-Planning Conference to guide work on a selected in-class project that requires planning, and to praise the child and provide a school point for using planning steps. Explain that the planning steps are introduced in sessions in sequential fashion, and that you will highlight the sections of the Task-Planning Conference that the child should use in class each week.

If the teacher does not believe that task planning will be relevant to the child for in-class work, you may continue to suggest that the teacher praise and award points for the use of time management skills. Alternatively, you may decide, with the teacher, that the child could use additional reinforcement for skills learned earlier in treatment, such as getting Ready to Go or keeping track of assignments, and you may add those skills to the list of target behaviors for the DAR. Keep in mind that target behaviors should be those that have a good probability of occurring on a given day; the child should not be returning home, more days than not, with a DAR that has "N/A" noted in the column for the teacher points. This will decrease the child's motivation for earning those points, and will make it difficult for the parent to award points and rewards at home.

Plan for the End of Treatment

Tell the teacher when treatment is scheduled to end, and review how the child and parent will be encouraged to continue using OST skills and routines after the end of treatment. Indicate that the parent will be advised to continue using reinforcement procedures at home, to encourage maintenance of learned behaviors. Encourage the teacher to continue prompting, monitoring, praising, and providing points, to support the child's continued use of OST tools that have been helpful in the classroom. Discuss how the teacher can continue using the DAR to select and reinforce two target behaviors each day, and help the teacher think about how to select appropriate behaviors for reinforcement. Remind the teacher that clear, specific prompts and reminders can help the child apply useful organizational skills and improve classroom functioning, and that praise and positive attention from the teacher can motivate the child to show continued improvement.

Ask the teacher if there are any questions about how to maintain positive gains that have resulted from treatment, and thank the teacher for collaborating with you and the family in helping the child improve OTMP skills. If you plan to request any posttreatment assessment of the child's status, find out whether the teacher is willing to complete any formalized assessment scales, at this time or in the future.

PART II

SESSION-BY-SESSION GUIDELINES

SESSION 1

Introduction
Parent and Child Orientation

============ **GOALS FOR THE SESSION** ============

You, the therapist, will:

- Orient the parent and child to the treatment rationale, content, and objectives.
- Understand how specific difficulties with organizational skills affect the child and family life.
- Understand the family's typical schedule.
- Contact the child's teacher and schedule a meeting (Teacher Contact 1), to be conducted before Session 4 (which will be within a week and a half).

The parent and child will understand:

- How people with attention-deficit/hyperactivity disorder (ADHD) are prone to problems in organization, time management, and planning (OTMP) behaviors.
- That organizational skills training (OST) is designed to overcome OTMP lapses, which are portrayed as mischievous "Glitches" that interfere with school success and family relations.
- That skills will be built through learning and practice in session, as well as through between-session use of tools and routines.
- That use of the new tools and routines will be supported by parents and teachers.

============ **MATERIALS NEEDED** ============

For the parent:

- Handout 1, Overview of Session Content
- Handout 2, Treatment Expectations
- One two-pocket folder

For you:

- Therapist Form 1, Session Points and Notes—Session 1
- Therapist Form 2, Interview Record of Problems in Organization, Time Management, and Planning
- Therapist Form 3, Interference and Conflict Rating Scales
- Therapist Form 4, Interview Form for Family's Schedule and Activities

For the child:

- Handout 3, Guide to the Glitches (two copies for the session)
- One two-pocket folder

SESSION SUMMARY CHECKLIST FOR SESSION 1

Item	Item Completed
Describe the treatment program and its rationale	
Explain the rationale for a focus on organizational skills	Yes/No
Overview of the skills taught (Handout 1)	Yes/No
Explain how skills are taught	Yes/No
Overview the treatment schedule and session format	Yes/No
Describe the teacher's role	Yes/No
Describe the use of rewards in session (Therapist Form 1)	Yes/No
Obtain the parent's understanding of the treatment schedule	
(Handout 2)	Yes/No
Set a schedule for regular twice-a-week meetings	Yes/No
Review the child's OTMP difficulties	Yes/No
Introduce the Guide to the Glitches (Handout 3)	Yes/No
Conduct a functional assessment of the child's OTMP problems (Therapist Forms 2 and 3)	Yes/No
Review the family's routines (Therapist Form 4)	Yes/No
Wrap up the session	
Provide the Guide to the Glitches and a folder apiece to the parent and child	Yes/No
Reward the child (Therapist Form 1)	Yes/No
Conclude the session	Yes/No

ABOUT THIS SESSION

In the first part of this session, you will orient the parent and child to the treatment, including its rationale, its content, the number of sessions, and the timing and format of sessions; you will then obtain the parent's commitment to the treatment. You will next briefly review the child's OTMP difficulties, based on the previous assessments, and introduce the Guide to the Glitches (Handout 3), before turning to a functional assessment of the child's OTMP difficulties. Finally, you will obtain information on the family's typical schedule and routine.

Note: The review of the Guide to the Glitches and the functional assessment of OTMP problems may not be completed by the end of the session. If you are unable to complete all of these tasks in this session, you may conduct the review of the family's schedule in the next session.

IN PREPARATION FOR THIS SESSION

To prepare for this session, you should have a basic understanding of the child's difficulties with OTMP behaviors from previous assessment interviews and measures (see Chapter 2 on assessment), as you will review these difficulties with the parent and child in this session.

DETAILED SESSION CONTENT

Describe the Treatment Program and Its Rationale

Explain to the parent and child that this first session will focus on a general overview of the treatment, and that you will be giving them a lot of information about what they will be doing over the next 10–12 weeks in OST. You may want to point out, especially to the child, that it may be difficult to sit and listen to all of this information, but that you will be paying attention to the child's attempts to listen and participate, and will be rewarding her for these behaviors at the end of the session.

Begin by explaining that this is a treatment designed for children who have been diagnosed with ADHD *and* have problems with organization that keep them from functioning well at school, at home, and in social situations. This treatment will show the child some new organizational tools and routines and teach the child the skills to use them, through in-session learning and practice and between-session, supported practice at home and in school.

Explain the Rationale for a Focus on Organizational Skills

Explain that inadequate organizational skills seem to hinder adjustment in children with ADHD. Many children with ADHD do not learn these skills well under typical circumstances, which is why this treatment tries to teach these skills in a very specific, supportive way. Tell the parent and child that improved organizational skills may result in fewer conflicts with parents and teachers and in lower levels of distress, in addition to preparing the child for the future.

Overview the Skills Taught

Explain that this program focuses on teaching children better OTMP skills. Give the parent Handout 1 (Overview of Session Content) and briefly review it, noting that the program includes these four modules:

- Tracking Assignments—using assignment records and calendars.
- Managing Materials—organizing papers, books, backpacks, and desks.
- Time Management—understanding time requirements; consulting with parents and teachers to set a schedule; organizing tasks in relation to time.
- Task Planning—learning the steps in planning; consulting with parents and teachers to develop effective plans that result in tasks that are neat, complete, and done on time, without rushing.

Explain How Skills Are Taught

Explain that several basic methods will be used to teach the child skills. In the sessions, the child will learn the skills and practice them. The methods used to guide the child's learning in session include discussing the skills with you, watching you demonstrate the skills, and practicing the skills while you provide praise and constructive feedback. Between sessions, the parent will help the child practice the skills and reward practice at home. In addition, the child's teacher will keep track of the child's skills practice at school.

Overview the Treatment Schedule and Session Format

Explain that there will be sessions twice a week over 10–12 weeks. State that there will also be regular contacts with the teacher, to describe what organizational skills the child is practicing, and that the teacher will provide a daily report on whether or not the child has used the skills in the classroom.

Describe the Use of Rewards in Sessions

Tell the child:

"You will be able to earn points in each session, which you can trade in for prizes." Points can be awarded for:

- Completing home practice between sessions and bringing the needed materials to our meetings.
- Listening to instructions.
- Practicing the steps taught.
- Accurately describing the steps to your parent.
- Packing required materials.

Show Therapist Form 1, and review the specific behaviors for which the child can earn points in this session. Note that this form is different from the general points form that will be used for regular sessions.

HELPFUL HINT: The points can be provided at the times suggested in the session outline. However, you can be flexible in providing points as you observe positive behaviors in session. If a child has been fully cooperative, the goal is to reach 10 points. Multiple points can be provided for each category. When giving points, provide praise to the child for showing the behavior. Of course, the points should be provided contingently. They should be used to encourage cooperation and engagement while discussing concerns about which the child may be quite sensitive.

Obtain the Parent's Understanding of the Treatment Schedule

Make certain that the family is able to engage in a twice-a-week therapy schedule. Verbally review Handout 2 (Treatment Expectations) with the parent. Ask whether the parent understands the treatment requirements and agrees to follow this plan as closely as possible.

If the parent is hesitant about agreeing to the commitment required for treatment, engage in problem solving to see whether any issues can be addressed. If they cannot be resolved, suggest an alternative to OST for consideration. For most cases, it is not recommended that OST be offered in piecemeal fashion (see Chapter 1).

Set a Schedule for Regular Twice-a-Week Meetings

Set times for regular twice-weekly sessions based on the child's schedule. *It is important to include a gap between sessions.* A gap of 2 days between sessions is ideal. Building skills requires practice for at least 1 day before presenting another skill. Suggest two session times a week, ideally on either Monday and Thursday or Tuesday and Friday. If a 2-day gap is not possible, you may work with a different schedule, as long as two sessions are scheduled each week on nonconsecutive days.

Review the Child's OTMP Difficulties

Describe the child's overall status (in relation to other children of the same age/grade) in OTMP behaviors. This should be based on your previous interview with the parents and teacher, and on the results of the BRIEF, COSS, or other assessment scales.

If the COSS was used, a simple statement should indicate that the child has scored above the cutoff for the Parent and Teacher COSS, the Parent COSS, or the Teacher COSS (whichever applies). For example, you might say to the child, "Your teacher let us know that you are having some trouble with organization in certain situations at school," or "Your parent also reported that you are having trouble staying organized at home." Finally, indicate how the child sees himself, based on the Child version of the COSS (e.g., "It looks like you also see yourself as having some trouble staying organized").

If other methods have been used to determine the child's organizational difficulties, refer to that information to establish why this treatment is appropriate for the child, in light of those difficulties.

Conclude the brief review of the formal scale results used or the intake interview by saying to the child:

"So it appears that some problems with getting and staying organized are tripping you up at home and at school. Fortunately, we have some special steps and tools that we can teach you how to use. For many children, learning to use these steps and tools has helped them get organized and avoid problems and conflicts at home and at school."

If the child has been cooperative to this point, award a point on Therapist Form 1, and indicate why the child has earned a point (e.g., "I am going to give you a point because you have been calm and listening carefully while we were talking about some difficulties you have being organized"). If the child has not paid attention or presented some challenging behaviors, this should be pointed out to the parent and child. For example:

"As we move along, I will have a chance to give you a point for listening carefully and cooperating with our discussion. Let's see if we can get some of those points in the next parts of our meeting."

Introduce the Guide to the Glitches

Use the Guide to the Glitches (Handout 3) to describe the approach you will be using to address OTMP problems. You should have two copies of the Guide to the Glitches. Give one to the child to keep. Have a two-pocket folder ready for the child, and another folder for the parent; let them know that they will use these folders for the materials they will be given in treatment. Keep the other copy of Handout 3, and make sure that you have one in your materials so that you can refer to it later in treatment.

Look at the pictures of the Glitches with the parent and child. Read the first few pages of text together, and look through the pictures of the four Glitches and the Mastermind. Details about each Glitch will be reviewed in other sessions.

Answer any questions. Determine whether the child and parent like the model, and check to see whether the ideas about Glitches make sense to them. If necessary, discuss and clarify any concerns or questions. Be tuned in to the possibility that they do not understand the Glitch metaphor or do not like this idea. If they are not receptive, describe the metaphor as just a way of thinking about OTMP difficulties. Let the child and parent know that it reflects the fact that organizational difficulties are often associated with ADHD, which makes them hard to control. Initiate a brief discussion to illustrate how the Glitches can get anyone into trouble.

(To the child) "Let's see if you have noticed that the Glitches have tricked anybody you know. I know that if I am rushing to leave my house, the Go-Ahead-Forget-It Glitch sometimes gets me when I leave my lunch on the kitchen counter. Maybe you have noticed when a Glitch has bothered one of your parents."

(To the parent) "Do you have any examples?"

(To both) "This is great. You see that the Glitches get to everyone. [Child's name], you have been listening really well. I think it's time to give another point for that [Therapist Form 1]. Now we are going to find out exactly how the Glitches mess with you at home and at school."

HELPFUL HINT: Give one copy of the Guide to the Glitches to the child to keep. Keep a copy of the Guide to the Glitches in your treatment materials, as you will refer to it frequently throughout treatment.

Conduct a Functional Assessment of the Child's OTMP Problems

The goal of the functional assessment is to determine exactly how difficulties with organizational skills affect the child and the family. After this review is completed, you should have a clear understanding of when, where, and in what situations the child struggles with organizing materials, managing time, and organizing the individual steps needed to complete tasks. You should also have an understanding about the level of conflict and stress that the child and family experience when the child encounters organizational skills problems.

Use Therapist Form 2 (Interview Record of Problems in Organization, Time Management, and Planning). The detailed information obtained in this interview reviews all of the areas addressed in four OST modules: Tracking Assignments, Managing Materials, Time Management, and Task Planning. While your initial pretreatment assessments have already yielded information on areas that the teacher and/or parent have endorsed as problematic, this interview will allow you to get a fuller picture of the child's OTMP struggles. Although all OTMP domains are the focus of treatment, the interview will help determine whether special attention (and perhaps extra practice) will be needed in domains that are identified as particularly problematic. The discussion below and Therapist Form 2 provide suggested questions for review from each of the OTMP domains.

HELPFUL HINT: This assessment needs to be conducted carefully and with a high level of support for the child. Throughout treatment, you will utilize an honest, direct approach that recognizes the child's difficulties without discouraging or blaming the child. During the interview, you need to gauge the tone of the discussion so that the child does not experience it as critical or distressing. Some children may argue with the information presented by their parents or may deny that they have any OTMP problems. If the child looks upset, let the child know that an honest discussion now will help overcome the conflicts that are occurring and reduce any distress that the child is experiencing at home and school. Praise the child for being brave in listening. Also, try to keep externalizing the problems as examples of the Glitches' being very crafty and getting the child into trouble.

Tell the child:

"Now we are going to discuss some difficulties you have staying organized. This will let us know how we can help you get better organized. It may be hard to listen to parts of this discussion, but we can use the information to help make things better at home and at school. I will keep giving points while you listen and participate in the discussion."

Use the Interview Record of Problems (Therapist Form 2) to guide your discussion for each organizational area. To review problems because of "Lapses in Memory and Materials

Management," you will review the area in general and then ask specific questions about common situations, such as keeping track of supplies, papers, and assignments, and other problematic areas (e.g., forgetting books in school). Ask the parent to describe what problems are noted at home in each area, and what problems the teacher has noted in the classroom related to these situations. For each situation discussed, you will ask the parent (with the child's help) to estimate how much the problems interfere with the child's functioning, as well as how much conflict the family experiences because of the problems (use Therapist Form 3 for rating the degree of interference and conflict experienced). The information that you gain on levels of interference and conflict will help you determine how much difficulty you and the child might encounter in overcoming problems in each area. Knowing that a particular area is associated with a high level of interference and/or conflict will help you anticipate when therapy may be particularly challenging for the child and family. For those particular areas, you will probably have to boost your enthusiasm, encouragement, and support.

As you go through the interview questions with the parent and child, focus on specific problems that the child experiences in each area, and try to gain an understanding of how those problems are manifested in the child's daily life. In addition, ask questions to determine whether the parent and/or teacher have already taken any steps to address these problems, and (if so) how successful these methods have been. The following is a sample discussion that might occur during the course of this functional assessment:

> THERAPIST: I would like to understand a bit more about concerns you've noted about Alex's difficulty remembering assignments and keeping track of supplies and papers. Can you tell me a little more about these kinds of problems?
>
> PARENT: It just feels like Alex is constantly misplacing his things. I can't keep reminding him to put his things away, but if I don't, he won't do it. Also, half the time, he doesn't have the things he needs to do his homework; he'll leave them in school or on the bus. It's just exhausting.
>
> THERAPIST: It sounds like the Go-Ahead-Forget-It Glitch is really causing trouble for you, Alex. Do you feel like there are certain times when this Glitch really pops up and makes it hard for you to remember things?
>
> ALEX: I guess I have a hard time remembering my homework stuff. Like, sometimes I forget to bring the books I need home, and then my mom gets really annoyed when I don't have them. I just have so many books at school, and sometimes I forget to put one or two in my backpack before I leave.
>
> THERAPIST: That must be frustrating. What happens when you realize you don't have the books you need for homework?
>
> ALEX: My mom yells at me, and then makes me call my friends to see if I can borrow theirs. Sometimes we drive back to school to get them. Sometimes my mom says she's not going to help me, so I just have to tell the teacher I couldn't do my homework.
>
> THERAPIST: OK, so it sounds like remembering books for homework is something that really causes problems for you at home. How much do you both think this problem with keeping track of supplies interferes with Alex's ability to do what he needs to do? Let's look at this Interference Rating Scale [on Therapist Form 3]. Would you say this problem interferes not at all, slightly, pretty much, or very much?
>
> PARENT: I would say that's a 4 on the scale. This is a serious problem for us, and comes up all the time.

THERAPIST: And how much conflict would you say this causes at home? Let's use the Conflict Rating Scale for this. Would you say none, a small amount, pretty much, or very much?

PARENT: Again, I would put that at a 4.

THERAPIST: And it looks like you agree with that, Alex. OK, so this is obviously one of the Glitch's tricks that is causing trouble for you. Have you tried anything to help Alex remember his things?

PARENT: I remind him every day, before he leaves the house, to bring home all his books for homework and really pay attention while he's packing up. But that doesn't seem to help. He says it's so crazy at the end of the day in school that he "just forgets."

THERAPIST: I understand. Lots of kids have the same kinds of problems with packing up their stuff and making sure they have what they need for schoolwork. This is one of the things we'll be working on together. We're going to teach you some ways to get that Go-Ahead-Forget-It Glitch under control, Alex, so that you can do what you need to do and not get into so much trouble with your mom and other grownups. Now I'm going to give you a session point, Alex, for staying calm while listening to your mom talk about your problems, and for giving me some really important information about the way the Glitches get in the way. [The therapist then moves on to the next area of concern in Lapses in Memory and Materials Management, perhaps asking about difficulties with keeping track of assignments next.]

For each area of "Lapses in Memory and Materials Management," you will guide the discussion similarly, focusing on the way the problem is experienced by the parent and child, the situations that are most problematic for the child, and the levels of interference and conflict this problem causes. You may not go through the Interview Record of Problems (Therapist Form 2) in order or ask all the questions, but should use that form flexibly, to record the concerns that are most prominent for the child and family.

To review "Problems in Time Management and Task Planning," review issues in that domain next, focusing on problems the child has with completing work and other activities on time, doing things carefully, and planning ahead for work or other activities. Ask the parent and child to provide specific examples of when these problems are noticed, and how often they occur. You might want to review specific items that the parent or teacher has endorsed on the COSS or BRIEF (if those measures were administered), or specific comments made during the initial interview, to get a better sense of the problems experienced in this area. Again, for each situation discussed, ask the parent to provide ratings of the degree of interference and/or conflict experienced because of these problems (Therapist Form 3). Finally, ask the Special Questions on Telling Time to determine the child's ability to tell time. Take another opportunity to provide the child with points.

To determine how well the child uses proactive organizational skills, review the area of "Problems with Organized Actions," asking about the child's use of special tools to record important information (e.g., assignments, due dates) or to store things. Get a sense of the kinds of organized actions the child takes to keep track of materials and responsibilities (e.g., calendar, school planner, folders, binders, storage boxes), and of the extent to which the child uses each tool properly.

Finally, ask about any other organizational areas that may create problems outside school. These problems may include managing equipment for sports, music lessons, other lessons, and clothes and toys or other items at home. Also, if the child moves from one parent's house to another in the case of separation or divorce, review problems that might occur because of this circumstance, such as leaving books or special toys at one house. Get interference and conflict ratings on the specific problems described. Award the child with points for good listening and comments throughout the discussion, and thank the child for being an active participant in this process.

Review the Family's Routines

The next interview is used to gain a better understanding of the family's and child's typical routines and schedules. It should reveal the family's rhythms and show how members of the family interact with one another. It can also provide a sense of how organized or chaotic the family environment is. Use Therapist Form 4 (Interview Form for Family's Schedule and Activities) to guide discussion and record responses. Explain that by reviewing the child's typical day during the week, you will be able to get to know the family a little better.

When the interview is finished, thank the parent and child for providing useful information. If appropriate, provide the child with another point.

Wrap Up the Session

Provide the Guide to the Glitches and a Folder Apiece to the Parent and Child

Give the child and parent a folder apiece to store session materials. The parent can store Handouts 1 and 2 in the folder, and should be instructed to bring the folder to future sessions. Tell the child to store the Guide to the Glitches (Handout 3) in the other folder, and to bring it to future sessions as well. Give the child a session point for storing the Guide to the Glitches in the folder.

Reward the Child

Sum the points earned. Let the child know that these behaviors resulted in earning 10 points, and that points can be used to obtain small prizes. Remind the child that points will be given for involvement in future sessions as well; if the child would prefer to save the points in a point bank, she can choose a larger prize in future sessions. If the child wants to select a prize at this point, either let the child pick a prize or provide the child with a 10-point prize (e.g., small toys or collectible items of interest to children in this age group). Most children should have no trouble earning this number of points. However, if the child was uncooperative and did not demonstrate the behaviors listed frequently enough to obtain 10 points, provide the child with praise for the behaviors that were observed and provide a smaller reward, such as a sticker or two. Alternatively, you could indicate that the child could have the points put into a point bank to be used at a later time.

Conclude the Session

Indicate that the next meeting is only with the parent. Check appointment time and schedule. Remind the child to bring the Guide to the Glitches to Session 3.

Introduction

Using Social Learning Strategies to Motivate Skills Building (for Parents Only)

You will:

- Provide an overview of the treatment goals and activities.
- Teach the parent the rationale and procedures for prompting, monitoring, praising, and rewarding the child's behaviors.

The parent will:

- Understand how ADHD puts a child at risk for developing OTMP difficulties.
- Understand that children with ADHD require extensive prompting and frequent, explicitly labeled praise.
- Learn how to track specific positive behaviors.
- Learn how to prompt, monitor, praise, and reward behaviors.
- Agree to complete a reward menu for homework.

For the parent:

- Handout 4, Helping Your Child Use Organizational Skills
- Handout 5, Interview for Developing a Reward Menu
- Handout 6, Homework: Let's Consider Possible Rewards
- Handout 7, Home Behavior Record: Behaviors to Prompt, Monitor, and Praise
- Handout 8, OTMP Checklist: Things to Remember for Session 3

For you:

- Materials for in-session practice with using praise:
  - Paper, markers/crayons, and containers
  - Blocks/Legos/small puzzles
  - Backpack with books, loose worksheets, and labeled folders (by subject)

ABOUT THIS SESSION

This session is held with the parent only. It is designed to prepare the parent for full participation in treatment by teaching how to prompt, monitor, praise, and reward the child's use of organizational skills. To encourage the parent, it is important to explain why parents need to participate so actively, be consistent in using the procedures described, and be patient as the child learns new OTMP skills.

SESSION SUMMARY CHECKLIST FOR SESSION 2

Item	Item Completed
Provide Information on ADHD and OTMP Problems	Yes/No
Discuss teaching organizational skills and turning them into habits	
Describe the skills and how they will be taught	Yes/No
Describe the therapist's role	Yes/No
Describe the parent's role (Handout 4)	Yes/No
Explain why parents need to prompt, monitor, praise, and reward	Yes/No
Explain when and how to use prompts	Yes/No
Describe what and how to monitor	Yes/No
Describe when and how to give labeled praise	Yes/No
Explain the system for positively rewarding the child	Yes/No
Conduct in-session practice: Use of praise	Yes/No
Interview the parent to develop a list of possible rewards (Handout 5)	Yes/No
Assign parent homework	
Create possible reward menus (Handout 6)	Yes/No
Prompt, monitor, and praise two non-OTMP behaviors (Handout 7)	Yes/No
Preview the next session (Handout 8)	Yes/No
Provide session points (if child waited while the parent was in session)	Yes/No

You will present a brief review of core ADHD symptoms and discuss why children with ADHD often have difficulty with organizational skills. If you believe a parent requires more time to understand the nature of ADHD (e.g., if a child has just received the diagnosis), then you should plan a separate instructional session to review all of the questions that may be raised.

One of the primary objectives of this session is to teach the parent the rationale and procedures for prompting, monitoring, praising, and rewarding the child's behaviors. This session is essential to gain the parent's cooperation in facilitating the child's practice of new organizational skills between sessions. The treatment does not focus on helping the parent create a behavior modification program for all problematic behaviors related to ADHD. Instead, the parent will learn techniques and procedures to encourage and facilitate the child's use of OTMP tools and routines.

DETAILED SESSION CONTENT

Provide Information on ADHD and OTMP Problems

This section of the session can vary in length. You can gauge the amount of time different families need by reviewing the parents' knowledge about ADHD. If parents are well versed, the time can be relatively short (about 5–10 minutes). If parents' knowledge is limited, briefly review the core ADHD symptoms of impulsivity, restlessness, and inattention. Review the subtypes, and indicate which subtype applies to the child. Then emphasize the deficits in executive functioning that hinder the child's ability to control behavior and attention at times, even though the child is capable of effectively regulating behavior and attention when highly motivated. Once you have explained this point, indicate how deficits in executive functing hinder the child's capacity to show organized behavior in response to day-to-day routines.

This information is intended to provide the parents with a rationale regarding why the treatment asks children to practice simple routines and why only selected, critical areas are stressed for school and home changes: tracking assignments, managing materials and supplies, managing time, and planning actions for projects and activities. Finally, explain that self-awareness and willingness to address one's problems is also lacking in most children with ADHD. Therefore, this treatment is designed to help the child address organizational problems gradually and with a great deal of support. In so doing, the treatment teaches skills in manageable chunks, so that the child is not overwhelmed and discouraged.

Explain that ADHD is believed to result from problems in brain systems that regulate behavior and attention:

> *Attention problems* show up in a variety of ways, including distractibility, difficulty sustaining attention long enough to complete tasks, not attending to detailed instructions at school, and so on.
> *Behavior problems* include being impulsive, being restless, having trouble waiting, and failing to keep track of time.

These difficulties, coupled with other symptoms of ADHD, make it hard for children to know what materials they need for working on projects, to remember what items to put in their backpacks or gym bags, to know how long it will take to complete assignments, or to plan a systematic approach to completing tasks.

A child is not to blame for these problems. On their own, children with ADHD often have difficulties with organization. However, they often can accomplish their required tasks when they are prompted by an adult. Thus, parents and teachers may wonder why the children do not simply stay organized independently. People often believe that children with ADHD are just being oppositional or lazy, when in reality the children require outside prompting because they cannot consistently activate the brain's "internal supervisor." OST is based on the idea that the brain's "internal supervisor," or the "Mastermind" from the Guide to the Glitches (Handout 3), is often missing in action for children with ADHD.

Discuss Teaching Organizational Skills and Turning Them into Habits

Explain that this treatment is designed to teach a child the skills necessary for getting and staying organized. Children with ADHD may not develop these skills on their own, or they may not use them consistently. The goal of OST is to make these skills part of a child's regular routine. To meet this goal, important adults, including parents, other caregivers, and teachers, need to help the child learn the skills and turn them into habits. They can do this by supporting the child in practicing these skills consistently, between sessions.

Describe the Skills and How They Will Be Taught

Review that the child will be taught skills in these four modules:

- Tracking Assignments—using assignment records and calendars.
- Managing Materials—organizing papers, books, backpacks, and desks.
- Time Management—understanding time requirements; consulting with parents and teachers to set a schedule; organizing tasks in relation to time.
- Task Planning—learning the steps in planning; consulting with parents and teachers to develop effective plans.

Describe the Therapist's Role

Explain that in each session, you will:

- Introduce a skill to the child.
- Show the child how the skill can be useful.
- Teach each skill as a series of steps.
- Have the child practice the skill's steps in the session.
- Discuss with the child where and when, at home and at school, she will practice the skill.
- Talk with the child about how to deal with potential problems that might make it difficult to use the skill.

At the end of each session, the child will tell the parent about the skill learned that day, demonstrate the skill for the parent, and explain how to use it. Together, you and the parent will arrange a schedule for practice of the new skill between sessions.

Describe the Parent's Role

Explain that the parent's role is to help the child practice each skill and incorporate it into the daily schedule. To do this most effectively, the parent needs to learn to:

1. *Prompt.* Remind the child when the skill should be used.
2. *Monitor.* Keep track of when and how often the child uses the skill.
3. *Give labeled praise.* Praise the child and say what the praise is for (i.e., attach a label to the praise by telling the child exactly which behavior was good).
4. *Reward.* Reinforce the child for successfully using the skill.

Explain to the parent: "We expect that the child will require time and practice to master these skills, so we will work slowly and patiently." Make it clear that you do not expect that simply telling the child what to do will work. You do not expect, for example, that you can tell the child how to keep track of papers and that the child will be able to apply that instruction consistently. Instead, you will work with the parent and child to develop an appropriate routine for keeping track of papers; teach the child the steps that must be followed to use that routine; and develop a method for the child to practice those skills repeatedly, with prompting from you, the parent, and the teacher.

Explain that a parent's help is essential to ensure that a child's practice is consistent and effective. This is why it is important for parents to learn why, how, and when to implement the behavioral techniques reviewed in this session, so that they can use them throughout this treatment to support their children's acquisition of new organizational skills.

Explain Why Parents Need to Prompt, Monitor, Praise, and Reward

> **HELPFUL HINT:** The following materials present parents with a short course in behavior modification. The usual ABC model has been translated into a "prompt, monitor, praise, and reward" model. These are the four behaviors that parents need to understand and utilize well. The model emphasizes consequences rather than stimulus control, although the treatment does present expectations regarding which behaviors should be performed in specific situations, so there is some attention to antecedents.

Explain to the parent that you, the parent, and the teacher will use basic behavior modification techniques (prompt, monitor, praise, and reward) to motivate skills practice and skills development. To begin with, the parent should understand a few basic principles related to the rationale for prompting, monitoring, praising, and rewarding new skill performance:

1. To learn a new behavior, children need to learn *when* to perform the new behavior; thus they need prompting from a responsible adult.
2. Children also need to learn that positive things will happen right after they demonstrate the new behavior; this makes it more likely that the behavior will be incorporated into their regular routines.
3. Positive things that motivate children include praise/attention from adults, a chance to participate in pleasurable activities, getting to play with special toys, having a special snack, going to a special place, or receiving points toward prizes.
4. Children with ADHD learn best when they get clear prompts (reminders), get praise for cooperation and effort, and obtain rewards for desired behaviors.

Tell the parent:

"When you prompt your child, you tell her [or him] exactly what behavior you expect to see. When you monitor your child, you know whether or not the behavior has been performed. When you praise your child, it is likely that the child will continue to use the behavior. And when you reward your child, your child is even more motivated to continue using the behavior at the appropriate time in the future."

Provide the parent with Handout 4 (Helping Your Child Use Organizational Skills), and indicate that it summarizes this discussion about how parents can help children improve their behavior.

Explain When and How to Use Prompts

Explain that during OST, the child will learn how to use skills in specific situations where organization is useful. For example, the child will be asked to check his backpack before school for items that will be needed for the day. This would be an appropriate time for the parent to prompt the child by asking him to go through the process of checking that items are present. Prompting is best done by:

- Moving close to the child.
- Gaining the child's attention, perhaps by making eye contact.
- Asking for one thing at a time.
- Being clear and concise.
- Using a pleasant voice.

Prompting should not involve repeated requests in a "nagging" tone of voice. The parent may need to repeat the prompt, but this should be done in a matter-of-fact, calm voice.

Here are some examples of effective prompts:

"Please put your books in your backpack."
"It is time to start your homework. Please get your desk ready by clearing off the extra materials."
"I think you need to plan your afternoon. Tell me how long you think it will take to finish your homework."
"Please look at the clock. You have 15 minutes before we have to leave for soccer. I want you to get the rest of the math problems on this sheet done before we leave."

Describe What and How to Monitor

Describe how charts will be used to monitor the child's performance of new organizational skills that are learned in sessions. The parent and teacher will use the charts to keep track of whether and how often the child performs the organizational skills. They will prompt, monitor, and praise/reward use of a new skill as it is being learned. After the child has mastered a skill, the parent and teacher will continue to praise the child's use of that skill, but will move on to monitor and reward newly learned skills. However, if questions arise about whether a child is still using a previously mastered skill, it may be necessary to add the previous skill back to the chart and monitor its occurrence.

Describe When and How to Give Labeled Praise

Explain that the parent should praise the child for listening to the prompt/instruction, praise again for initiating the behavior, and remind the child that points will be received for completing the requested behavior. In praising the child, the parent should describe the behavior that is being praised. Make certain that the parent knows that praise can be provided in the parent's personal style. The parent does not have to be a cheerleader or super-sweet, just honest and positive. Here are some examples:

> "Good job! You carefully checked to make sure all of your papers were put in your binder."
> "Great! You cleared your desk for homework."
> "Wow. You have all of your things in your bag."
> "Nice job. Your homework supplies are all out and ready."
> "This is wonderful; you have all of your homework listed on your assignment sheet."
> "OK, you wrote down all of the steps you need to take to complete your report."
> "Thank you. You helped by putting your toys back in the storage bin."

Explain the System for Positively Rewarding the Child

Explain that immediate praise is rewarding and important. In addition, a point system for earning more tangible rewards is important to motivate the child. The point system will be set up to work as follows:

1. For learning and practicing skills, the child can earn points that count toward rewards.
2. Rewards can be provided at the end of each day when a set number of points are earned.
3. Rewards can also be provided at the end of each week for accumulated points.

For the system to work, the rewards need to be activities and/or items the child finds genuinely enticing. Some rewards can be created by restricting desired items or activities that a child now receives for "free" (without any requirements) and making the child earn those things by accumulating points for using the new organizational skills. For example, the child may "earn" 20 minutes of video game time if she uses the newly learned skills to organize materials.

Conduct In-Session Practice: Use of Praise

Tell the parent:

> "Now that we have gone over the general concepts involved in motivating improved organizational skills, I want to work with you to practice praising your child for small, desired actions. By reinforcing the smaller actions that make up a new skill, you can encourage your child to incorporate that new skill into daily routines."

Select an activity you can ask the parent to do that will allow you to demonstrate how to focus on small, positive actions on a frequent basis. When you provide labeled praise to the parent, do it often, at a rate of once every 20–30 seconds or so.

Here are our suggested options for in-session practice:

1. Have a supply of paper, markers, and/or crayons. Ask the parent to make a drawing of a house, car, or animal. As the parent draws, comment on the positive actions you observe. Examples of comments:

    "I like how you are concentrating on your drawing."
    "You seem to be thinking carefully about your drawing. That's great."
    "What an interesting choice of colors. That looks really nice."
    "I like your straight lines."
    "Your drawing is very creative."
    "You are putting in a great effort to get this done."
    "Thank you for listening to my request to make a drawing."

2. Provide some blocks, other construction toys, or a small jigsaw puzzle, and ask the parent to make something out of the pieces. Comment on positive actions. Examples of comments:

    "I liked how you looked at me when I gave the directions."
    "Thank you for following the directions to make something."
    "You made a very nice start on your design."
    "You are picking up the pieces carefully."
    "I like how you are concentrating on your play."
    "You are staying nicely focused on what you are doing."
    "You are making a very good effort to put the pieces together."

3. Have a backpack, books, papers, and folders available. Ask the parent to pack the backpack with all of the books, and to put papers that are labeled by subject in the correct folder (also labeled). Comment on positive actions. Examples of comments:

    "Very good listening to my request!"
    "You are showing me that you remembered what I said. That's great."
    "I like how you are looking at the labels on the folders. That is a good way to decide where to put the papers."
    "You are putting all of the books in the backpack. That's a very good way to get organized."
    "I like how you are working carefully to make sure you get everything in the bag."
    "That was good, when you looked at the paper to know which folder it goes into."
    "You are going at a good pace, but you are not rushing."
    "You are putting things in the bag carefully and neatly. I like that."

4. Have the parent put away markers and paper. Provide a container for the markers and a folder for the papers. Leave some of the tops off the markers. Examples of comments:

    "I am glad that you looked at me when I gave you the directions."
    "You are doing a good job picking up the markers."
    "You are putting the right color cap on each marker. That's great."
    "I see you are using the folder for the papers, like I asked. Thank you. You are doing well."

"It looks like you have almost all of the markers in the container. It's nice to see how carefully you're working."

"It is nice to see you do this with a smile."

"You are still going at it. I like how you are staying focused on picking up markers."

After the practice, summarize what you did as you praised the parent:

"I hope that you noticed that I provided positive comments. I also noticed and commented on small actions. Finally, I made comments often. All of these strategies will help motivate your child to get started on an activity and continue working on that activity. Providing such labeled praise also helps keep your relationship with your child positive. It makes your child more interested in pleasing you. When you take these actions, they go a long way to help children build skills, including getting better organized."

You should now switch roles with the parent, engaging in the activities and asking the parent to provide you with labeled praise. Suggest that the parent can use the tips listed in the "Praise" section of Handout 4 to provide appropriate praise, as you role-play a child engaging in an activity. At times, step out of your role as a child to provide feedback and any corrections. Make certain that the parent understands that the praise does not have to be "fake." Again, the parent can develop a personal style, which does not have to be syrupy-sweet. Help the parent observe closely and select positive behaviors to praise, even if the statements are short in duration. In particular, guide the parent in the process of finding brief instances of positive behaviors, even when your behavior as the "child" is challenging and not matching the parent's expectations exactly.

In your role play, demonstrate some mild misbehavior. For example, say, "I don't want to do that now." Then step out of the role play and ask the parent to ignore what you have just said. For instance, tell the parent that she could say, "I like that you listened to me and know what I asked you to do. Please get started."

If there is time, demonstrate two different activities. It can be very useful to use the backpack activity to help the parent practice providing labeled praise for organizational skills.

After the practice, ask the parent to consider how his child reacts to praise. Some children do not enjoy praise. In this case, suggest that the parent just thank the child for engaging in the behavior.

Interview the Parent to Develop a List of Possible Rewards

If time permits, conduct a brief interview with the parent about the things the child enjoys, using Handout 5 (Interview for Developing a Reward Menu). Inform the parent that this information will help her in selecting appropriate rewards that will motivate the child to perform the new behaviors learned in this treatment.

If you complete this interview in session, make a copy of the information gathered for your records. You can then refer to it in the next session, when you will help construct a reward menu. If you do not have time to complete this interview in session, you may instruct the parent to do this for homework. Make sure to check that the parent understands the instructions, and ask whether the parent has any questions about how to use the form at home.

Assign Parent Homework

Create Possible Reward Menus

If you have completed Handout 5 in session, give the parent the filled-in handout and ask him to select which items on that form can be used as daily rewards and which can be used as weekly rewards. The parent should record those selections on Handout 6 (Homework: Let's Consider Possible Rewards). Otherwise, the parent will complete Handout 5 as a brainstorming exercise at home, and use what is written there to fill in Handout 6.

Emphasize that it is important for the parent to follow through on the process of creating a reward menu, which should take about 10–20 minutes. Emphasize that this is crucial, as the treatment cannot move forward appropriately unless a home behavior management program is in place.

Prompt, Monitor, and Praise Two Non-OTMP Behaviors

Help the parent select two behaviors from the list below (or two other behaviors of concern to the parent) to prompt, monitor, and praise for the week. Make sure the parent does not select behaviors that reflect the child's major problems with OTMP behaviors. The behaviors selected should be ones on which the child can show improvement easily, as the parent begins to practice the use of praise after this session and add point rewards after the next session. The experience should both encourage the parent and be motivating to the child. The selected behaviors below are not as complicated as OTMP behaviors. Directly addressing organizational problems at this time may cause the child to become antagonistic or defensive.

Suggested Behaviors to Prompt, Monitor, and Praise (Choose Two)
- Picking up clothes off floor
- Brushing teeth
- Putting toys away
- Clearing table after meal
- Feeding a pet
- Hanging up coat
- Turning off lights
- Laying out clothes for the morning
- Making bed
- Others: _____

_____

To document that he has prompted, monitored, and praised the two behaviors, the parent should fill out Handout 7 (Home Behavior Record: Behaviors to Prompt, Monitor, and Praise). Explain that the parent will have to show successful and consistent attempts to prompt, monitor, and praise these two behaviors before turning to prompting, monitoring, praising, and rewarding the child for completing important OTMP behaviors. So completion of this homework is essential in order to address the Glitches that impair the child's organizational functioning. This expectation ensures that the parent is engaged in fulfilling the parental role in treatment.

Preview the Next Session

Give the parent Handout 8 (OTMP Checklist: Things to Remember for Session 3), inform the parent that the next session will include the parent and the child. The first part of the session will review the parent's homework assignment to prompt, monitor, and praise the two non-OTMP behaviors selected. Then the menu of rewards will be reviewed, and the parent will be provided with guidelines for rewarding the non-OTMP behaviors. Finally, the child will begin to receive instruction in the first OTMP skill.

Provide Session Points

If the child waited while the parent was in session, you may call the child into session at this point and give up to 10 points for waiting patiently. Allow the child to select a reward or save the points for future use. Tell the child that you will start your work together in the next session, and remind the child to bring the folder from Session 1 to the next meeting.

Tracking Assignments

*Implementing Behavior Management Procedures
and Getting It All Down*

GOALS FOR THE SESSION

You and the parent will:

- Develop a simple point program, which provides the child with daily and weekly rewards for target behaviors.

The parent will:

- Demonstrate an understanding that she must change her routine (i.e., implement behavior-monitoring procedures) to help her child control the Glitches.
- Agree to prompt, monitor, praise, and/or reward specified target behaviors on a daily and weekly basis.
- Demonstrate understanding of how she can monitor the child's use of the Daily Assignment Record (Handout 10).

The child will:

- Understand why it is important to keep track of assignments and avoid the Go-Ahead-Forget-It Glitch.
- Share information about how he is informed about homework assignments, and how he currently keeps track of that information.
- Practice writing down assignments and listing materials needed for completing assignments on the Daily Assignment Record (Handout 10).

MATERIALS NEEDED

For the parent:

- OTMP parent's folder
- Handout 9, Reward Menu
- Handout 13, Home Behavior Record: Behaviors to Prompt, Monitor, and Praise

For you:

- Whiteboard or blackboard, with markers or chalk/eraser
- Therapist Form 5, Session Points and Notes
- Therapist Form 6, Interview Form for Tracking Assignments

For the child:

- File folder with 20 copies of the Daily Assignment Record (Handout 10) stapled to the right side, and an Assignment and Test Calendar (Handout 11) for the current month stapled to the left side
- Handout 10, Daily Assignment Record (three to five copies for in-session practice)
- Handout 12, Reminder for the Daily Assignment Record
- Handout 14, OTMP Checklist: Things to Remember for Session 4

ABOUT THIS SESSION

This session represents the start of the skills-building sessions with the child. The session emphasizes the first skill module, Tracking Assignments. It focuses on teaching the child a new method for tracking assignments and keeping track of items needed to complete those assignments—namely, the Daily Assignment Record (often referred to as the DAR). In addition, you will work together with the parent, at the start of this session, to develop a simple point program that will be used to reward specific target behaviors. This point program will be used to reinforce and support the child's between-session practice of all the target behaviors learned over the course of the treatment; thus you must work with the parent to develop a point program that is simple to use and acceptable to both parent and child. Some parents may have more difficulty developing and implementing an appropriate point program. In such a case, it may be necessary to spend additional time helping the parent understand, create, and agree to cooperate with an appropriate behavior modification system.

IN PREPARATION FOR THIS SESSION

The first teacher contact should have been held prior to this session, so you should know what procedure for tracking assignments is acceptable to the teacher. The preferred method is the development of a personalized DAR (as detailed in the session content). However, a teacher may already have a method, such as a specific planner, that can be adapted if the teacher is uncomfortable with the idea of allowing the child to use a different method from

SESSION SUMMARY CHECKLIST FOR SESSION 3

Item	Item Completed
Review implementation of behavior monitoring, and develop a simple point program (with parent/child)	
Review questions about behavior modification steps (Handout 7)	Yes/No
Discuss and problem-solve challenges to implementation	Yes/No
Review list of rewards that may be used to reinforce target behaviors (Handout 6)	Yes/No
Develop a simple point program (Handout 9)	Yes/No
Conduct skills building with the child alone: The Daily Assignment Record	
Discuss the need to track assignments	Yes/No
Review how the Go-Ahead-Forget-It Glitch can cause problems (Handout 3)	Yes/No
Gather information from the child about the nature of homework assignments/materials, and methods used for keeping track of these (Therapist Form 6)	Yes/No
Show sample of the Daily Assignment Record (Handout 10) and personalize with the child's subjects	Yes/No
Conduct in-session practice: Recording assignments with the DAR	Yes/No
Wrap up the session (with parent/child)	
Support the child in explaining the use of the DAR to the parent (Handouts 10, 12)	Yes/No
Describe the home exercise; review how the parent will prompt, monitor, and reward two non-OTMP target behaviors, and prompt, monitor, and praise use of the DAR (Handout 13)	Yes/No
Reward the child (Therapist Form 5)	Yes/No
Conclude the session (Handout 14)	Yes/No

the other students in the class. Before working with the existing method, make certain that you know how successful the child is in tracking assignments, turning in assignments, and having necessary materials for assignments when using that method. It is imperative that you speak with the teacher before the child uses the DAR (or other method) at school, so that the teacher knows how to prompt, monitor, praise, and record school points for the child's use of new organizational steps. If a teacher does not find that the DAR is an acceptable approach, please turn to the "Alternative Procedures" section, which follows the "Detailed Session Content," to obtain ideas for an adaptation. For most children, having a reliable method for tracking assignments is critical, so we do not advise dropping this component of treatment.

DETAILED SESSION CONTENT

Review Implementation of Behavior Monitoring, and Develop a Simple Point Program (with Parent/Child)

The discussion with the parent on the use of behavior management procedures is crucial. It may not be possible to complete all of the material in this session. The work with the child can be cut short and rolled over into the next session. There is enough room in sessions later on to make up for the delayed content. Therefore, make sure to take the time to obtain parental compliance in implementing prompting, monitoring, and praising for target behaviors. Also, make sure that the parent understands how to set point goals for the day and for the week. Finally, take the time to make certain that the parent has a list of desired rewards for the target behaviors that will be provided on a daily basis and a weekly basis. All of these steps are outlined below in detail.

Review Questions about Behavior Modification Steps

Review the Home Behavior Record from the previous session (Handout 7) with the parent, asking him to discuss the two behaviors that he was asked to prompt, monitor, and praise in the previous session. Ask the parent about the methods used for prompting the behaviors, and note whether he indicated in the specified box on the Home Behavior Record whether or not the behavior occurred. Ask both the parent and child to describe what happened when the behaviors were praised. Also, ask them both whether they have any questions about how to use the Home Behavior Record or, more generally, how to implement the prompt–monitor–praise sequence with target behaviors.

Discuss and Problem-Solve Challenges to Implementation

Prompting, monitoring, and rewarding behaviors with praise and points are crucial parts of the program. It is important to make certain that parents know how to use these steps and agree with the use of these steps. If a parent is confused by the process, take the time to clarify the procedures and explain how to integrate the procedures into the daily routine. If necessary, provide a brief review of the material introduced in the previous session, so that the parent understands the use of the simple behavior modification procedures involved in the program.

If the parent has not completed the Home Behavior Record, it may be necessary to spend some time reviewing how the parent can change the daily routine to incorporate prompting, monitoring, and praising target behaviors (see Handout 4). *Do not allow the parent to begin awarding points and rewards for OTMP target behaviors until the parent has demonstrated successful attempts to prompt, monitor, and praise the two non-OTMP behaviors.*

If the parent has not been effective in tracking the behaviors of concern, it is appropriate to find out what factors hindered the completion of this homework. For example, a parent might indicate difficulty with remaining calm and matter-of-fact when delivering prompts. Alternatively, a parent might admit that she was unable to remember to use the Home Behavior Record, or that she left it at home instead of bringing it to the session.

Use a patient, problem-solving approach to determine what got in the way of implementation and to develop some ideas on how to overcome those barriers. Below is an example of a problem-solving approach that might be taken with a parent who has forgotten the Home Behavior Record at home.

> PARENT: I was so busy rushing out of the house to get here that I forgot the chart at home.
>
> THERAPIST: It can be difficult to remember all the things you need when you're trying to get somewhere with young children. Let's see if we can think of a way to make it easier for you to remember your papers for these sessions. Where did you keep the Home Behavior Record? Was it in the treatment folder? On a bulletin board or fridge?
>
> PARENT: I had it on the fridge, so I could remember to do it. But then I forgot to take it down and put it back in my folder.
>
> THERAPIST: What if you set up an alert on your phone that reminds you, on the morning of the days we meet, to put the Home Behavior Record back in your folder and put the folder in your car? Would that help?

Review List of Rewards That May Be Used to Reinforce Target Behaviors

Ask both the parent and child about the list of rewards that they have compiled (Handout 6), obtaining feedback from the child to determine how motivating the listed rewards are to him. Based on this feedback, and a consideration of practical issues (e.g., the parent's assessment of how easy it will be for her to distribute specific rewards), help the parent compile a brief menu of rewards, from which the child will be able to choose (see Handout 9). If the parent did not complete Handout 6 and is having difficulty thinking of possible rewards for the child, you may spend some time helping the parent and child think together of rewards that are realistic and motivating. Use the interview questions on Handout 5 to guide this discussion. The following rewards may be helpful as suggestions for parents who are "stuck" in trying to think of rewards.

Daily Rewards

- Special time with parent (e.g., reading, puzzles, games, outside time)
- TV/computer/music player/video game time (less time for fewer points and more time for more points)
- Art/drawing materials
- Staying up 15–30 minutes past bedtime (depending on the number of points earned)
- Choosing dessert
- Riding bike

Weekly Rewards

- Dinner or lunch at a restaurant
- Trip to a park/zoo/bowling alley/other special destination
- Seeing a movie in a theater
- Having a friend over for a sleepover
- Being excused from doing a chore
- Small toys/collectibles
- Credit for iTunes

Develop a Simple Point Program

For most parents participating in this treatment, a simple point program is best; overly elaborate systems will only overwhelm parents and make follow-through less likely. The main objective in developing the point program is to help a parent and child establish daily and weekly goals for the target behaviors. Daily rewards will be given for completion of selected target behaviors each day, and weekly rewards will be given for cumulative performance over the course of the week (i.e., for the sum of points from all days of the week).

At this point, the parent is learning to consistently prompt, monitor, and reward only two behaviors—namely, the non-OTMP behaviors selected in Session 2. One simple option for developing this system is to follow the guidelines below (see Handout 9):

- Each target behavior on the Home Behavior Record is worth 1 point; thus, on the current Home Behavior Record (Handout 13), the child can earn a maximum of 2 points. The daily goals can be set at 50% and 100% of the points that can be earned for performing the target behaviors. The child can select from Level One on the Reward Menu for performing one of the behaviors (i.e., earning 1 point), and from Level Two (more valued prizes/activities) for performing both of the behaviors (i.e., earning 2 points).
- For weekly rewards, suggest that the parent set a goal of approximately 60% of the possible points over the days on which the behaviors are possible, to earn a Level One reward. That goal is likely to be 6 out of 10 possible points for performance over the 5 weekdays. If the child earns 80% or more of the weekly points, the child may choose from the Level Two rewards.

HELPFUL HINT: The guidelines for calculating weekly points, outlined above and on Handout 9, are based upon a situation in which the parent is monitoring target behaviors that are only observed on weekdays (e.g., performing a chore that is only required on weekdays), so that the total possible points that could be earned is 10. If the parent is monitoring target behaviors for all 7 days of the week, adjust the total possible weekly points accordingly on Handout 9.

Make certain that the parent understands how to use the simple point program and when to provide the rewards (at the end of each day *and* at the end of the week). Present the parent with a hypothetical situation that illustrates use of the point program.

Tell the parent:

"For now, you will be monitoring two behaviors for your child at home—picking up clothes off the floor, and clearing the table. Let's pretend that on Monday, your child picks up her clothes, but does not clear the table when prompted. You would give her 1 point for the day, and let her choose from the choices under Level One on the Reward Menu. If she picks up her clothes and clears the table on Tuesday, you would give her 2 points for the day, and let her choose a reward from Level Two on the Reward Menu. Now let's say that on Wednesday, Thursday, and Friday, your child performs both of these behaviors, earning 2 points each day. On Friday, you would praise your child for earning 9 points for the week, and tell her to choose a weekly reward from Level Two on the Reward Menu."

If you know that the family schedule is very tight, you may decide to allow parents to provide rewards only once a week. However, this decision should only be made under the following conditions: (1) if the child is showing good progress; (2) if the parents are providing a high level of praise on a daily basis; and (3) if the child agrees to this provision (i.e., if the weekly reward is motivating enough). If you believe that the child needs more concrete, immediate feedback daily, you may suggest that the parent provide the child with a nominal item daily, such as a sticker, temporary tattoo, or stamp.

Inform the parent and child that you will briefly review implementation of the point program at the beginning of each session; thus the parent should be prepared in each session with the Home Behavior Record and a report of which rewards were used to reinforce positive performance. Ask whether the parent has any questions about how to implement this program at home, and review any questions or concerns carefully.

Remind the parent and child that points will also be used to reward positive behaviors during the sessions. Let the child know that the behaviors he uses to control the Glitches will be rewarded with points during the sessions, and that he will be able to select a small prize for accumulated points at the end of each session.

Indicate that the session will now focus on work with the child. Politely excuse the parent, and begin the work with the child.

Conduct Skills Building with the Child Alone:
The Daily Assignment Record

Praise the child for listening carefully and/or contributing to the discussion with the parent regarding the point program. You may award the child points on the Session Points and Notes form (Therapist Form 5) at this time. Then explain to the child that you will be speaking today about why it is important to keep track of assignments and the items needed to complete those assignments.

Discuss the Need to Track Assignments

Initiate a discussion with the child about the reasons why we need to keep track of our assignments, or of the things we need to get done. Explain that sometimes when people forget their assignments, they can get into trouble. You can ask whether this has ever happened to the child; for example, ask what happens when the child goes back to school without homework.

Next, consider, with the child, some real-life problems that might happen if a person forgets assignments. You may draw from the following examples for this discussion, or make up your own, based on the child's interests.

If the child likes sports . . ."

"Do you know that professional teams have equipment managers?"

"Let's pretend that the equipment manager for the New York Yankees [or another favorite team] had to remember to put new shoelaces in Derek Jeter's [or another favorite player's] spikes before a big game. Let's pretend that he forgot to do it, and Jeter was all ready to play but he could not, because he could not lace his spikes. What would happen to the equipment manager?"

"Let's pretend that the coach of the U.S. Gymnastics team for the Olympics has asked the equipment manager to order new gloves and wrist supports for the team. The equipment manager has many things to do and forgets to order the new gloves. When the competition starts, the gymnasts do not have the new gloves they need to perform on the parallel bars. What will happen to the equipment manager?"

"Think about Hope Solo, the goalie for U.S. Women's Soccer [or another favorite player for a favorite team]. Imagine she needed new goalie gloves and asked the equipment manager to get them. But the Go-Ahead-Forget-It Glitch got in the way. A big game was starting, and Hope asked for her gloves. The manager said she forgot them. What would they do?"

If the child likes music . . .

"Famous singers go on tour. Who is your favorite singer? Well let's pretend that singer has a new song. The tour organizer is told to type out the words so the singer can memorize the words while traveling to the show. What would happen if the tour organizer forgot that assignment?"

"Let's pretend that the person who has to check all of the microphones forgets that he was supposed to replace the battery on one of the cordless microphones. The famous singer goes to start the show, and no one can hear her. What will happen then?"

Then tell the child:

"These are just some examples of problems that can happen when people forget their assignments. These problems can develop very easily when the Go-Ahead-Forget-It Glitch is around. Today we are going to start helping you keep track of your assignments at school, because even though we all try to remember everything we're supposed to do, sometimes we have to help ourselves out by doing special things. We want you to always make sure you know what you are supposed to do and what you are supposed to have with you. Our approach will help keep the Go-Ahead-Forget-It Glitch under control."

Review How the Go-Ahead-Forget-It Glitch Can Cause Problems

Tell the child:

"Let's look at the Guide to the Glitches [Handout 3] for a moment, to remind ourselves of the problems the Go-Ahead-Forget-It Glitch can cause when we don't keep it under control."

Review the description of the Go-Ahead-Forget-It Glitch in detail, paying special attention to the ways that the Glitch tries to get the child in trouble by convincing the child that she does not need to write down her assignments. Give the child session points (Therapist Form 5) for listening to the discussion thus far, and for giving examples of ways in which the Go-Ahead-Forget-It Glitch has gotten the child into trouble by making him forget important assignments or materials.

*Gather Information from the Child about the Nature of Homework
Assignments/Materials, and Methods Used for Keeping Track of These*

Using Therapist Form 6 as a guide, discuss what homework the child usually gets, what materials are usually needed to complete the homework, how the child is told about homework, and what method the child uses to remember the homework assignments and materials. To keep the child engaged in this discussion, provide praise and session points for examples and answers that the child provides.

*Show Sample of the Daily Assignment Record, and Personalize
with the Child's Subjects*

Tell the child:

> "So now we've talked about why it's important to have a way of keeping track of our assignments—to make sure that the Go-Ahead-Forget-It Glitch doesn't get us in trouble. We've also discussed how you keep track of your homework assignments, and we've talked about some times when that method hasn't worked out perfectly for you [you can refer specifically to any issues the child has noted].
>   "It seems like the most important things to have, when we think about keeping track of our assignments, are (1) a place to write down the assignments and (2) a way of making sure that you know which materials to take home for those assignments."

Explain that you are going to give the child an assignment record that has been very useful for other children, because it helps the child keep track of the assignments *and* the items that are needed for those assignments. Show the child the Daily Assignment Record (Handout 10), and describe why it is a helpful record for keeping track of assignments. Highlight the following components of the DAR:

- The subject listed on the side
- The place for writing the assignment for the day
- The place for checking off needed materials
- The place to write down assignments that are not due the next day
- The place for teachers to mark that the child has filled in the information accurately

HELPFUL HINT: You will need the child to help you personalize the subjects listed. Thus it is best if you can conduct this session with access to a computer and printer, so that you can type in the appropriate subjects and print out accurate copies for the child. If this is not possible, you may also cross out and write in the appropriate subjects for the first few forms, and have blank copies ready for the next session.

Tell the child:

> "I think that using this Daily Assignment Record, or DAR (as we often call it), could make it less likely that you will forget any assignments or items that you need to complete your

assignments. Let's practice using it, and then we can see if we should change it at all to fit what you need."

Conduct In-Session Practice: Recording Assignments with the DAR

Provide the child with *three* different situations that simulate the number and type of assignments the child receives. Have the child complete the DAR for each of these practice situations. Include some trials in which assignments are stated orally, and some in which the assignments are written down on the whiteboard or blackboard.

The following are some examples that can be used for practice. You may also use examples that more closely fit the child's typical homework assignments.

Examples

1. A math assignment with a worksheet on multiplication, a spelling assignment to do p. 16 in a spelling workbook, and a science assignment to review facts on a handout.
2. A math assignment with a worksheet and two review pages from a math workbook, a reading assignment to write a reading journal entry, and a social studies assignment to color in a map.
3. A social studies assignment to create a family tree, a science assignment to come up with an idea for the science fair, and a math assignment requiring the use of a workbook and a protractor.
4. A spelling assignment to write sentences using 10 of the week's spelling words, a math assignment to study for tomorrow's quiz on averages (using the math workbook and class notes), and a reading assignment to read two chapters in a book.

Act as the teacher, giving example assignments, and instruct the child to use the DAR to write down the assignments and check off the items needed. Do not provide corrective feedback during the time that the child is writing down assignments; give the child feedback only after she has completed each practice example. Provide praise for the act of writing, for writing down information accurately, for checking off items needed, and for listening to any corrective feedback.

After the child has completed three rounds of practice with the DAR, show the child the DAR folder that he will take home. Show the child that 20 copies of the DAR are stapled together on the right side of the folder, and the left side of the folder has two pages that contain school-day calendars for the current month and the next month. Indicate that one DAR can be used each day. Inform the child that she will be leaving with one of these folders to use, as her new method for keeping track of assignments.

HELPFUL HINT: You can decide, with the child, how she will manage use of the DAR sheets in the folder. Some children prefer to tear off the top page after each day's homework is completed, leaving a fresh sheet on top for filling in the next day's assignment. However, only allow the child to do this if she is able to reliably save those old sheets in a folder, as she will need to bring those old sheets to each session to review with you. Alternatively, the child should be instructed to leave all sheets stapled in and flip to the next blank sheet when she needs to write down a new day's assignments. You can tear out and review the old sheets at each session meeting, so that the folder does not become cluttered with too many papers. This latter method should only be used at the very beginning of treatment. Later, the child should have only the most recent DAR on top, so that she can see the calendar and the day's assignments in one viewing.

Provide the child with another *two or three* simulated situations in which he is required to write down assignments, check what is needed, and list any longer-term assignments. (It is important to have the child practice in session with the method approved by the teacher.) Review the accuracy of responses after the child has completed each example, and award session points for good practicing. Note any mistakes (e.g., omissions, mismatches, etc.) after each trial, and encourage the child to increase accuracy on the next trial.

Adjust the number of practices based on several factors, including how much time is left, how slowly the child writes, and your assessment of two of the important treatment goals for children:

1. Has the child obtained enough practice to indicate understanding and comfort with the "boring" procedure?
2. Is the child proficient in using the DAR or planner to record assignments and materials needed?

Stop the session in the allotted time period. However, do not consider that the child has met criteria for moving on to the next skill until the child has successfully completed two trials with 100% accuracy. Thus you might decide to present additional practice opportunities with the DAR in the next session, if the child is struggling with the practices in this session.

Wrap Up the Session (with Parent/Child)

Support the Child in Explaining the Use of the DAR to the Parent

Ask the child to show the DAR folder to the parent and to explain how the DAR can be used to keep track of assignments and materials. Provide any necessary corrections to the explanation, and ask the child to describe again how the DAR will be used. Praise the child for accurate descriptions about how to use the DAR.

Provide a brief summary of how the DAR folder will be used, indicating that the child will write down homework assignments on the DAR pages and can keep track of tests and other long-term assignments on the Assignment and Test Calendar. Note that the teacher will provide a check on the DAR. For now, the teacher will give the child a check if he makes an effort to fill in the DAR; in the future, the teacher's check will be given for accurate completion of the DAR. Provide the child with the Reminder for the Daily Assignment Record (Handout 12), which summarizes all of the steps in using the DAR.

Indicate that the Assignment and Test Calendar (Handout 11) can be completed by the parent, with the child's help, before the next session, though this is not necessary (use of the Assignment and Test Calendar will be reviewed and practiced in more detail in Session 4).

HELPFUL HINT: At the end of each session, you must fill in the two blank spaces in the far right column of the DAR with the two OTMP target behaviors that the teacher should prompt, monitor, and praise. The teacher will put a check for each behavior performed in school, and the parent will provide the child with the number of points that matches the number of checks when the child arrives home. You will need to fill in these target behaviors at the end of each session, on a blank copy of the DAR in the child's DAR folder. You may do this yourself, perhaps when the child leaves to get the parent from the waiting room, or have the parent and child do this together, as a way of reinforcing the behaviors that the child must perform in school.

Describe the Home Exercise; Review How the Parent Will Prompt, Monitor, and Reward Two Non-OTMP Target Behaviors, and Prompt, Monitor, and Praise Use of the DAR

Provide the parent with a Home Behavior Record (Handout 13). Point out that two spaces on this sheet are for non-OTMP behaviors, and the third space is to indicate the use of the DAR. Remind the parent to prompt, monitor, and praise all target behaviors listed. Emphasize that for now, the parent should only base points and give rewards on the child's performance of the non-OTMP target behaviors. While the child is acclimating to using the DAR, the parent should only monitor and praise its use.

Reward the Child

Review the Session Points and Notes (Therapist Form 5) with the child, and praise the child for the positive behaviors that earned points in the session. Add up the total points earned for this session, and indicate that the child may select a prize as a reward.

HELPFUL HINT: You can decide how to structure the session point and prize system. One option is to have different prize baskets, containing 10-, 20-, and 30-point prizes, respectively. The child can then be instructed that he may "spend" the session points earned at the end of each session or "save" them, if he is interested in earning a larger reward in future sessions. This multilevel prize system can increase motivation in some children to earn session points. However, you should point out to the parent that the same system will not be used for home rewards; when the child earns points for target behaviors on the Home Behavior Record, he will earn a daily reward *and* can still add those daily points to the weekly total, to earn a weekly reward.

CONCLUDE THE SESSION

Confirm the next session appointment. Give the child and parent the OTMP Checklist (Handout 14). Remind the parent to bring the current version of the Home Behavior Record (Handout 13), and the child to bring the DAR folder, to the next session.

ALTERNATIVE PROCEDURES

As noted earlier, some teachers may not be comfortable with the idea of allowing children to use a different method for tracking assignments from the method their peers are using. For example, a teacher may insist that a child use a standard planner to write down homework assignments. In that case, you would not want to give the child extra work by having her write down assignments in the planner and the DAR. Below are two options that can be suggested as variations on the DAR:

Suggested Option 1

You might get permission from the teacher to add a small checklist of items needed for homework, listed by subject, which could be paper-clipped or taped into the child's planner. You would then have the teacher and parent monitor and praise the child for writing down assignments in the planner and using the small checklist.

Suggested Option 2

Some planners have enough room on them for children to write a list of items at the bottom of the page. These planners also often have a place for teacher comments, where a checklist of items needed may be inserted. This extra space has been used successfully by some children as a substitute for the DAR.

These options are, of course, just two possible adaptations. You should be creative and flexible in working with the teacher, child, and parent to construct a method for keeping track of assignments and materials that works for all of them. Always keep in mind, however, that any method must include (1) a place to write down the assignments and (2) a way of making sure that the child knows which materials to take home for those assignments.

SESSION 4

Tracking Assignments

The Daily Assignment Record and the Assignment and Test Calendar

===== GOALS FOR THE SESSION =====

You will:

- Confirm the parent's commitment to and understanding of the home point program for target behaviors.
- Contact the teacher before the next session to check on use of the DAR and discuss the upcoming use of the accordion binder (see Chapter 3, Teacher Contact 2).

The parent will:

- Share efforts to prompt, monitor, praise, and reward target behaviors, using the Home Behavior Record (Handout 13).
- Demonstrate understanding of how to monitor the child's use of the Daily Assignment Record (Handout 10) and the Assignment and Test Calendar (Handout 11).
- Agree to prompt, monitor, praise, and/or reward specified target behaviors between sessions, using the Home Behavior Record (Handout 15 or 15a).

The child will:

- Learn how to use the Assignment and Test Calendar (Handout 11).
- Demonstrate awareness of the number of papers provided at school (Therapist Form 8).
- Recognize problems with managing papers.
- Practice separating papers into categories for storage and transfer.

83

▨▨▨▨▨▨▨▨▨▨▨ MATERIALS NEEDED ▨▨▨▨▨▨▨▨▨▨▨

For the parent:

- Handout 15, Home Behavior Record: Behaviors to Prompt, Monitor, Praise, and Reward
  Or
- Handout 15a, Home Behavior Record: Behaviors to Prompt, Monitor, Praise, and Reward
- Handout 9, Reward Menu
- Handout 18, Home Point Bank

For you:

- Whiteboard or blackboard, with markers or chalk/eraser
- Six file (or two-pocket) folders
- A selection of grade-appropriate papers for the child to practice filing in folders (see "In Preparation for This Session")
- Therapist Form 3, Guide to the Glitches
- Therapist Form 5, Session Points and Notes
- Therapist Form 7, Sample Assignments for DAR and Assignment and Test Calendar Practice
- Therapist Form 8, Interview Record Form for School Materials
- Therapist Forms 9–12 (Optional), Trekking Adventure . . . forms

For the child:

- Child's DAR folder (child should bring this to the session for review)
- Handout 10, Daily Assignment Record (three copies for in-session practice)
- Handout 11, Assignment and Test Calendar (two copies for in-session practice)
- Handout 16, Keeping Track of School Papers
- Handout 17, OTMP Checklist: Things to Remember for Session 5

ABOUT THIS SESSION

In this session, you will continue to work with the child on keeping track of assignments and materials, with a new focus on keeping track of long-term assignments and tests. In addition, you will introduce the concept of paper organization and storage. At the beginning of the session, you will assess the parent's completion of the Home Behavior Record and ensure that the point program is being implemented appropriately. If there are any problems with implementation of the home program, you can spend some time at the beginning of this session, working with the parent to fine-tune that program.

The session activities focus on giving the child practice with several simple sets of behaviors: (1) tracking homework assignments with the Daily Assignment Record (DAR); (2) tracking long-term assignments and tests with a calendar; and (3) using a rudimentary

SESSION SUMMARY CHECKLIST FOR SESSION 4

Item	Item Completed
Review implementation of the behavior-monitoring and point program (with parent/child)	
Review the parent's use of the Home Behavior Record and point program (Handout 13)	Yes/No
Discuss and problem-solve challenges to implementation	Yes/No
Discuss the Home Behavior Record to be used, based on a review of parental implementation (Handout 15 or 15a)	Yes/No
Conduct skills building with the child alone: DAR review, Assignment and Test Calendar, and paper storage	
Review the child's use of the DAR folder since the previous session	Yes/No
Teach the child to use the Assignment and Test Calendar (Handout 11)	Yes/No
Conduct in-session practice: Assignment and Test Calendar (Handout 11; Therapist Form 7)	Yes/No
Introduce the characteristics of the Go-Ahead-Lose-It Glitch (Handout 3)	
Discuss the number and type of papers typically received at school (Therapist Form 8)	Yes/No
Critically review the child's current method for storing and transferring papers	Yes/No
Conduct in-session practice: Paper organization and storage	Yes/No
Optional: Practice paper storage for an imaginary trekking adventure (Therapist Forms 9–12)	Yes/No
Wrap up the session (with parent/child)	
Support the child in explaining the use of the Assignment and Test Calendar and paper storage to the parent (Handout 11)	Yes/No
Describe the home exercise: DAR, Assignment and Test Calendar, and record of papers received in school (DAR folder; Handouts 10, 11, 16)	Yes/No
Review the Home Behavior Record and the plan for prompting, monitoring, praising, and rewarding the target behaviors (Handouts 15/15a, 9, 18)	Yes/No
Add new target behaviors to the DAR folder	Yes/No
Reward the child (Therapist Form 5)	Yes/No
Conclude the session (Handout 17)	Yes/No

categorization and filing system to store and retrieve papers. Multiple instances of practice are used to decrease the child's discomfort in using these routines, increase the child's speed in performing the behaviors, and help the child recognize the utility of these routines.

IN PREPARATION FOR THIS SESSION

During the in-session practice, the child will sort and file an assortment of papers. You will need to provide the child with a selection of papers that the child might receive in school, including announcements/informational papers (e.g., permission slips, notices about after-school activities); math worksheets; brief stories to read; small packets on science or social studies with accompanying questions; maps; and lists of spelling words. You may find these materials online on educational websites (e.g., *www.tlsbooks.com*; *www.jumpstart.com*) or create sample worksheets of your own, keeping in mind the grade level of the child with whom you are working.

DETAILED SESSION CONTENT

Review Implementation of the Behavior-Monitoring and Point Program (with Parent/Child)

By this time, it is *essential* that the parent has monitored the frequency of the three target behaviors (two non-OTMP behaviors and the DAR); has provided you with evidence that he has prompted the responses appropriately (i.e., gave the child needed reminders and did not expect the child to recall the behaviors independently); and has shown that he has provided praise for all three behaviors and points/rewards for use of the DAR. If the parent has failed to do so—because of confusion regarding implementation, because of disorganization, or because he does not understand the importance of this process—use time at the beginning of this session to resolve these issues. If this is necessary, you may shift practice in activities that are not addressed with the child today to later sessions. There is flexibility in Sessions 5–8 to allow time for catching up.

Review the Parent's Use of the Home Behavior Record and Point Program

Discuss the two non-OTMP behaviors that the child was asked to perform, and review the filled-in Home Behavior Record for these (Handout 13). Determine how many opportunities there were for the behaviors to occur, and how many times the child performed the behaviors. Ask the parent about the methods used to prompt the behaviors. Ask the parent and child what happened when the behaviors were praised. Review what daily and/or weekly rewards were used to reinforce the behaviors. Praise all efforts to perform this behavior-monitoring plan effectively.

Determine whether the parent has been prompting, monitoring, and praising the child's completion of the DAR. If the parent worked with the child to transfer information to the Assignment and Test Calendar, review that briefly.

Discuss and Problem-Solve Challenges to Implementation

If the parent has not completed the Home Behavior Record or provided points/rewards for the two non-OTMP targets, discuss what factors hindered implementation.

If the parent is confused about how to use the Home Behavior Record or the point/reward program, review the instructions for using those tools carefully.

- Make sure that the parent understands where to write down points for the child on the Home Behavior Record (Handout 13).
- Review how to set point goals for the day and the week (e.g., the child could have earned 2 points each day and 14 points each week) and how to give rewards accordingly (Handout 9).
- Make sure that the parent has an acceptable list of desired rewards (Handout 9) for daily and weekly performance of the target behaviors.
- Go through some simulated situations with the parent of how the child might perform on a given day, and how the parent would praise the child and award points and rewards accordingly.

If the parent forgot to complete the Home Behavior Record or forgot to bring it to the session, take some time to help the parent come up with a system for organizing these new procedures. Given that many parents of children with ADHD may have difficulties with organization themselves, you may need to work with such parents on managing the procedures that they will need to employ as part of this treatment. Provide appropriate support to these parents and praise them for commitment to the program, while acknowledging the difficulty that many parents have in adding a new routine to an already hectic schedule. Use problem solving to find out what barriers prevented implementation and what can be done to overcome those barriers. For example, a parent might report that checking the child's DAR was forgotten and that the schedule was too tight to put a check down on the Home Behavior Record at the end of the day. In this case, you would praise the parent for engaging in the process of reviewing the DAR and reinforcing the child. Then work with the parent to see how you can make the notation system more manageable. For example, perhaps the parent can leave the Home Behavior Record on a nightstand, inside a book that is read before bed, and make appropriate notes at the end of the day.

Discuss the Home Behavior Record to Be Used, Based on a Review of Parental Implementation

If the parent has been consistent in prompting, monitoring, praising, and rewarding the non-OTMP behaviors, she can move on to use points and rewards for the OTMP target behaviors as well. The next version of the Home Behavior Record (Handout 15) contains five child behaviors to be prompted, monitored, praised, and rewarded: two non-OTMP behaviors (most parents will want to continue with the two targets that have been used thus far); completing the DAR; completing the Assignment and Test Calendar; and writing down a list of papers received at school each day.

If the parent *has not* completed the Home Behavior Record and provided points and rewards for the two non-OTMP targets, ask her to prompt, monitor, and praise/reward the two non-OTMP targets only. She will then prompt, monitor, and just praise the completion of the DAR at school and the other two OTMP target behaviors that will be taught in this session (Handout 15a). Indicate that only when the home behavior management system is solidly established will OTMP behaviors be focused on exclusively. It is imperative for the parent to be consistent in following through with reinforcement.

Conduct Skills Building with the Child Alone: DAR Review, Assignment and Test Calendar, and Paper Storage

Begin by awarding the child session points (Therapist Form 5) and praising him for good listening and any contributions he made to the discussion with the parent. Explain that you will be working together in this session on some more tools that will help with controlling the Go-Ahead-Forget-It Glitch and the Go-Ahead-Lose-It Glitch.

Review the Child's Use of the DAR Folder since the Previous Session

If the child has brought the DAR folder to the session, praise her for doing so (and provide points on Therapist Form 5). Praise her also for any efforts she made to complete copies of the DAR since the last session.

If the child did not bring the DAR folder to the session, use a problem-solving approach to determine why it was forgotten and how the child can remember the folder for future sessions. Refer to the Go-Ahead-Forget-It Glitch, and remark that the Glitch seems to have gotten in the way again, making the child forget something that she needed. Ask what the Glitch did to "mess things up" this time, and determine how the child can use the Mastermind to battle the Glitch next time. Below is an example of a dialogue in which these sensitive issues are discussed in a constructive, humorous way:

THERAPIST: So how did the Glitch get in the way of your bringing the DAR folder to the session today? What tricks did it pull to mess you up?

CHILD: Well, I took the DAR folder out of my bag to check my homework after school, and I left it on my desk, in my room. I guess I forgot to put it back in my bag. I really meant to put it back—but I finished my homework early and wanted to go play video games with my brother.

THERAPIST: Ah, yes, that's one of the Glitch's favorite tricks. It loves to convince kids that they don't have to put things back where they belong right away, because they'll remember to do it later. And it loves it when you get distracted by something else that's more fun . . . because then it knows you'll probably forget! So what do you think you can do next time, to make sure the Glitch doesn't make you forget the DAR folder again?

CHILD: I guess I should put the DAR folder back in my bag as soon as I finish my homework, and not leave it lying around.

THERAPIST: Great idea! I'm going to give you a session point for thinking of that; I really think that will be a good way to control the Go-Ahead-Forget-It Glitch and remember your DAR folder for next session.

If the child has brought the DAR folder to the session, ask the child about his experience with using the DAR to record assignments in school, and ask whether he has any questions about how to use the DAR properly. Review the copies of the DAR that were completed, and assess whether the child needs to modify his use of the DAR in any way. Here are some points to consider and review:

- Does the child have enough room to write in all of the homework assignments for each subject? If not, you may need to modify the form electronically, to allow more room for writing. Remember that children with ADHD often have difficulty with handwriting, and you don't want the experience of using the DAR to be frustrating for the child.
- Did the child write the assignments in the correct subject rows? Were there any assignments that did not belong to a particular subject? If so, should the DAR be modified to include a new subject, or is this an infrequently assigned item that can be placed in a row labeled "Other"?
- Did the child check off all of the items needed to complete the assignments?
- Did the child write down long-term assignments/tests in the correct column?
- Did the teacher sign the DAR?
- Did the child write the date in the top right-hand corner?

If the child is still not completely comfortable with the procedures involved in using the DAR, or if the DAR folder has been left at home, engage in *two to three more rounds of practice* with the DAR—providing simulated assignments and asking the child to write them down on the DAR, as was done in Session 3. Otherwise, if the child has been effective in using the DAR appropriately, you may move on to the next activity.

Teach the Child to Use the Assignment and Test Calendar

The child may have already filled in the Assignment and Test Calendar (Handout 11) with the parent after the previous session. Even so, use some time in this session to explicitly review and practice the use of this handout. Indicate that the child will use the Assignment and Test Calendar to keep track of long-term assignments and tests. Discuss, briefly, why this type of calendar is useful: It can show the child, at a glance, what assignments are due in the next month, and can help the child anticipate what is coming up and what work has to be done for those upcoming projects or tests.

Show the child how to set up the Assignment and Test Calendar for each month. The calendar is set up as a shell, with boxes provided for the 5 school days in each week. The child and/or the parent can write in the dates in their appropriate place for the current month and the next month, and can then keep track of assignments that are due during that 2-month period. As you set up copies of the Assignment and Test Calendar with the child in session, describe each step you take, so that the child becomes familiar with the use of this calendar.

Conduct In-Session Practice: Assignment and Test Calendar

Take out some blank copies of the DAR and of the Assignment and Test Calendar for practice.

- Create some sample lists of assignments that are due immediately and some that are due in the future (within the week, later in the month, and during the next month). You may refer to the Sample Assignments for DAR and Assignment and Test Calendar Practice (Therapist Form 7) or create your own sample assignments.
- Use the whiteboard/blackboard to write down a list of short- and long-term assignments that a child might receive in school. Direct the child to use the DAR to record the short-term assignments by subject, and to write down the long-term assignments in two places: (1) on the DAR, under the heading "Other Assignments and Due Dates"; and (2) on the Assignment and Test Calendar, by due date.
- Repeat this process *two to three times*, praising the child for writing down assignments and tests first on the DAR, and then on the Assignment and Test Calendar (for long-term assignments and tests).
- Provide any corrective feedback, and adjust the number of practices according to the child's demonstrated proficiency with this new method of recording assignments.

Introduce the Characteristics of the Go-Ahead-Lose-It Glitch

Tell the child:

> "We have been talking a lot about the Go-Ahead-Forget-It Glitch, and have learned how to use some tools that will help us control that Glitch better, like the DAR and the Assignment and Test Calendar. Now I want to talk to you a little about the Go-Ahead-Lose-It Glitch, because we want to make sure that we can learn some ways to control that Glitch too."

Take out the Guide to the Glitches (Handout 3) and turn to the section on the Go-Ahead-Lose-It Glitch. Review the material on this Glitch in detail, pointing out specifically how the Go-Ahead-Lose-It Glitch can trick people into losing papers that they need by making sure that they don't put them away properly.

Discuss the Number and Type of Papers Typically Received at School

The next skill that you will introduce to the child pertains to the management of papers for schoolwork. The ultimate objectives of this discussion are for you and the child to understand (1) what papers are used during a typical day and week at school; and (2) how the child currently stores and transfers those papers between home and school.

To this end, you will conduct a brief interview with the child to get a sense of the number and types of papers that she typically uses for school. You can use Therapist Form 8 to facilitate this discussion, although you do not need to ask each question on the interview form. You can also use the information recorded on the copies of the DAR completed thus far to determine the types of assignments the child must complete, and what materials those assignments require (textbooks, workbooks, handouts, etc.).

Critically Review the Child's Current Method for Storing and Transferring Papers

Once you have gathered information about what papers are typically used and how they are stored, discuss the child's success in using the current method (however haphazard) for organizing papers from school. You can use some of the following questions to identify what issues might need to be addressed in this area:

"Have your parents and teachers ever said anything about the way you keep your homework sheets, announcements, or other papers? For example, have you heard that they are wrinkled, or torn, or shoved into the bottom of your bag?"

"Do you ever have problems finding papers when you need them—for example, when you have to complete your homework or when you have to return papers to your teacher in class?"

"Have you ever forgotten papers in school that were supposed to go home, or vice versa?"

You may be able to gather some "data" regarding how the child manages papers by asking the child to show you her backpack and to find selected papers that are listed on her DAR for that day's assignments. Note how quickly the child can find those papers, and how neatly the papers are kept. You will not be able to take this step, of course, if there are no papers for the child's homework that evening.

In a constructive and nonjudgmental tone, engage the child in a brief discussion of the paper organization methods being used, and ask the child to consider some alternative ways for managing any problems that have been mentioned (e.g., losing papers, taking a long time to find papers). If the child is defensive at all, end the discussion and indicate that you will be experimenting with some different ways of organizing papers in this and the next session. Provide the child with session points for providing useful information and attending throughout this discussion.

Conduct In-Session Practice: Paper Organization and Storage

The aim of the following practice activity is to help the child learn to separate and categorize papers, to label them appropriately, and to select a location to store them, so that the child can find them quickly and reliably. Using the papers you have gathered (see "In Preparation for This Session"), engage the child in a number of different practice activities, intended to provide a demonstration of specific key skills related to paper organization and storage. The child will not complete the worksheets, but will simply need to practice organizing them, using different folders.

Filing Papers for Later Use
- *Key skills: separating papers into categories, labeling, and storing*
- Show the child the assortment of papers that you have collected for this practice exercise. Ask him to pretend that these papers were given out in school and that he must store these papers somewhere, so they can be taken home.
- Give the child the papers one at a time and ask him to separate the papers by category (e.g., math papers, announcements, science papers, etc.).
- Show the child the six folders you have, and ask how he might use these folders to organize the papers. You can guide the child in this process, suggesting that he might want to label the folders by subject and/or purpose (one folder for announcements, one for math, etc.).

- Ask the child to file the papers into the folders, using the categorization system he has developed.
- Review with the child how he would know where a paper is when he uses this system (e.g., by using the labels on the folders).

Retrieving Papers for Completing Homework
- *Key skills: finding papers needed for homework, putting back other papers, and returning papers to their storage location after task completion*
- Provide simulated assignments with the papers given. For example, you may tell the child that she must complete a math worksheet that was among the practice papers.
- Ask the child to find the needed paper, as if she was getting ready to complete it for homework.
- Have the child pull out the needed paper and put back other, unnecessary papers.
- Have the child return the paper to its proper folder after it has been used. (*Note:* The child does not actually have to complete the worksheet at this time, but can pretend that she has done so.)

Handling Papers at School
- *Key skills: finding needed papers, turning in homework, using and storing other papers in class*
- Acting as the teacher, request that the child find and hand in a specific homework paper from the batch of practice papers.
- Then ask the child to take out a worksheet (e.g., a science packet) and pretend to work on it in class.
- Finally, ask the child to put the paper back in the appropriate folder, so it can be worked on again at a later time.

Provide the child with session points and generous praise as he practices the various paper management exercises above.

Note: The aim of this paper practice with folders is to help the child become comfortable with sorting and categorizing papers. However, the child will not use folders in this way to organize school papers. Instead, the child will be taught to use an accordion binder for paper storage and organization, and this tool will be introduced in Session 5.

Optional: Practice Paper Storage for an Imaginary Trekking Adventure

If time permits and you think the child might enjoy and/or benefit from additional practice with paper storage for an imaginary adventure, you can engage the child in storing needed papers for a trekking adventure. On the adventure, the child must have a set of instructions for using a special instrument, directions for finding a certain spot, a list of supplies needed to continue the adventure after arriving at the adventurers' general store, and a special code to decipher a message from the leader of the adventurers (Therapist Forms 9–12, respectively). Have the child separate the papers and store them in folders, as she did for the practice with school papers. Then talk the child through the various steps in the adventure, and ask the child to find papers as they are needed, noting how easily the papers are retrieved during the simulated adventure.

You may use this opportunity to discuss with the child how paper organization is important not only in a school setting, but in other life situations, where being able to store and retrieve materials effectively can have practical importance.

Wrap Up the Session (with Parent/Child)

Support Child in Explaining the Use of the Assignment and Test Calendar and Paper Storage to the Parent

Guide the child in explaining what he did in session to the parent:

- Ask the child to explain how he will transfer information about long-term assignments and tests from the DAR to the Assignment and Test Calendar (Handout 11).
- Ask the child to explain why it is helpful to do this.
- Ask the child to discuss how he learned to separate papers into categories and store them in folders.
- Provide any additional explanation that may be needed, if the child's discussion of these areas is incomplete.

Describe the Home Exercise: DAR, Assignment and Test Calendar, and Record of Papers Received in School

Review, with the parent and child, the actions that the child will practice at home and school:

- The child will continue to use the DAR (Handout 10) to track homework assignments.
- The child will use the Assignment and Test Calendar (Handout 11) to keep track of long-term assignments.
- The child will keep a list of papers received at school each day (Handout 16) and bring that list to the next session.

Review the Home Behavior Record and the Plan for Prompting, Monitoring, Praising, and Rewarding the Target Behaviors

Show the parent the Home Behavior Record (Handout 15 or 15a), and review which behaviors the parent will prompt, monitor, praise, and/or reward. As noted above, if the parent has successfully completed the previous session's homework, the version of the Home Behavior Record to be used (Handout 15) contains five child behaviors to be prompted, monitored, praised, and rewarded:

1. One non-OTMP behavior
2. A second non-OTMP behavior
3. Completing the DAR
4. Completing the Assignment and Test Calendar. (*Note*: If there are no long-term assignments to be recorded on a given day, instruct the parent to award a point if the child cooperatively responds to the question "Did you learn about any long-term assignments or test dates today?")
5. Writing down a list of papers received at school each day

The parent will continue to use the point program that was developed in Session 3. You may review Handout 9 briefly with the parent at this point, pointing out that, while the number of possible daily points has changed from 2 to 5, the parent can continue to use the percentage-based system for allocating rewards from a two-tiered reward menu. As is explained on the Reward Menu, the child can choose from Level One of the reward menu for earning 60% (e.g., 3 out of 5) of the daily points, and choose from Level Two for earning 80% or more (e.g., 4 or 5 out of 5) of the daily points. For weekly rewards, the child will have to earn at least 60% of the weekly points (e.g., 15 out of 25) to choose a reward from Level One, and can choose from Level Two for earning 80% (e.g., 20 out of 25) or more of the total possible points for the week.

If the parent *did not* complete the previous session's homework, the version of the Home Behavior Record to be used (Handout 15a) asks the parent to prompt, monitor, and praise the following behaviors, providing rewards as instructed in Session 3:

1. One non-OTMP behavior
2. A second non-OTMP behavior

In addition, the parent will prompt, monitor, and just praise:

1. Completing the DAR
2. Completing the Assignment and Test Calendar
3. Writing down a list of papers received at school each day

You may give the parent the Home Point Bank (Handout 18), and indicate that this handout can be used to keep track of daily and weekly point totals over the course of the month.

Add New Target Behaviors to the DAR Folder

The target behavior for which the teacher will provide a school point is "Completed the DAR." You may write this target behavior in on the next few DAR forms in the child's DAR folder, so that the teacher will know what to check for in the days before the next session.

Reward the Child

Review the Session Points and Notes (Therapist Form 5) with the child, and praise the child for the positive behaviors that earned points in the session. Add up the total points earned for this session, and indicate that the child may spend or save the points.

Conclude the Session

Confirm the next session appointment. Give the child and parent the OTMP Checklist (Handout 17). Remind the parent to bring the current versionof the Home Behavior Record (Handout 15 or 15a), and the child to bring the DAR folder and the list of papers received at school (Handout 16), to the next session.

SESSION 5

Managing Materials
Managing Papers for School

━━━━━━━━━━ **GOALS FOR THE SESSION** ━━━━━━━━━━

You will:

■ Confirm the parent's ongoing implementation of the home point program for target behaviors.

The parent will:

■ Describe efforts to prompt, monitor, praise, and reward target behaviors, using the Home Behavior Record (Handout 15 or 15a).
■ Demonstrate understanding of how she can monitor the child's use of the accordion binder and DAR folder.
■ Agree to prompt, monitor, praise, and/or reward specified target behaviors between sessions, using the version of the Home Behavior Record that will be used from now on (Handout 19).

The child will:

■ Provide information about papers received at school (Handout 16).
■ Learn how to use the accordion binder.
■ Set up a personalized binder and practice its use with a collection of sample papers.

━━━━━━━━━━ **MATERIALS NEEDED** ━━━━━━━━━━

For the parent:

■ Handout 19, Home Behavior Record

95

For you:

- Sample accordion binder, set up with labels for different subjects (see Chapter 2)
- New accordion binder, for child to personalize
- Materials for decorating the binder (e.g., permanent markers, stickers, self-adhesive jewels, glitter glue, stamps)
- A selection of grade-appropriate papers for the child to practice filing in binder (see "In Preparation for This Session," below)
- Therapist Form 5, Session Points and Notes

For the child:

- Child's DAR folder (child should bring this to the session for review)
- Handout 10, Daily Assignment Record (three blank copies for in-session practice)

SESSION SUMMARY CHECKLIST FOR SESSION 5

Item	Item Completed
Review implementation of the behavior-monitoring and point program (with parent/child)	
Review the parent's use of the Home Behavior Record and point program (Handout 15 or 15a)	Yes/No
Review the parent's and child's understanding of how to use the DAR and the Assignment and Test Calendar	Yes/No
Conduct skills building with the child alone: Using the accordion binder to manage school papers	
Conduct OST homework review: DAR folder, Keeping Track of School Papers (Handout 16)	Yes/No
Introduce the accordion binder	Yes/No
Set up the child's personal binder	Yes/No
Conduct in-session practice: Using the DAR to track assignments (Handout 10) and the binder to file papers (Handout 20)	
Wrap up the session (with parent/child)	
Support the child in explaining the use of the binder to the parent	Yes/No
Describe the home exercise: DAR, Assignment and Test Calendar, and binder	Yes/No
Review the Home Behavior Record (Handout 19)	Yes/No
Add new target behaviors to the DAR folder	Yes/No
Reward the child (Therapist Form 5)	Yes/No
Conclude the session (Handout 21)	Yes/No

- Handout 20, Accordion Binder Instructions
- Handout 21, OTMP Checklist: Things to Remember for Session 6

ABOUT THIS SESSION

In this session, the child will learn a new method for storing papers in an accordion binder, which will allow for improved management of school papers and increased control of the Go-Ahead-Lose-It Glitch. The session activities focus on (1) introducing the child to the idea of using an accordion binder for storing school papers; (2) helping the child set up and personalize a binder; and (3) guiding the child in integrating tracking of assignments (using the DAR) and management of papers (using the binder).

Note: If there are any practice activities that need to be completed as carry-overs from the previous session (e.g., practice with the DAR and Assignment and Test Calendar; practice with filing papers by category), there should be enough time to insert those activities in this session.

IN PREPARATION FOR THIS SESSION

You will need to have some materials prepared in advance for this session, to facilitate the child's use of the accordion binder. Before the session, you should:

1. Prepare a sample accordion binder, with tabs for each section labeled (in permanent marker, directly on the section tabs) with a subject name (e.g., Math, Social Studies, Writing, Science). You should also have tabs with these labels: DAR Folder, Announcements, Notes for Parents, and OTMP papers.
2. Prepare a collection of sample papers, to be used for in-session practice with storing papers in the binder. You can find a wide selection of academic worksheets and handouts online, organized by grade level, and should print out a selection that represents the subjects the child typically studies in school. You may also create your own handouts, if necessary. In addition, you will want to create some simple announcements (e.g., letting parents know about an upcoming bake sale) and permission slips, such as the child would typically receive in school.

DETAILED SESSION CONTENT

Review Implementation of the Behavior-Monitoring and Point Program (with Parent/Child)

At this point in treatment, it is anticipated that the parent has become more comfortable using the home behavior management system, and that a brief review at the beginning of each session of how the parent was able to prompt, monitor, praise, and reward target behaviors should suffice. However, some parents will continue to require more support in carrying out this home component, and there is time at the start of each session to problem-solve any issues that may arise.

Review the Parent's Use of the Home Behavior Record and Point Program

Review the Home Behavior Record (Handout 15 or 15a) with the parent assessing whether the parent was successful in prompting, monitoring, praising, and rewarding the specified target behaviors. Determine whether there were any problems in the implementation of any of these steps, and provide guidance and advice if necessary.

Troubleshooting Note: Although some parents will adhere to all aspects of the home behavior program (i.e., completing Home Behavior Records accurately, prompting behaviors, awarding points consistently, giving rewards appropriately), other parents may be less consistent in following through with this part of the program. By the fifth session, most parents should be comfortable with the home behavior program. However, some parents, especially those with organizational difficulties of their own, may continue to require coaching in the use of this program. It is preferred that, by the fifth session, all children be given the chance to earn home points and rewards for using organizational behaviors. Therefore, you will have to be especially attentive to a parent who is inconsistent in following through on the home behavior program. Encourage such a parent to use points and rewards to reinforce organizational behaviors, while you carefully monitor the parent's use of the program.

You should make every attempt to simplify the home points program for parents who have difficulty with these procedures, making sure that rewards are simple and easy to provide. For example, privileges (e.g., extra time on the computer or iPod) are easier to give and require less organization than tangible items (e.g., stickers, small toys, treats). Furthermore, you should continue to offer advice on how the parent can remember to keep track of points, relying on knowledge of the parent's routines to suggest the most seamless integration of the points system into that routine.

If, after several sessions of monitoring and support, the parent remains unable to follow through with a daily point and reward system, you may propose a simplified home points program. In a simplified system, the parent should continue to provide prompts, praise, and points daily, with one reward given at the end of each week for points earned over the course of that week. Although this system is not ideal, as it does not provide more immediate reinforcement for the child's use of newly learned behaviors, it may be necessary for some parents who are not able to provide daily rewards consistently. If a parent does use a simplified, weekly reward schedule, you must monitor implementation of this system closely to ensure that the parent is providing the promised weekly reward, and that proper praise and attention are given daily.

Review the Parent's and Child's Understanding of How to Use the DAR and the Assignment and Test Calendar

Ask the parent and child to describe their experiences using the DAR and the Assignment and Test Calendar thus far. If they express any misunderstanding regarding how the tools are to be used, provide clarification and review the steps for use. If they report problems in using these tools, encourage them to work with you to come up with solutions. For example, some children might report that they find it difficult to flip to the appropriate DAR sheet in the folder; you might suggest that they use a paper clip to mark the spot for noting assignments each day. Other children might report that they are embarrassed about having to use a different method for recording assignments from the method their classmates use; you can talk with the children about what to say when classmates ask why they are using a different folder, or about ways to make the DAR folder less conspicuous.

Conduct Skills Building with the Child Alone: Using the Accordion Binder to Manage School Papers

Begin by awarding the child session points (Therapist Form 5) and praising her for good listening and discussion with the parent present. Explain that you will be working together in this session on a new tool that will help with controlling the Go-Ahead-Lose-It Glitch.

Conduct OST Homework Review: DAR Folder, Keeping Track of School Papers

If the child has brought the DAR folder to the session, praise her for doing so (and provide points on Therapist Form 5). Briefly, review the copies of the DAR that have been completed since the previous session, as well as the Assignment and Test Calendar. Note any problems with how the child has recorded assignments, and provide guidance if necessary on how to correct those problems in the future.

For example, you might need to remind the child to record the date at the top of each form, or to add a long-term assignment to the Assignment and Test Calendar. You should also check to ensure that the teacher has provided points in the far right column on the DAR for each day; if those points are missing, ask the child why this occurred. Although teacher absences can contribute to an understandable gap in DAR points provided, a pattern of missing teacher points can indicate a problem, which should be addressed with an additional teacher contact (see the "Troubleshooting . . ." section of Chapter 3).

Then ask the child to take out Keeping Track of School Papers (Handout 16), provided last session, where he should have listed the papers he received at school. Provide points for bringing in this form. Briefly review the list of papers the child has made, and discuss whether this list is typical for a given week at school.

Introduce the Accordion Binder

Tell the child:

> "Today we are going to talk more about how to control the Go-Ahead-Lose-It Glitch. Last time, we talked a lot about papers, and we practiced ways of separating and storing papers. We also talked about how easy it is for you to find papers you need for school-work, and whether you sometimes get into trouble because you can't find some of your papers."

After this introduction, review the list of school papers that the child completed, and comment in one of the following ways, depending on how many papers are listed:

> "From what we discussed last time and the list of school papers you brought back with you today, it seems like you get a lot of papers at school."

Or

"From what we discussed last time and the list of school papers you brought back with you today, it seems like you get only a few papers, but you have a lot of workbooks that you need to have with you for getting homework done."

Then continue:

"We learned last time that it is helpful to separate papers into categories and to have a special place to keep those papers. We used different folders to store papers last time, but we think that keeping track of lots of folders can be difficult for kids. Instead, we are going to show you a different kind of binder, called an 'accordion binder,' which can be used to store lots of papers in separate sections. You can also use this binder to store your workbooks, if they are thin enough, so you will always be sure to have what you need for your homework."

Show the child the binder and say:

"We think this accordion binder is a great way for kids to store papers, because it has pockets for different subjects, sides that close, so papers can't escape, and a flap that closes, so papers don't fall out. Because there are no openings, it will keep the Go-Ahead-Lose-It Glitch from getting to your papers. You can keep all of your papers in this binder, including your DAR folder. If you put papers in this binder as soon as you receive them, in the right pockets, you will be able to find them easily when you need them for doing homework. Then, if you put them back in the same places after you're done, you'll be able to find them easily and turn them in."

Note: If the child's teacher has told you that an accordion binder will not be an acceptable option or if the child strongly objects to its use, please turn to the "Alternative Procedures" section at the end of this chapter for ideas on alternative paper storage methods.

Set Up the Child's Personal Binder

Show the child the sample binder that you have prepared. Then give the child a new binder, and tell the child that you will now work together to set it up so that it works best for her school subjects.

Help the child create labels for each section of the binder, writing the names of the different subjects directly on the binder tabs with permanent marker (paper labels can easily fall out). If the child has difficulty with handwriting, you may want to write the subject names on the tabs. Create labeled tabs for each subject listed on the child's DAR, and for the following sections: DAR Folder, Announcements, Notes for Parents (e.g., permission slips, notes from the teacher), and OTMP Papers (for treatment handouts). Give the child session points for listening to instructions and participating in setting up the binder.

HELPFUL HINT: Most children enjoy the act of setting up their binders. You should spend some session time allowing the child to decorate the binder, using materials like glitter glue, stickers, self-adhesive jewels, stamps, and/or permanent markers. The more personalized the binder, the more likely the child will be to use the binder.

Conduct In-Session Practice: Using the DAR to Track Assignments and the Binder to File Papers

You will now help the child add the new routine of storing papers in the binder to the previously taught routine of tracking assignments with the DAR. The child will practice the following steps for managing assignments involving papers:

1. Use the DAR to record assignments for each subject, checking off the correct box for "Handout" in the "What Do I Need to Take?" column.
2. Place the papers in the correct sections of the binder, according to subject or use.
3. Place the DAR folder in the correct section of the binder, and close the binder.
4. When it is time to do homework, pull out the DAR folder, and check the list of assignments.
5. Pull out the appropriate paper(s) for each assignment and complete work.
6. Put each paper back in the correct section of the binder before moving on to the next assignment.
7. When homework is completed, put the DAR folder back in the binder, check that all papers are in the correct location, and close the binder.

Practice the use of these steps with a selection of grade-appropriate sample assignments and papers. For example, if you give the child a math worksheet, a science worksheet, and a permission slip, the child will write "Do worksheet" and check off "Handout" in the rows for both math and science on the DAR, and "Sign permission slip" in the row for "Announcements or Special Papers." The child will then place the worksheets in the appropriate section of the binder according to subject, the permission slip in the "Notes for Parents" section, and the DAR folder in its section of the binder. You could then walk the child through the steps he would follow at home, asking him to take out what he needs for each assignment and put it back after simulating completion.

For the first practice trial, praise the child for placing papers in the binder, disregarding accuracy in using the correct sections. For the second practice trial, provide praise for correct placement of papers in sections, giving feedback on accuracy as needed.

Next, show the child the Accordion Binder Instructions (Handout 20), and review the steps for the binder. Guide the child through two more practice trials, working until the child reaches 100% accuracy on two trials. Provide points and praise for these practice exercises. Indicate that from now on the child will use the binder, as practiced in this session, to store all school papers.

HELPFUL HINT: If the child is a slow writer, you may want to have her go through the process of writing assignments on the DAR only once, and provide previously filled-out DARs to go along with the rest of the papers. The main objective of this practice exercise is to increase proficiency in using the binder.

Wrap Up the Session (with Parent/Child)

Support the Child in Explaining the Use of the Binder to the Parent

Guide the child in explaining what he did in session to the parent:

- Ask the child to show the binder to the parent, and explain how the binder is used to store papers. The child may refer to the Accordion Binder Instructions (Handout 20), if that helps.
- Provide any additional explanation that may be needed, clarifying that from now on the child will use the binder, as practiced in session, to store all school papers.

Describe the Home Exercise: DAR, Assignment and Test Calendar, and Binder

Review, with the parent and child, the actions that the child will practice at home and school:

- The child will use the binder to store and transfer school papers. The teacher will check for use of the binder and give a point if the child puts papers in the binder. The parent will check whether papers are stored in the binder when the child arrives home, and when the child completes homework. At this point, the child will receive teacher and parent points for having all papers in the binder. After the next session, the child will only receive points if the papers are in the correct sections of the binder. This allows for a gradual adjustment to this new method for storing papers.
- The child will continue to use the DAR and the Assignment and Test Calendar to track assignments.

Review the Home Behavior Record

Show the parent the Home Behavior Record that will be used from now on (Handout 19), and review which behaviors the parent will prompt, monitor, praise, and reward, as described in the home exercise. The Home Behavior Record should contain five child behaviors to be prompted, monitored, praised, and rewarded:

- *School behavior 1*: Completed the DAR. (*Note:* The parent should check the DAR each day for the teacher points, located in the last column.)
- *School behavior 2*: Put papers in the binder.
- *Home behavior 1*: Brings home the DAR folder.
- *Home behavior 2*: Put papers in the binder.
- *Home behavior 3*: Completed the Assignment and Test Calendar.

Note: The non-OTMP behaviors will no longer be monitored or rewarded with the Home Behavior Record. However, you can encourage the parent to continue prompting and praising those behaviors, to ensure maintenance.

HELPFUL HINT: From this session forward, you will use the same template (Handout 19) for the Home Behavior Record, which contains spaces in the first column for writing in the two school behaviors for which the teacher provides a check and the three home behaviors that the parent must prompt and monitor at home. You will need to write in the appropriate school and home behaviors at each session meeting before giving the Home Behavior Record to the parent; use the numbered list that is provided at the end of each session, under "Review the Home Behavior Record." You may fill in these behaviors either before the session, or at the end of the session, as you review the behaviors to be monitored with the parent.

Add New Target Behaviors to the DAR Folder

The target behaviors for which the teacher will provide school points are these:

1. Completed the DAR accurately.
2. Put papers in the binder.

Reward the Child

Review the Session Points and Notes (Therapist Form 5) with the child, and praise the child for the positive behaviors that earned points in the session. Add up the total points earned for this session, and indicate that the child may spend or save the points.

Conclude the Session

Confirm the next session appointment. Give the child and parent the OTMP Checklist (Handout 21). Remind the parent to bring the Home Behavior Record (Handout 19), and the child to bring the DAR folder and accordion binder, to the next session.

ALTERNATIVE PROCEDURES

Some children may object to using the accordion binder because they do not want to be different from their classmates. If a child is not comfortable with using the accordion binder, or if a teacher will not allow use of the binder, find out what method is being used and determine how that approach might be altered. In many cases, either the approach will be too simple (e.g., the child has no clear routine), or the approach may be too complicated. Work to develop a routine that is systematic, but can be easily completed by a child with attention problems. The following two options may be helpful.

Option 1: A Single Folder

If the child does use folders, determine whether the child has a separate folder for each subject. Although the use of separate folders is often suggested by parents, this is often too complicated for children with attention problems. Instead, consider the use of a single large folder with two sides—one side for papers "To Go Home," which would include homework sheets and announcements; and one side for papers "For School," which would include completed homework, signed permission slips, and so forth. Make certain that the folder is sturdy and that the parent and child keep checking the folder's integrity, as folders do not last long. Having replacements on reserve is sometimes necessary.

Option 2: Papers Pasted into Composition Books

The second method is being used more often by teachers in many schools: Children have a bound composition book for their notes, and they are asked to tape or paste handouts into the book. If this method is being used, make certain that the child has a routine for actually putting the papers in the book. Many children skip this step and lose papers. Adding a single folder as an addition to the routine can be helpful. Any paper that has to be pasted or taped into the composition book can be placed in the folder and then added to the composition book at home. Doing this at home is often necessary, because teachers may not provide enough time for children to complete this process at school.

SESSION 6

Managing Materials

*Review of Routines for Tracking Assignments
and Managing Papers*

GOALS FOR THE SESSION

You will:

- Review and assess the child's use of the methods learned thus far for managing school assignments and papers (DAR, Assignment and Test Calendar, and accordion binder).

The parent will:

- Describe efforts to prompt, monitor, praise, and reward target behaviors, using the Home Behavior Record from the previous session (Handout 19).
- Understand how the child will continue to use the DAR, Assignment and Test Calendar, and accordion binder.
- Agree to work with the child to "weed out the binder" to be discarded/filed.
- Agree to prompt, monitor, praise, and reward specified target behaviors between sessions, using the Home Behavior Record from this session (Handout 19).

The child will:

- Discuss how she has been using the DAR, Assignment and Test Calendar, and accordion binder, and problem-solve any issues with the therapist.
- Learn how to "weed out the binder" and decide which papers to discard and which papers to store.
- Learn how to file old papers that are still needed in a file box.

MATERIALS NEEDED

For the parent:

- Handout 19, Home Behavior Record

105

For you:

- Sample accordion binder
- A selection of grade-appropriate papers for the child to use for practice in weeding out the binder and in short-term storage (see "In Preparation for This Session")
- Handout 3, Guide to the Glitches
- Therapist Form 5, Session Points and Notes

For the child:

- Child's DAR folder (child should bring this to the session for review)
- Child's accordion binder
- Small file box
- Handout 22, OTMP Checklist: Things to Remember for Session 7

SESSION SUMMARY CHECKLIST FOR SESSION 6

Item	Item Completed
Review implementation of the behavior-monitoring and point program (with parent/child)	Yes/No
Conduct skills building with the child alone: Review and training in short-term paper storage	
Review use of the accordion binder	Yes/No
Review use of the DAR	Yes/No
Review use of the Assignment and Test Calendar	Yes/No
Provide training in short-term storage of papers	Yes/No
Conduct in-session practice: Weeding out the binder	Yes/No
Wrap up the session (with parent/child)	
Review any changes in the routines for tracking assignments and managing papers	Yes/No
Support the child in explaining how to weed out the binder and store papers in a file box	Yes/No
Describe the home exercise: DAR, Assignment and Test Calendar, binder, and weeding out the binder	Yes/No
Review the Home Behavior Record (Handout 19)	Yes/No
Add new target behaviors to the DAR folder	Yes/No
Reward the child (Therapist Form 5)	Yes/No
Conclude the session (Handout 22)	Yes/No

ABOUT THIS SESSION

In this session, you will conduct an in-depth review of the child's use of the methods already taught for tracking assignments and managing papers: the DAR, Assignment and Test Calendar, and accordion binder. You will also introduce a related skill: "weeding out the binder," deciding which papers should be discarded, and storing old papers that may be needed in a file box.

Note: The activities in this session may not require the use of an entire session. If the child is doing well with the methods for tracking assignments and managing papers, the review of these tools should not take very long. If there is time left over, you may move on to the material for the next session—introducing the idea of a backpack checklist.

IN PREPARATION FOR THIS SESSION

You will need to have some materials prepared in advance for this session, to facilitate the child's practice of "weeding out the binder" and storing old papers that should be kept in a file box. You may use the sample papers that were used in Session 5, and mark each paper with a date—including some that are due in the future, some that have been completed recently, and some that are several weeks old. You should also add some papers that a child might want to save (e.g., study guides, reference materials like a 100's chart or multiplication table for math, completed book reports, or tests with high grades). Also include some old announcements for activities that have already occurred. It is not necessary to create elaborate sample papers; even a blank sheet of paper with a title that indicates what it is intended to represent (and a date) will suffice for the practice trials.

DETAILED SESSION CONTENT

Review Implementation of the Behavior-Monitoring and Point Program (with Parent/Child)

Review the Home Behavior Record (Handout 19) with the parent, and discuss the child's performance of the OTMP behaviors between sessions.

- Discuss the behaviors that were observed, noting how frequently the child used the DAR, Assignment and Test Calendar, and accordion binder correctly.
- Ask the parent about his methods for prompting the behaviors.
- Review what rewards were used to reinforce the child's performance of the behaviors.
- Help the family manage any problems with implementation (e.g., problems with prompting, recording points, or providing rewards).

Conduct Skills Building with the Child Alone: Review and Training in Short-Term Paper Storage

Begin by awarding the child session points (Therapist Form 5) and providing praise for good listening and discussion with the parent present. Explain that you will be using this session to review the skills the child has been using so far to control the Go-Ahead-Forget-It and Go-Ahead-Lose-It Glitches, and to teach one more skill for managing papers. Let the child know that you will start by reviewing how the child has been doing with the accordion binder (the tool most recently introduced), the DAR, and the Assignment and Test Calendar. Indicate that this review will help you and the child make sure that the first steps for controlling the Go-Ahead-Forget-It and Go-Ahead-Lose-It Glitches are in place, before you add more skills for controlling the other Glitches. As you review each of the following behaviors, provide session points and praise for cooperative discussion and practice.

Review Use of the Accordion Binder

Review the child's use of the accordion binder (or alternative method) for storing and transferring school papers since the previous session. Check the DAR folder and the Home Behavior Record (Handout 19) to determine whether the child received a school point for using the binder appropriately and a home point for having all papers in the binder upon arrival at home. (See the "Troubleshooting . . ." section in Chapter 3 for steps to take if the teacher is not providing points appropriately.) Look through the child's binder to see whether papers are in the correct sections. Praise the child for using the binder correctly.

Determine whether the child has had any problems using the binder, and problem-solve accordingly:

- Was the binder used consistently, or were there some days when a school or home point was not earned? Remember that the child will probably need some time to get used to this new method for storing papers. Take some time in this session to practice using the binder again, giving the child sample papers to file in the binder and reinforcing accurate performance. Work until the child is 100% accurate on two consecutive practice trials.
- Did the child remember to separate papers into the correct sections? Some children report that they do not have enough time at the end of the school day to separate homework papers into different sections. If this is the case, you may want to modify the procedure for using the binder: Instruct the child to put all homework papers into one section of the binder at school, and to sort them into the correct sections at home. This will alleviate some of the pressure on the child, while still ensuring that all papers arrive home in good condition.
- Did the binder break? Some children may overstuff their binders with papers and workbooks, causing them to crack. Discuss with the child how to use the binder with care, deciding which papers/workbooks should be stored in the binder and which should be placed elsewhere in the backpack.
- Did the child refuse to use the binder? Although most children enjoy using the binder, some children may express embarrassment about using a different type of folder than their peers are using. You can try to work with the child to determine how to answer classmates' questions about the binder (e.g., "I found it in the store with my mom and thought it looked cool," or "My folder kept ripping, and I wanted to make sure no papers fell out"). However, if the child is truly uncomfortable using the binder, you can suggest an alternative paper storage method (see "Alternative Procedures" at the end of Session 5).

Review Use of the DAR

Review how the child has been using the DAR, and use problem solving to address any issues.

- Has the child been writing down all assignments and checking what materials are needed for assignments? If the child is forgetting to do either of these tasks, review the steps for using the DAR again, and practice with sample assignments if necessary until the child is 100% accurate on two consecutive practice trials.
- Has the child been accurate in recording assignments and materials needed? Has the child had any difficulties completing homework because of incomplete assignment information or missing materials? If this is the case, ask the child to describe how she records homework assignments. Does she copy assignments from the board, or are assignments given orally? Is the child pressed for time when writing down assignments and checking off materials? If so, perhaps an alternative arrangement can be made with the teacher, so that the child has more time to record assignments.
- Has the child's teacher been checking the DAR daily and giving points for its use? If there are points missing on certain days, ask the child whether the teacher prompts him to show the DAR to the teacher each day. If the teacher is not reminding the child to provide the DAR for review and points, it is unlikely that the child will remember to do this on his own. It is difficult for children with ADHD to recall independently when they are supposed to execute certain behaviors, especially newly learned behaviors. Thus it is important for teachers to prompt such children to use this new skill. You may need to call the child's teacher to discuss this, and to encourage her to continue prompting the child to present the DAR for review and points.

Review Use of the Assignment and Test Calendar

Review how the child has been using the Assignment and Test Calendar, and use problem solving to address any issues. Has the child used the calendar consistently, or is she still relying on memory to keep track of long-term assignments? Has the child forgotten any assignments or tests, or had to rush to complete projects, because the due dates were not recorded on the Assignment and Test Calendar? If there have been any problems with using the calendar consistently, ask the child what has prevented her from using the calendar. If she reports that she sometimes forgets to record things on the calendar, you may need to speak with the parent, to make sure that the parent prompts the child to complete this routine daily. If the child is unclear about how to use the calendar, review the procedures for use again and practice with sample assignments, making sure that the child is 100% accurate on two consecutive trials before moving on.

Provide Training in Short-Term Storage of Papers

Tell the child:

"You have been doing well so far with using the DAR, the Assignment and Test Calendar, and the accordion binder. Now I want to teach you one more step that can help you keep your binder in good shape and make sure you don't have too many papers in it that you don't really need. We call this step 'weeding out the binder.' Every few days, you will look through the papers in your binder and decide which papers need to stay in the binder (such as papers for assignments/projects that you are still working on), which papers can be thrown away (such as old announcements or completed homework sheets that you don't need any more), and which papers you want to hold on to because you might need them later (such as review sheets that might be used for studying for tests, old book reports that you want to save, or reference papers that you might use again). If you have papers in your binder that you don't need to use right now, but that you might need later, you can store them in a file box like this one [show a small file box, with hanging file folders]. We can label the folders in this box, and you can put your old papers in here, so that you will be able to find them when you need them later on."

Discuss with the child how to organize the file box, thinking about what kinds of papers the child might need to save for later use. For example, you might create hanging file folders for "Reports," "Study Materials," or "Reference Papers." Alternatively, you might create folders labeled by subject, if the child anticipates that there will be multiple papers in each subject that might need to be saved. Demonstrate how the child can file papers in the file box, using the categorization system that you and the child select.

Conduct In-Session Practice: Weeding Out the Binder

Use a sample accordion binder, filled with the first batch of papers marked with dates of completion (there should be at least four papers in each practice trial; reserve some papers for the next trials). Explain that some papers in the binder are due soon and that some have already been completed. Instruct the child to separate the papers into those that should be kept in the binder (e.g., assignments that have yet to be completed), those that should be thrown out, and those that should be stored in the file box.

Tell the child:

"Remember, it's OK to throw out papers if you don't need them any more. This helps you stay organized by making sure your binder doesn't get overstuffed with papers you don't need. If you find papers that can be thrown out, this is a good time to let the Go-Ahead-Lose-It Glitch do what it loves to do. So if there's an old announcement in your binder, go ahead and lose it . . . because you don't need it any more!"

Guide the child in two to three rounds of practice with weeding out the binder. Praise the child and award session points for keeping new papers in the binder, throwing out papers that are not needed, and filing old papers in the correct folders in the file box.

Wrap Up the Session (with Parent/Child)

Review Any Changes in the Routines for Tracking Assignments and Managing Papers

Tell the parent that you have spent some time reviewing the use of the DAR, the Assignment and Test Calendar, and the accordion binder, and summarize your discussion with the child regarding any modifications to the routines. If it was determined that the child needs more prompting to use any of the OTMP behaviors, ask the parent to increase prompts accordingly. If no issues were noted with the use of the OTMP behaviors, indicate that the child is doing well with the use of these methods, and ask the parent to continue supporting the child's use of those behaviors.

Support Child in Explaining How to Weed Out the Binder and Store Papers in a File Box

Guide the child in explaining how to weed out the binder, and ask the child to explain why this process is important. Have the child show the parent the file box, and explain to the parent how it will be used to store papers that do not need to stay in the binder. Indicate that the child will take this file box home and use it from now on, as part of the paper management routine.

Describe the Home Exercise: DAR, Assignment and Test Calendar, Binder, and Weeding Out the Binder

Review, with the parent and child, the actions that the child will practice at home and school:

- The child will continue to use the DAR and the Assignment and Test Calendar to track assignments.
- The child will use the binder to store and transfer school papers. The child will receive points from the parent and teacher if the papers are in the correct sections of the binder.
- The parent and child will work together to weed out the binder at the end of each day, deciding which papers should be kept in the binder, which should be discarded, and which should be stored in the file box. After the next session, this weeding-out process will only be performed once a week; however, it should be practiced daily for the first few days, to ensure skill acquisition.

Review the Home Behavior Record

Show the parent the Home Behavior Record (Handout 19), and review which behaviors the parent will prompt, monitor, praise, and reward, as described in the home exercise. The Home Behavior Record should contain five child behaviors to be prompted, monitored, praised, and rewarded:

- *School behavior 1*: Completed the DAR accurately.
- *School behavior 2*: Put papers in the binder.
- *Home behavior 1*: Completed the Assignment and Test Calendar.
- *Home behavior 2*: Papers in binder upon arrival at home and put back into the binder after homework.
- *Home behavior 3*: Weed out the binder.

Note: The non-OTMP behaviors will no longer be monitored or rewarded with the Home Behavior Record. However, you can encourage the parent to continue prompting and praising those behaviors, to ensure maintenance.

Add New Target Behaviors to the DAR Folder

The target behaviors for which the teacher will provide school points are these:

1. Completed the DAR accurately.
2. Put papers in the binder.

Reward the Child

Review the Session Points and Notes (Therapist Form 5) with the child, and praise the child for the positive behaviors that earned points in the session. Add up the total points earned for this session, and indicate that the child may spend or save the points.

Conclude the Session

Confirm the next session appointment. Give the child and parent the OTMP Checklist (Handout 22). Remind the parent to bring the Home Behavior Record (Handout 19), and the child to bring the DAR folder and binder, to the next session.

Managing Materials
Introducing a Backpack Checklist

GOALS FOR THE SESSION

You will:

- Determine what materials the child needs to take back and forth between school and home.
- Understand the child's current method for checking that all needed materials are in the backpack.
- Work with the child to develop a personalized backpack checklist, to facilitate management of needed materials.

The parent will:

- Describe efforts to prompt, monitor, praise, and reward target behaviors, using the Home Behavior Record from the previous session (Handout 19).
- Understand how the child should use the backpack checklist and "Check It Out" procedures daily.
- Agree to prompt, monitor, praise, and reward specified target behaviors between sessions, using the Home Behavior Record from this session (Handout 19).

The child will:

- Indicate which items must be carried back and forth each day between school and home.
- Learn a new method for making sure that needed items are in the backpack—the backpack checklist.

113

MATERIALS NEEDED

For the parent:

- Handout 19, Home Behavior Record

For you:

- Materials to create the backpack checklist: index cards, markers/crayons/colored pencils, scissors (to trim the index cards to fit), plastic name tag holder, large safety pins
- Cardboard luggage tags (see Chapter 2)
- Colored paper (to serve as sample papers for practice)
- Handout 10, Daily Assignment Record (three copies, filled in with sample assignments)
- Therapist Form 5, Session Points and Notes
- Therapist Form 13, Interview on School Materials

SESSION SUMMARY CHECKLIST FOR SESSION 7

Item	Item Completed
Review implementation of the behavior-monitoring and point program (with parent/child)	Yes/No
Conduct skills building with the child alone: Backpack checklist	
Conduct OST homework review: DAR, Assignment and Test Calendar, accordion binder, weeding out the binder	Yes/No
Conduct interview on school materials (Therapist Form 13)	Yes/No
Explain the rationale for using a checklist	Yes/No
Demonstrate how to use the backpack checklist	Yes/No
Create a personalized backpack checklist	Yes/No
Conduct In-Session Practice: Check It Out	Yes/No
Wrap up the session (with parent/child)	
Support the child in explaining how to use the backpack checklist	Yes/No
Describe the home exercise: DAR, binder, calendar, backpack checklist	Yes/No
Review the Home Behavior Record (Handout 19)	Yes/No
Add new target behaviors to the DAR folder	Yes/No
Reward the child (Therapist Form 5)	Yes/No
Conclude the session (Handout 24)	Yes/No

For the child:

- Child's DAR folder, accordion binder, and backpack
- Handout 23, Check It Out: Steps
- Handout 24, OTMP Checklist: Things to Remember for Session 8

About This Session

In this session, you will teach the child another skill for controlling the Go-Ahead-Forget-It Glitch. You will work with the child to create a personalized backpack checklist, which will help the child remember all needed materials when packing the backpack. In the next session, the child will be able to create checklists for other activities or bags (e.g., sports bags, dance bags, sleepover bags).

In Preparation for This Session

You will need to have some materials prepared in advance for this session, to help the child create and practice using a backpack checklist. The backpack checklist is a list of items that the child must carry between school and home. It is pinned to the inside of the backpack, so that it is visible when the bag is opened and can be used as a visual reminder of what should be inside the bag. The list should be created in a durable format, so that it will not become crumpled with excessive use. We have recommended using a plastic name tag (or badge) holder, with a trimmed index card inside, pinned to the inside of the bag with a safety pin. Other formats may also work, as long as the format meets the following criteria: (1) The checklist is short and easy to read; (2) the list is placed in a protective holder, so it is not damaged; and (3) the list is attached to the backpack in a place where it is visible as the child is packing the bag.

You should create a sample backpack checklist before the session, so that you can show the child what such a list looks like and demonstrate how it can be pinned into the backpack. The sample checklist should contain the following questions, in list format:

1. Do I have my DAR folder in my binder?
2. Are all my papers in the binder?
3. Do I have my binder?
4. Do I have the books I need?
5. Do I need anything else special today?

You will also need to create a second, coded checklist, to tie onto the backpack zipper. For this purpose, we recommend using a blank cardboard luggage tag, with strings that can be tied to the zipper. Again, you can be creative in using alternative materials for this purpose. The coded checklist might have the numerals 1, 2, 3, 4, and 5 written on it, to represent the five questions above; different colors for each of the five questions; or even a diagram or pictures to represent the steps that must be followed in packing the backpack.

DETAILED SESSION CONTENT

Review Implementation of the Behavior-Monitoring and Point Program (with Parent/Child)

Review the Home Behavior Record (Handout 19) with the parent, and discuss the child's performance of the OTMP behaviors between sessions.

- Discuss the behaviors that were observed, noting how frequently the child used the DAR, Assignment and Test Calendar, accordion binder, and weeding-out routines correctly.
- Ask the parent about how she prompted the behaviors.
- Review what rewards were used to reinforce the child's performance of the behaviors.
- Help the family manage any problems with implementation (e.g., problems with prompting, recording points, or providing rewards).

Conduct Skills Building with the Child Alone: Backpack Checklist

Begin by awarding the child session points (Therapist Form 5) and providing praise for good listening and discussion with the parent present.

Conduct OST Homework Review: DAR, Assignment and Test Calendar, Accordion Binder, Weeding Out the Binder

Review the Home Behavior Record (Handout 19) and DARs from the last few days, and note whether the child is using the DAR, Assignment and Test Calendar, binder, and weeding-out routines consistently. Examine the child's backpack and accordion binder, noting whether all papers are in the binder, and whether papers are stored in the correct sections of the binder. If papers are not in the binder, or are not in the correct sections, point that out and ask the child to self-correct any misplacements. If necessary, review the steps for using the binder again, and give additional practice by having the child remove the papers from the binder and put them back again in the correct sections. Finally, ask the child how the weeding-out process worked between sessions. Ask the child whether there were any papers that needed to be thrown out or stored in the file box. Provide session points (Therapist Form 5) for this review.

Conduct Interview on School Materials

Tell the child:

"In the last few sessions, we have been working on learning a new way to store the papers you need for school. You have been using the accordion binder [or alternative method] to separate and carry your papers, and you have a file box at home to store papers that you don't need to carry back and forth to school. Now we want to add one more step that will help you control the Go-Ahead-Forget-It Glitch. We will work together to create a checklist that will go in your backpack, with a list of all the things you have to remember to pack. This checklist will help you make sure that you know which materials you need to have with you when you pack your backpack in school and at home. It will also help you be sure that you don't forget anything. Before we do this, I want to talk with you about what you usually have to carry back and forth between school and home, and about any problems you might have with moving your stuff from one place to another."

Ask the child about the things that have to be packed in the backpack for school/home use. You can use the interview questions on Therapist Form 13, although you may already know the answers to some of them from past discussions with the child. Do not repeat questions if they have been asked and answered in the past; instead, you can ask the child to confirm the information you already know (e.g., "So most days you have to take your spelling notebook home, right?" or "You told me that you have music lessons after school most days; what do you need to pack for that?"). You can jot down notes on the interview form, so that you know what items to include on the backpack checklist.

Explain the Rationale for Using a Checklist

After the child has shared information on the things that need to be carried in the backpack and on any problems encountered with remembering needed materials, you should discuss why a checklist for needed items can be useful. You want to develop this new routine with as much input as possible from the child, to increase the child's motivation for using it. Thus a brief discussion, in which you use directed questions to help the child see the merits of a checklist, is an important part of this process.

Tell the child:

"So it seems like you have to remember to pack a lot of things in your backpack every day, which means that there are a lot of opportunities for the Go-Ahead-Forget-It Glitch to play tricks on you. How do you think you can make sure that you have all the things you need in your backpack? Do you think a checklist could help, by reminding you what you need each day? You have been using a checklist on your DAR, to help you remember the items you need for each homework assignment. Has this been useful? Let's think about it, though; there is still a chance for the Go-Ahead-Forget-It Glitch to get you while you pack up at the end of the day. What if you write down all the materials you need on your DAR, but then you forget your DAR folder inside your desk? What if you put your DAR folder in your bag, but forget your accordion binder at school, so you don't have your homework sheets?

"Would it help if you made a list to remind you what you need to pack each day, and if that list was displayed somewhere you could see, as you pack up your bag? Where could you keep that list so that you could see it as you pack your bag at school and at home?"

Demonstrate How to Use the Backpack Checklist

Show the child a sample backpack checklist, and demonstrate how it can be pinned into the inside of the backpack, so that it hangs from the top of the inside compartment and is visible when the bag is being packed. Point out its essential features: (1) It is a short, simple checklist of all the things the child needs to pack in the school bag; and (2) it is visible as the child packs the bag, so the child can use it as a step-by-step packing guide to make sure that nothing is forgotten.

In addition to this comprehensive checklist, you will also show the child a shorter, coded checklist on a cardboard luggage tag, which can be tied onto the backpack zipper. This highly visible second checklist acts as a visual reminder to the child to consider whether everything has been packed in the bag. This checklist can use a diagram, pictures, numerals to delineate the number of things the child must pack, or a color-coded list.

Demonstrate how you can use the two checklists. First, remove the binder, DAR folder, and any books from the backpack. Then, with the backpack open, look at the checklist, which contains the following four questions:

1. Do I have my DAR folder in my binder?
2. Are all my papers in the binder?
3. Do I have my binder?
4. Do I have the books I need?

Say each question out loud, and demonstrate how you should check for each item before placing it into the bag. Once everything is in the backpack, zip up the bag and look at the luggage tag, which is tied to the outside zipper, with a code written on it (e.g., 1, 2, 3, 4, to represent the four questions above). Show how you can use this numbered code as a final check that you used all of steps for packing up appropriately. For example, hold up one finger at a time and say, "I have my DAR folder in the binder; I have the binder in the bag; all my papers are in the binder; and I have my books").

Create a Personalized Backpack Checklist

Tell the child that you will now work together to create a backpack checklist for the inside of the backpack and a coded tag for the outside zipper. Take out the needed materials, and ask the child for input in forming the list of questions to go on the checklist. The four questions above should be on the checklist, because if the child has the items on that list, she should be able to complete all homework. However, you should also ask the child whether any other items need to be included on the checklist, based on your earlier discussion about what needs to be taken between home and school. For example, the child might need to carry a bus pass, musical instrument, or sports equipment daily or almost daily; these items could be added to the checklist. After you have created the backpack checklist for inside the backpack, you can help the child create a coded luggage tag to attach to the outside zipper, which will act as a final check that all the steps for packing the bag have been followed.

HELPFUL HINT: You can be flexible in creating a backpack checklist that works for the child; however, you want to keep the checklist reasonably simple. You should try to avoid creating multiple checklists for different days of the week or different situations (e.g., days with extracurricular activities or different specialty subjects). Instead, try to find a way to include alternatives on a basic checklist that can be used every day (e.g., you might add a fifth question: "Do I have materials for extracurriculars?"). Sometimes a general fifth question can be "Anything else?" to refer to those items that are not needed every day, such as instruments for in-school music lessons or sneakers for gym class.

Conduct In-Session Practice: Check It Out

Tell the child:

"Now that you have your own backpack checklist, you can use a new routine, which we will call 'Check It Out,' to make sure that you have all the things you need when you're packing up your bag in school and at home. First, you will look at your DAR and see what items you need for homework. You will put all your papers in your binder, and all of the books you need in your backpack. Then you will put the DAR folder in the binder and put the binder in the backpack. Finally, you will 'Check It Out,' using your backpack checklist. Ask yourself each of the questions out loud as you check that you have followed each step. Then you can zip up your backpack and use the code on the zipper tag to make sure that you've followed all of the steps. Let's practice these steps now, using your DAR from today."

Attach the child's backpack checklist to the inside of the child's backpack with a safety pin, and tie the coded luggage tag to the outside zipper. Instruct the child to unpack the backpack, take out the DAR folder, and look at the DAR for the day. Have the child follow the steps described above, using the Check It Out procedures to pack the backpack with what is needed. Provide praise and any necessary feedback on this first round of practice.

Then guide the child through two to three more rounds of practice, using sample materials. Use the sample DARs (Handout 10), filled in with practice assignments, and colored sheets of paper with simple headings on them, to correspond to the homework papers needed for the sample DAR assignments. (*Note:* Colored paper is used so that it is easier to remove from the child's binder after the practice is completed.) For each practice trial, instruct the child to unpack the backpack and practice the Check It Out steps with the DAR and materials that are provided. Provide session points for all practice trials.

Give the child Handout 23, which lists the Check It Out steps. Review the steps for packing the backpack at school and at home, using the checklists. Tell the child that he can use this handout to help explain these steps to the parent.

Wrap Up the Session (with Parent/Child)

Support the Child in Explaining How to Use the Backpack Checklist

Tell the child to show the parent the backpack checklist and coded zipper tag, and to describe how they are used in making sure that all needed items are in the backpack. Ask the child to review the steps on the Check It Out guide (Handout 23) with the parent, explaining how these steps can help to control the Go-Ahead-Forget-It Glitch.

Describe the Home Exercise: DAR, Assignment and Test Calendar, Binder, Backpack Checklist

Review, with the parent and child, the actions that the child will practice at home and school:

- The child will continue to use the DAR and the Assignment and Test Calendar to track assignments.
- The child will use the binder to store and transfer school papers. The child will

receive points from the parent and teacher if the papers are in the correct sections of the binder.

- The child will use the backpack checklist at home, after homework is completed, when packing the backpack for school.
- The child should also use the backpack checklist when packing up at school, but will not receive school points for this behavior yet.

Review the Home Behavior Record

Show the parent the Home Behavior Record (Handout 19), and review which behaviors the parent will prompt, monitor, praise, and reward, as described in the home exercise. The Home Behavior Record should contain five child behaviors to be prompted, monitored, praised, and rewarded:

- *School behavior 1*: Completed the DAR accurately.
- *School behavior 2*: Used the binder and turned in all papers.
- *Home behavior 1*: Completed the Assignment and Test Calendar.
- *Home behavior 2*: Papers in binder upon arrival at home and put back into the binder after homework.
- *Home behavior 3*: Used the backpack checklist when packing the bag for school.

Add New Target Behaviors to the DAR Folder

The target behaviors for which the teacher will provide school points are these:

1. Completed the DAR accurately.
2. Used the binder and turned in all papers.

Reward the Child

Review the Session Points and Notes (Therapist Form 5) with the child, and praise the child for the positive behaviors that earned points in the session. Add up the total points earned for this session, and indicate that the child may spend or save the points.

Conclude the Session

Confirm the next session appointment. Give the child and parent the OTMP Checklist (Handout 24). Remind the parent to bring the Home Behavior Record (Handout 19), and the child to bring the backpack, DAR folder, and binder, to the next session. In addition, tell the parent and child that you will be working on creating checklists for other bags in the next session. If the child has to pack other bags regularly (e.g., sports bags, dance bags), the child should bring those bags to the next session, so that you can work on creating checklists for those bags.

SESSION 8

Managing Materials
"Other Stuff" and Other Bags

GOALS FOR THE SESSION

You will:

- Contact the child's teacher prior to the next session to describe the Ready to Go procedures, which are introduced in the next session (Teacher Contact 3).

You and the child will:

- Discuss other items that the child must carry in the backpack.
- Create a new backpack checklist, including other items that have been discussed.
- Discuss different options for organizing items in the backpack.
- Create a checklist for a bag used for other activities.

The child will:

- Practice organizing and packing the backpack, using an updated backpack checklist.
- Practice using an activity bag checklist to pack a bag.

The parent will:

- Describe efforts to prompt, monitor, praise, and reward target behaviors, using the Home Behavior Record from the previous session (Handout 19).
- Understand how the child should use the backpack checklist daily and the activity bag checklist as needed.
- Agree to prompt, monitor, praise, and reward specified target behaviors between sessions, using the Home Behavior Record from this session.

121

MATERIALS NEEDED

For the parent:

- Handout 19, Home Behavior Record

For you:

- Index cards, markers/crayons/colored pencils, scissors (to trim the index cards to fit), plastic name tag holder, large safety pins, blank luggage tags
- Organizational tools/containers (rubber bands, folders, pencil cases/pouches, Ziploc bags)
- Sample gym clothes (sneakers, shorts, t-shirt) for packing practice

SESSION SUMMARY CHECKLIST FOR SESSION 8

Item	Item Completed
Conduct review and discussion (with parent/child)	
Review implementation of the behavior-monitoring and point program	Yes/No
Discuss items that must be packed in the backpack/activity bag	Yes/No
Conduct skills building with the child alone: Packing "other stuff"	
Conduct OST homework review: DAR, Assignment and Test Calendar, accordion binder, Check It Out	Yes/No
Discuss "other stuff" the child must pack for school	Yes/No
Create a new backpack checklist with other items	Yes/No
Discuss backpack organization	Yes/No
Conduct in-session practice: Packing the backpack	Yes/No
Discuss "stuff" needed for other activities	Yes/No
Create an activity bag checklist	Yes/No
Wrap up the session (with parent/child)	
Support the child in explaining how to use the new backpack checklist and activity bag checklist	Yes/No
Determine a routine for packing up at home	Yes/No
Review the Home Behavior Record (Handout 19)	Yes/No
Add new target behaviors to the DAR folder	Yes/No
Reward the child (Therapist Form 5)	Yes/No
Conclude the session	Yes/No

- Therapist Form 5, Session Points and Notes
- Therapist Form 14, Photos of Backpacks
- Video recorder (optional)

For the child:

- Child's DAR folder, binder, and backpack
- Handout 25, OTMP Checklist: Things to Remember for Session 9

ABOUT THIS SESSION

In this session, you will expand upon the Check It Out steps that were learned in the previous session. The child will add other items to the backpack checklist that are needed for school/home (e.g., bus pass, keys, lunch box, calculator). In addition, the child will learn how to organize the backpack more effectively and pack all of the necessary items in an efficient manner. Finally, the child will learn how to create a checklist for packing other bags (e.g., bags for extracurricular activities, sleepovers).

IN PREPARATION FOR THIS SESSION

You will need to have the same materials that were used in the previous session—this time, for creating a new backpack checklist, and for creating a checklist for an activity bag. In addition, you should be prepared with items that can be useful in organizing the interior compartments of a backpack (e.g., rubber bands, folders, pencil cases/pouches, Ziploc bags). Some children's backpacks may contain built-in compartments for organization of materials, but others may not, so you should be prepared to provide the child with some tools for organizing the smaller items in the backpack.

DETAILED SESSION CONTENT

Conduct Review and Discussion (with Parent/Child)

Review Implementation of the Behavior-Monitoring and Point Program

Review the Home Behavior Record (Handout 19) with the parent, and discuss the child's performance of the OTMP behaviors between sessions.

- Discuss the behaviors that were observed, noting how frequently the child used the DAR, Assignment and Test Calendar, accordion binder, and Check It Out routines correctly. Problem-solve any issues with implementation of these routines.
- Ask the parent how he prompted the behaviors.
- Review what rewards were used to reinforce the child's performance of the behaviors.
- Help the family manage any problems with implementation (e.g., problems with prompting, recording points, or providing rewards).

Discuss Items That Must Be Packed in the Backpack/Activity Bag

Tell the parent and child that after this session, the child will use the backpack checklist at home and at school, and will receive points from the parent and teacher for doing so. Indicate that you will be working with the child on adding other items to the backpack checklist that are usually taken to school (e.g., bus pass, keys, lunch box, calculator). Ask the parent for input regarding which items should be included on this list.

Also, tell the parent that you will create a checklist for other bags that the child must pack (e.g., activity bags, overnight bags for sleepovers). If the parent brought in an activity bag (as requested at the end of the previous session), examine it briefly, and discuss any issues that the child has had with packing this bag (e.g., items that are frequently forgotten).

> **HELPFUL HINT:** Many children spend their time in two households because of parental separation or divorce. For these children, it is important to review their methods for taking items back and forth between those households. Spending time helping these children create checklists for overnight bags can help reduce stress or conflicts that can result when a child forgets important items.

Conduct Skills Building with the Child Alone: Packing "Other Stuff"

Begin by awarding the child session points (Therapist Form 5) and providing praise for good listening and discussion with the parent present.

Conduct OST Homework Review: DAR, Assignment and Test Calendar, Accordion Binder, Check It Out

Review the Home Behavior Record (Handout 19) and DARs from the last few days, and note whether the child is using the DAR, Assignment and Test Calendar, binder, and Check It Out routines consistently. Examine the child's backpack and accordion binder, noting whether all papers are in the binder, and whether papers are stored in the correct sections of the binder. Finally, ask the child how the Check It Out process worked between sessions. Provide session points (Therapist Form 5) for this review.

Discuss "Other Stuff" the Child Must Pack for School

Tell the child:

> "You have been working hard to control the Go-Ahead-Forget-It Glitch, and you've been doing a great job keeping your school papers organized, using the accordion binder. You also have a backpack checklist now, which helps you make sure that you have all your papers in your binder, the binder itself, and all the books you need for homework. Now we have to think about the 'other stuff' you need for school, like pencils and pens, rulers, erasers, and other things. I want to talk to you about how you store those other things in your backpack, and how easy it is for you to find those things when you need them."

Ask the child to help you make a list of all the things she must carry in her backpack. Other items might include pens, pencils, erasers, rulers, markers/colored pencils, glue stick, travel money/passes, house keys, cell phone, water bottle, library card, lunch money, and so on. Have the child think about days when special items are needed, such as musical instruments for days when the child has a music lesson; sports equipment or gym clothes for days when a sport is practiced; or days when the child has a play date after school and wants to bring a special toy. Jot down notes as the child describes these items, noting items that are needed every day and items that are needed only on special days. Award session points as the child engages in making this list.

Create a New Backpack Checklist with Other Items

Tell the child that you will now create a modified backpack checklist together. You will add some of the important items from this new list to the key four items that are already on the checklist (DAR in binder, papers in binder, binder in backpack, books in backpack). You should consider adding only one or two additional items, to keep the checklist manageable but comprehensive. For example, the child might add two more prompts:

5. Do I have _____ [important daily item or frequently needed item]?
6. Do I need any special items for today?

You can be flexible in creating these additional items, based on the specific demands that the child reports for packing items in the backpack. If there is space on the original backpack checklist, you may write these additional items in there; if not, you can create a new checklist, using the same materials as in Session 7. You can also modify the original zipper tag to include the new items, or create a new one. Attach the new checklist and zipper tag to the backpack. Indicate that the child will now use this checklist to pack the backpack, and that you will practice using it in just a few moments.

Discuss Backpack Organization

Tell the child:

> "Now that we've talked about all the stuff you have to keep in your backpack, let's talk about how your backpack usually looks. How would you describe your backpack? Do you think it's neat or messy? Have other people told you that it's a mess? Has stuff in your bag gotten ruined because it was crumpled, torn, or spilled on? [Wait for child's response.] Lots of kids who come in here have trouble keeping their backpacks organized. Sometimes it's difficult to store so much stuff in the backpack without having things get all mixed up. Let's think about how you store your stuff."

Ask the child to show you where he keeps the items on the list you made above. Look to see where the pens, pencils, markers, and so on are; are they in a pencil case or special compartment, or are they floating around at the bottom of the bag? Are there toys and personal items crammed into the main compartment, with books and folders? Are there crumbs from snacks or spills from drinks at the bottom of the bag? Does the child use smaller compartments for important items, like keys or passes, or are those items lost in larger compartments?

Show the child the photos of backpacks in Therapist Form 14, which represent varied levels of organization, from very disorganized to obsessively neat. Ask the child to select the photo that looks like her backpack most of the time. Then ask the child to select the photo of the backpack that she would like to have.

Tell the child:

"Let's think about how we can organize your backpack better, so it looks more like the last photo you pointed to. One of the best ways to organize your backpack and make sure stuff doesn't get lost inside your bag is to use compartments. Let's see if we can decide which things should go into which compartments of your bag."

Work with the child to determine where things should go, using the compartments that are provided in the bag. For example, you might put all of the books and folders in the largest compartment, or you might decide to put smaller books in one compartment and larger books in another. Show the child how to use smaller compartments for things that can get lost in the larger areas (e.g., pencils, glue sticks), and how to put cards and passes in special holders. Discuss why it makes sense to keep snacks and drinks separate from important items like books and papers, to make sure the important items don't get stained.

Next, consider whether containers (e.g., pencil cases) might be helpful, especially if the child's backpack does not have multiple compartments. If there is no room for a pencil case, even a simple trick like tying rubber bands around pencils to keep them together can be useful. Decide where any containers should be kept and what they should hold. Finally, summarize how the child can reorganize the backpack, using the tools and tips you have discussed.

Conduct In-Session Practice: Packing the Backpack

Instruct the child to unpack the backpack and spread items out on the desk. Next, tell the child to practice packing the bag, using the new tools you have discussed for organizing the items in the backpack. Tell the child to use the new backpack checklist for the Check It Out steps after packing up. If possible, use a digital video recorder to record the child packing the bag. After the child has finished packing, review the video or orally review what you observed, discussing how the child followed through on the new organizational plan. If there is room for improvement (e.g., it took the child a long time to fit all his books into one compartment, or the child forgot to use the containers appropriately), give constructive feedback and ask the child to unpack and practice packing again, focusing on developing the most effective procedure for packing the bag. Provide session points for practice and discussion.

As an extension of this practice with packing the bag, ask the child to pretend that she must pack the bag for a school day when extra items are needed (e.g., day with gym class, music lessons, gymnastics class, etc.). You can refer to the new backpack checklist, which includes a reference to "special items," and use one to two of those special items (e.g., gym clothes, clarinet, leotard) in these practice activities. If you do not have the actual items available, use pieces of paper with a drawing or words to represent the items. Guide the child in one to two practice rounds of unpacking and packing the bag, including a different special item in each round. Help the child think about how compartments or containers might be useful in storing these items. As the child practices packing the bag for each of the "special days," provide praise and session points for use of the backpack checklist, effective solutions for storing the items, and organized procedures for packing the bag. Emphasize that the child should use her eyes, and not her memory, when packing, so that she looks to see whether items are included as she goes over the list. This is a special reminder that helps control the Go-Ahead-Forget-It Glitch.

Discuss "Stuff" Needed for Other Activities

Tell the child:

> "If you keep using the procedures we just practiced for packing your backpack, you should have a more organized backpack and should be able to remember what you need for school. Now let's think about other kinds of bags you need to pack for other activities."

You may already know about activity bags that the child must pack, from your discussion with the parent and child. If so, you may focus on those activity bags for this exercise. If the parent and child have not mentioned any activities that require the packing of a bag with special items, you can ask the child to think about any time he might need to pack a bag; for example, he might go on a sleepover to a friend's house, or spend a long weekend at his grandparents' house, or need to pack a bag for a day at the beach or pool.

Create an Activity Bag Checklist

Ask the child what items are needed for the activity or outing selected, and work with the child to create a checklist for the bag she needs to pack for the activity or outing. Use the same format and materials as for the backpack checklist, and think about where the child can attach this new checklist in the activity bag.

If the child has brought in an activity bag with items, use this bag for in-session practice—unpacking the items and then having the child repack them, using the new checklist. If the child has not brought in an activity bag, go through the steps on the checklist, and suggest that he use these steps to practice packing the bag at home.

Provide praise and session points for discussion and practice. Remind the child to use her eyes, not her memory, when packing, to make certain that items on the list are in the bag.

Wrap Up the Session (with Parent/Child)

Support the Child in Explaining How to Use the New Backpack Checklist and Activity Bag Checklist

Tell the child to show the parent the new backpack checklist and coded zipper tag, and to explain the new items on the list. The child should also show the parent the new method for organizing the bag, point out the use of any compartments and/or containers, and explain why this new way of organizing the backpack will be helpful in controlling the Glitches (e.g., fewer crumpled items, greater ease in finding needed items). The child should also show the parent the checklist that was created for an activity or outing bag, and describe how this checklist can be used to make sure needed items are in that bag.

Determine a Routine for Packing Up at Home

Help the child break down the new routine for packing the backpack (developed in this session) into steps, so that this routine can be used at home and in school when the child packs the backpack. For example, you might break down a child's packing-up routine as follows:

1. Place DAR and all homework sheets in the binder, and place the binder in the largest compartment of the backpack.
2. Place all books needed for homework in the largest compartment of the backpack, in front of the binder.
3. Put pencils, markers, and glue stick into the pencil box, and put the pencil box in the second compartment of the backpack.
4. Put snacks and drink into the side compartment.
5. Check it Out on the backpack checklist.

The parent should prompt the child to follow the steps in this routine between sessions, allocating time each evening or morning to observe that the child has followed these steps and to give praise and points accordingly.

Review the Home Behavior Record

Show the parent the Home Behavior Record (Handout 19), and review which behaviors the parent will prompt, monitor, praise, and reward. At this point, the child has learned a number of behaviors that could be monitored and praised (completing the DAR, transferring information to the Assignment and Test Calendar, storing paper in the binder, and using the backpack checklist); however, the Home Behavior Record should only contain five behaviors to be prompted, monitored, praised, and rewarded. Based on your understanding of how the child is doing with regard to the organizational behaviors learned thus far, you may select five behaviors to include that require the most monitoring and reinforcement. The list should include the two newest behaviors learned (i.e., using the backpack checklist when packing the backpack, and using a checklist for packing bags for other activities/outings). The following is a suggested list of behaviors that might be appropriate for the Home Behavior Record, though variations might make sense for some children.

- *School behavior 1*: Used the binder and turned in all papers.
- *School behavior 2*: Used the backpack checklist at school when packing bag.
- *Home behavior 1*: Papers in binder upon arrival at home and put back into the binder after homework.
- *Home behavior 2*: Used the backpack checklist when packing the bag for school.
- *Home behavior 3*: Used checklist for activity/outing bag.

Add New Target Behaviors to the DAR Folder

The target behaviors for which the teacher will provide school points are these:

1. Used the binder and turned in all papers.
2. Used the backpack checklist at school when packing bag.

Reward the Child

Review the Session Points and Notes (Therapist Form 5) with the child, and praise the child for the positive behaviors that earned points in the session. Add up the total points earned for this session, and indicate that the child may spend or save the points.

Conclude the Session

Confirm the next session appointment. Give the child and parent the OTMP Checklist for the next session (Handout 25). Remind the parent to bring the Home Behavior Record (Handout 19), and the child to bring the backpack, DAR folder, and binder, to the next session.

Managing Materials
Getting Work Areas Ready to Go

You will:

- Introduce a routine for making work areas "Ready to Go."
- Learn about the child's workspaces at home and school, and develop a plan for using Ready to Go steps in each space.
- Send an e-mail reminder to the teacher to begin prompting the child to use Ready to Go in school (arrange for this before the session, so the teacher is ready to monitor this behavior the next school day).

The child will:

- Practice Ready to Go steps in session.
- Learn how to use Ready to Go steps at home and in school.

The parent will:

- Describe efforts to prompt, monitor, praise, and reward target behaviors, using the Home Behavior Record from the previous session (Handout 19).
- Understand how the child should use the Ready to Go steps at home.
- Agree to prompt, monitor, praise, and reward specified target behaviors between sessions, using the Home Behavior Record from this session.

════════ **MATERIALS NEEDED** ════════

For the parent:

- Handout 19, Home Behavior Record

For you:

- Materials for in-session practice with Ready to Go (see "In Preparation for This Session")
- Therapist Form 5, Session Points and Notes
- Therapist Form 15, Ready to Go: What's Up with That Desk?
- Therapist Form 16 (Optional), Ready to Go: Materials for Adventure Practice

For the child:

- Child's DAR folder, binder, and backpack
- Handout 26, Getting Ready to Go
- Handout 27, OTMP Checklist: Things to Remember for Session 10

SESSION SUMMARY CHECKLIST FOR SESSION 9

Item	Item Completed
Review implementation of the behavior-monitoring and point program (with parent/child)	Yes/No
Conduct skills building with the child alone: Ready to Go	
Conduct OST homework review: DAR, Assignment and Test Calendar, accordion binder, Check It Out	Yes/No
Discuss getting workspaces Ready to Go (Handout 26)	Yes/No
Conduct In-Session Practice: Ready to Go	Yes/No
Interview the child about home and school workspaces (Therapist Form 15)	Yes/No
Optional: Conduct Ready to Go practice with an imaginary adventure	
Wrap up the session (with parent/child)	
Support the child in demonstrating the Ready to Go steps	Yes/No
Determine a routine for using Ready to Go at home	Yes/No
Review the Home Behavior Record (Handout 19)	Yes/No
Add new target behaviors to the DAR folder	Yes/No
Reward the child (Therapist Form 5)	Yes/No
Conclude the session (Handout 27)	Yes/No

ABOUT THIS SESSION

In this session, the child will learn to get work areas "Ready to Go." The child will learn a quick routine for obtaining materials that are needed for the task at hand and putting away potentially distracting or unnecessary materials. The child will practice the steps in this routine in session with several simulated tasks, and will learn how this routine will be implemented at home and in school.

IN PREPARATION FOR THIS SESSION

To prepare for this session, you will need to have materials for the child to use in practicing making a workspace Ready to Go in session. The following is a list of suggested materials for this practice. If you do not have all of these materials on hand, you may substitute other available materials or use a representation of the item (e.g., a piece of paper with a drawing of a loaf of bread to represent a loaf of bread, or a cup with "peanut butter" written on it to represent a jar of peanut butter).

Suggested Items
- Materials for school assignments: markers, crayons, pencils, pencil sharpener, erasers, blank paper, ruler, plastic stencil, glue stick, tape, stapler, folders, workbooks, books, calculator, math worksheet (with grade-appropriate calculations; if possible, use a worksheet that requires the use of some tools aside from a pencil and paper)
- Materials for making a peanut butter and jelly sandwich: peanut butter, jelly, bread, knife, plate, napkins
- Materials that are considered inappropriate to the work (or distracting): workbooks from subjects that are not being studied, a box of paper clips, a magazine, video game, crossword puzzles, toys, comic books, a letter opener, a can of soda, a bottle of ketchup, a screwdriver, and so on.

Suggested Items for Optional Practice
- See Therapist Form 16.

DETAILED SESSION CONTENT

Review Implementation of the Behavior-Monitoring and Point Program

Review the Home Behavior Record (Handout 19) with the parent, and discuss the child's performance of the OTMP behaviors between sessions.

- Discuss the behaviors that were observed, noting how frequently the child used the DAR, Assignment and Test Calendar, accordion binder, and Check It Out routines (backpack checklist and checklist for another bag) correctly.
- Ask the parent how she prompted the behaviors.
- Review what rewards were used to reinforce the child's performance of the behaviors.
- Help the family manage any problems with implementation (e.g., problems with

prompting, recording points, providing rewards, or implementing organizational routines).

Conduct Skills Building with the Child Alone: Ready to Go

Begin by awarding the child session points (Therapist Form 5) and providing praise for good listening and discussion with the parent present.

Conduct OST Homework Review: DAR, Assignment and Test Calendar, Accordion Binder, Check It Out

Review the Home Behavior Record (Handout 19) and DARs from the last few days, and note whether the child is using the DAR, Assignment and Test Calendar, binder, and Check It Out routines consistently. Examine the child's backpack and accordion binder, noting whether all papers are in the binder, and whether papers are stored in the correct sections of the binder. Finally, ask the child how the Check it Out process worked between sessions (i.e., using the backpack checklist and the checklist for an activity or outing bag). Provide session points (Therapist Form 5) for this review, and problem-solve any issues with implementation of the routines.

Discuss Getting Workspaces Ready to Go

Tell the child:

> "Today we will be talking about how you can make your workspaces, especially your desk at school and your homework work area, neat and ready for work. If you want to do something as quickly and easily as possible, it helps to make sure that you have all the right materials ready before you start working. You should also make sure that your workspace is neat, so you can stay focused on your work and not get distracted by other things. We will learn some simple steps that will help you make sure you have what you need to get your work done and that you put away things that you don't need. We will call these steps getting 'Ready to Go.' We will practice the steps in session, so that you are ready to take on your desk at home and at school."

Show the child Handout 26, and review the steps that the child will take when getting ready to work on a school assignment or other task. The child should consider the following questions:

1. Do I have everything I need? (Consider everything, including the kitchen sink!)
2. What should I put away?
3. Is my work area clear?
4. Are there any things that could distract me? (If so, put them away.)

Point out that these steps can be used to prepare for a variety of situations, and give the child some examples (e.g., school assignment, art project, cooking, building project). Indicate that the child will now practice using these steps to get ready to work on some simulated tasks.

Conduct In-Session Practice: Ready to Go

Select a work area in the session room (preferably a desk or table). Set up the work area with a variety of items, including items that are needed for the task at hand, obviously inappropriate items, items that are slightly inappropriate, and items that could be highly distracting.

> **HELPFUL HINT:** The work area should be set up so that the child can engage in careful consideration of what is needed and what is not needed for the task. Thus you should have a wide variety of materials available, to highlight the decision-making process the child should engage in when getting Ready to Go. For example, in the first practice task, when the child is instructed to get ready to draw a picture, appropriate items would be markers, paper, and other art materials; obviously inappropriate items could be a screwdriver, a bottle of ketchup, or a can of soda; slightly inappropriate items could be a pencil sharpener, a protractor, lined paper, or a roll of tape; and highly distracting items could be a puzzle, a comic book, toys, or a magazine.

For each practice assignment, set up the work area as described above, and give the child the basic instructions for the suggested tasks as described below. Then tell the child to go through the Ready to Go steps out loud while putting away items that are not needed and neatly setting out items that are needed, so that the work area is ready. Next, instruct the child to begin working on the task. If the child realizes that he needs items that are not in the work area, point out that the Ready to Go steps may need to be reviewed again, and discuss how stopping to find needed materials slows the child down. If there are items that distract the child as he works, point out that perhaps these items should have been put away before work began. The child does actually not have to complete the assignments; the objective of the exercises is simply to help the child see the benefits of having a prepared, neat work area.

The following three activities are suggested for practicing the Ready to Go steps:

1. *Drawing a picture.* Ask the child to draw a picture of the session room. Indicate that the child should use straight lines when drawing furniture (so the child considers the need for a ruler) and that the drawing should be in color (so the child considers the need for crayons or markers).
2. *Completing a math worksheet.* Give the child a grade-appropriate math worksheet to complete. If possible, use a worksheet that requires the use of some tools aside from a pencil and paper (e.g., a ruler, stencil, calculator, etc.).
3. *Making a peanut butter and jelly sandwich.* Ask the child to take out all the necessary materials to make a peanut butter and jelly sandwich and then eat it.

Interview the Child about Home and School Workspaces

Because the child will be asked to use the Ready to Go steps both at home and at school, it is important for you to learn more about the child's workspaces in both locations, to help the child determine how the procedure will work. Use Therapist Form 15 to conduct a brief interview about the child's home workspace for completing homework. Then discuss how to use Ready to Go to prepare for doing homework. Give the child an example assignment from the DAR for the day, and ask how she would use Ready to Go steps at home to get ready to do that assignment.

Tell the child:

"Let's say you needed to do your _____ assignment [pick a subject from homework assigned on the DAR, or, if the child does not have any homework, a recent assignment that one of you remembers]. Think about the materials you usually have at your kitchen work area. Would you need to get any other supplies to make sure you were Ready to Go for this assignment—for instance, a pencil, paper, an eraser, a ruler? What would you want to put away?"

Next, ask about the child's school workspace, using the questions on Therapist Form 15, and ask the child how she would use the Ready to Go steps in school. Use an example or two of typical class assignments (e.g., preparing to take a spelling test, preparing to complete a science experiment).

Optional: Conduct Ready to Go Practice for Other Activities

If time permits, you may conduct an imaginary exercise with the child, for which Ready to Go steps can be implemented. This imaginary practice can help the child understand the steps better and provide extra practice with the steps. The activities do not involve a desk or workspace per se, but the main ideas of considering all items and removing distractions can be highlighted in this practice.

Refer to the optional materials listed in Therapist Form 16, and select one of the three imaginary work adventures: the Adventure to Mars, the Superstar Concert Adventure, or the Fashion Show Adventure. Review the selected adventure with the child, and ask the child to use the Ready to Go steps to prepare for the adventure. Emphasize again that being Ready to Go for different tasks can be helpful in many different situations, not only in completing school assignments.

Wrap Up the Session (with Parent/Child)

Support the Child in Demonstrating the Ready to Go Steps

The child should show the parent the handout on Ready to Go steps (Handout 26) and describe how to use the steps in preparing for an assignment or task. Next, the child will demonstrate the Ready to Go steps, using a sample assignment that you select. You may use an assignment from the child's DAR, or ask the child to complete a simple task, like writing sentences for a spelling list. Praise the child for explaining the steps and demonstrating how to use them, and provide any additional explanation and/or clarification to the parent as needed.

Determine a Routine for Using Ready to Go at Home

Tell the parent that the child will use Ready to Go at home and at school, before beginning work on assignments. Work with the parent and child to determine how they will use Ready to Go at home (e.g., the child tells the parent when he is ready to start homework, the parent prompts him to get Ready to Go, and then the parent checks the workspace to make sure the child has prepared it appropriately for the assignment). The parent can use Handout 26 to guide the child in completing all of the necessary steps for being Ready to Go. If the child misses some of the steps, the parent should praise the child for making an effort, and prompt the child to add any steps that have been missed. The parent will provide praise and points for use of the steps, even if corrective feedback is given, as long as the child cooperatively completes all of the steps and is Ready to Go.

Tell the parent and child that the teacher will be monitoring the child's use of Ready to Go in school, for a selected assignment each day. The teacher will select an assignment and prompt the child to get Ready to Go. The teacher will then note whether the child has completed the steps on the DAR.

Review the Home Behavior Record

Show the parent the Home Behavior Record (Handout 19), and review which behaviors the parent will prompt, monitor, praise, and reward. The following is a suggested list of behaviors that might be appropriate for the Home Behavior Record, though variations might make sense for some children.

- *School behavior 1*: Used the binder and backpack checklist, and turned in all papers.
- *School behavior 2*: Got the desk Ready to Go.
- *Home behavior 1*: Papers in binder upon arrival at home and put back in the binder after homework.
- *Home behavior 2*: Used the backpack checklist when packing the bag for school.
- *Home behavior 3*: Got work area Ready to Go for homework

Add New Target Behaviors to the DAR Folder

The target behaviors for which the teacher will provide school points are:

1. Used the binder and backpack checklist, and turned in all papers.
2. Got the desk Ready to Go.

Reward the Child

Review the Session Points and Notes (Therapist Form 5) with the child, and praise the child for the positive behaviors that earned points in the session. Add up the total points earned for this session, and indicate that the child may spend or save the points.

Conclude the Session

Confirm the next session appointment. Give the child and parent the OTMP Checklist for the next session (Handout 27). Remind the parent to bring the Home Behavior Record (Handout 19), and the child to bring the backpack, DAR folder, and binder, to the next session.

Time Management
Understanding Time and Calendars

████████ GOALS FOR THE SESSION ████████

You will:

- Review the child's use of steps for Tracking Assignments and Managing Materials, including the Assignment and Test Calendar.
- Discuss the rationale for using calendars and clocks.
- Help the child create a personal calendar to track activities and events.
- Teach the child how to estimate and record the length of time needed to accomplish tasks.

The child will:

- Understand why clocks and calendars are useful tools.
- Create a personal calendar to track activities and events.
- Learn how to estimate and record the length of time needed to accomplish tasks.

The parent will:

- Describe efforts to prompt, monitor, praise, and reward target behaviors, using the Home Behavior Record from the previous session (Handout 19).
- Agree to work with the child on creating a personal calendar.
- Agree to prompt, monitor, praise, and reward specified target behaviors between sessions, using the Home Behavior Record from this session.

■■■■■■■ MATERIALS NEEDED ■■■■■■■

For the parent:

 ■ Handout 19, Home Behavior Record

For you:

 ■ Stopwatch (to use in session and to give to child)
 ■ Therapist Form 5, Session Points and Notes
 ■ Therapist Form 17, My Personal Calendar: Crystal
 ■ Therapist Form 18, My Personal Calendar: Carl
 ■ Therapist Form 19, Time Detective Worksheet: In-Session Activities

For the child:

 ■ Child's DAR folder, binder, and backpack
 ■ Handout 28, Personal Calendar (two copies)

SESSION SUMMARY CHECKLIST FOR SESSION 10

Item	Item Completed
Review implementation of the behavior-monitoring and point program (with parent/child)	Yes/No
Conduct skills building with the child alone: Introduction to time management	
Conduct OST homework review: DAR, Assignment and Test Calendar, accordion binder, Check It Out, Ready to Go	Yes/No
Discuss clocks and calendars	Yes/No
Help the child develop a Personal Calendar (Handout 28)	Yes/No
Provide an introduction to time estimation	Yes/No
Conduct In-Session Practice: Being a Time Detective (Therapist Form 19)	Yes/No
Wrap up the session (with parent/child)	
Support the child in explaining the Personal Calendar (Handout 28) and the Time Detective Worksheet (Handout 29) to the parent	Yes/No
Review the Home Behavior Record (Handout 19)	Yes/No
Add new target behaviors to the DAR folder	Yes/No
Reward the child (Therapist Form 5)	Yes/No
Conclude the session (Handout 30)	Yes/No

- Handout 29, Time Detective Worksheet
- Handout 30, OTMP Checklist: Things to Remember for Session 11

ABOUT THIS SESSION

This session provides an introduction to the OTMP skills related to time management. In this and the next four sessions, the child will learn how to use clocks and calendars to organize tasks and activities, and to control the "Time Bandit." In this session, the child will work on creating a personal calendar and listing activities for a typical week. The child will also learn a new skill for estimating and recording how long activities take.

> **HELPFUL HINT:** As you begin to work with the child on time management, you should begin to consider whether it will be helpful to include a supplementary session to instruct the child in time telling. The skills related to time management will be performed more easily if the child is able to read both digital and analog clocks, and to tell how much time has passed from one clock reading to the next (e.g., how many minutes between 3:15 and 3:30, or, at a more difficult level, between 3:50 and 4:10). In this session, note how the child responds to the "Time Detective" work, and consider how the child performed on the suggested pretreatment assessment on time-telling skills. If you determine that instruction in telling time will be useful, it is best to add this lesson after Session 11. The child is likely to be more motivated to engage in this instruction after Sessions 10 and 11, which will help the child to see why time telling is relevant to many organizational tasks.

DETAILED SESSION CONTENT

Review Implementation of the Behavior-Monitoring and Point Program

Review the Home Behavior Record (Handout 19) with the parent, and discuss the child's performance of the OTMP behaviors between sessions.

- Discuss the behaviors that were observed, noting how frequently the child used the DAR, Assignment and Test Calendar, accordion binder, backpack checklist, and Ready to Go steps.
- Ask the parent how he prompted the behaviors.
- Review what rewards were used to reinforce the child's performance of the behaviors.
- Help the family manage any problems with implementation (e.g., problems with prompting, recording points, providing rewards, or implementing organizational routines).

Conduct Skills Building with the Child Alone: Introduction to Time Management

Begin by awarding the child session points (Therapist Form 5) and providing praise for good listening and discussion with the parent present.

Conduct OST Homework Review: DAR, Assignment and Test Calendar,
Accordion Binder, Check It Out, Ready to Go

Review the Home Behavior Record (Handout 19) and DAR from the last few days, and note whether the child is using routines to track assignments, manage papers and materials, and get workspaces Ready to Go. At this point in treatment, some of these behaviors have been faded from the list of behaviors reinforced on the DAR and Home Behavior Record. However, they should still be monitored and praised, and it is important for you to remain aware of how the child is using these routines at home and in school by checking on these behaviors in each session. If the child is not using these behaviors consistently, and as a result is experiencing problems completing tasks or managing materials, you should review the procedures with the child and parent, and consider adding the problematic behaviors to the list of behaviors to be rewarded on the DAR and Home Behavior Record.

Ask the child to discuss how the Ready to Go routine worked at home and school, since these steps are still relatively new, and provide clarification or problem solving if necessary. Provide session points (Therapist Form 5) for this review.

Discuss Clocks and Calendars

Tell the child:

> "So far, we've been working on learning tools and routines that help you keep track of your assignments and manage your papers and materials. For the next few meetings, we are going to talk about another organizational skill—time management. We will learn ways to keep the 'Time Bandit' under control, by helping you know your schedule, get things done on time, and have enough time to finish your tasks.
>
> "Today we will be talking about two tools that help us keep track of time—clocks and calendars. Clocks and calendars help us manage our schedules. They tell us what day and time school starts, or when our next soccer game is, or when our friend's birthday party is. They also tell us when to change activities. For instance, if it's 3:30 on a Monday [you should refer to the appropriate day and time of the week, corresponding to when the child is seen], you know that you have to stop what you are doing and get ready to leave, so you can meet with me. By using a clock, we can tell how long an activity has been going on and help us plan how much longer we have to complete the activity. For example, the clock in a basketball game tells us how much time is left to play, and by looking at the clock at school, you can figure out how much longer you have to finish a test. Calendars also help us know how much longer we have to do certain things—like how many days are left in our winter vacation. Some clocks tell us how much time has passed, so we know if we are fast or slow—like a stopwatch, which can tell a runner how quickly she finished a race. We will work with a stopwatch later today, and help you learn how to time activities, so you can start to figure out how much time you need to do certain things.
>
> "First, we will talk about how calendars can be used to keep track of your school assignments and other important activities. Calendars have been used for centuries. People created them because they needed to know when to plant and harvest their crops. We now use a Gregorian calendar, which was created in 1582. Calendars help us

plan many activities. Can you think of some activities that you might mark on a calendar?"

Help the child consider different uses for a calendar (keeping track of holidays and school vacations, knowing when assignments are due, knowing when a friend or family member's birthday is, knowing when big games or performances are coming up, etc.).

The child has already been using a calendar to keep track of school assignments—the Assignment and Test Calendar. Review briefly how this calendar has helped the child to keep track of long-term assignments and tests, and to prepare for due dates as they approach.

Help the Child Develop a Personal Calendar

Tell the child:

> "Calendars can be helpful for keeping track of other activities, in addition to school-related assignments. I know that you have a busy schedule every week—you have lots of different activities that occur on different days of the week. [Give examples from the child's life—e.g., soccer practice, piano lessons, band practice, OST sessions]. Let's look at two examples of other children's personal calendars. Each one lists the regular activities that make up the child's week."

Show the child Therapist Forms 17 and 18, pointing out how the personal calendar can help the child review his schedule for the week in one glance. Discuss why being able to keep track of the child's schedule can be useful: It can help him know what to expect on each day of the week and how to plan additional activities.

Tell the child that you will be working together to create a personal calendar, like these sample calendars, which lists the child's regular weekly schedule. Use one of the blank copies of Handout 28 to complete a rough draft of the child's personal calendar in session. Guide the child in completing this task, asking questions about each day of the week (e.g., "What do you have on Monday night? Do you have any activities on Thursdays after school? What days do you come to see me?") Reserve one blank copy to send home, so that the child can verify the schedule with the parent and create a final version.

Provide an Introduction to Time Estimation

Tell the child:

> "People who manage their time well have a good understanding of how long different activities take to complete. In order to know how much time you need to do homework, get dressed in the morning, or get ready for soccer practice, you need to be good at estimating (or guessing) how long it takes to actually do each of those tasks. We are going to teach you to be a good 'Time Detective,' by giving you practice in investigating how long it takes to do different activities. We will practice time estimation skills now, and you will also get some Time Detective homework. All of this will help you control the 'Time Bandit.' If you get better at knowing how much time you need to do your tasks, you'll be able to make sure you leave enough time to do your tasks, and you won't run out of time when you're trying to get something done."

Conduct In-Session Practice: Being a Time Detective

Give the child a stopwatch, and tell her that she can keep this stopwatch and use it for the Time Detective activities in session and at home. Show the child how to use the stopwatch, pointing out how to start the time running, how to stop, how to read the minutes and seconds displayed, and how to reset the time to 0 at the end of each practice round. Using Therapist Form 19, give the child an activity (e.g., throwing a ball back and forth 10 times) and ask her to estimate how long the activity will take. Record the child's estimate in the first column, next to the activity. Then tell the child to perform the activity and use the stopwatch to determine how long it actually takes to complete. Repeat this process with six to eight of the activities on Therapist Form 19, or with similar activities that the child wants to try. Try to make this activity fun, using some tasks that allow the child to get up and move around the room. Take turns using the stopwatch, and participate with the child. Give session points for completion of these practice exercises.

Now give the child the Time Detective Worksheet (Handout 29), and indicate that the child should practice these Time Detective skills more at home. The child should complete at least three activities from the handout each day, writing down an estimate of how long the activity will take to complete, and then using the stopwatch to find out and record the actual length of time for each activity.

Wrap Up the Session (with Parent/Child)

Support the Child in Explaining the Personal Calendar and Time Detective Worksheet to the Parent

Guide the child in explaining how a personal calendar is used, and have the child show the parent the personal calendar you created together in session. Give the child and parent a blank copy of the Personal Calendar (Handout 28), and ask the parent and child to work together to create a complete and accurate calendar at home and bring it to the next session. Next, ask the child to show the parent the Time Detective Worksheet (Handout 29) and describe how to estimate and then record the length of time each activity takes to complete. Describe how the child will be asked to use the Time Detective Worksheet daily to practice time estimation and recording skills.

Review the Home Behavior Record

Show the parent the Home Behavior Record (Handout 19), and review which behaviors the parent will prompt, monitor, praise, and reward. The following is a suggested list of behaviors that might be appropriate for the Home Behavior Record, though variations might make sense for some children. You have flexibility in deciding which behaviors need the most reinforcement, and can modify the home and school lists accordingly.

- *School behavior 1*: Turned in all assignments.
- *School behavior 2*: Got the desk Ready to Go.
- *Home behavior 1*: Had all materials for homework.
- *Home behavior 2*: Worked on Time Detective Worksheet.
- *Home behavior 3*: Conducted a Personal Calendar interview or review.

Add New Target Behaviors to the DAR Folder

The target behaviors for which the teacher will provide school points are these:

1. All assignments are turned in.
2. Got the desk Ready to Go.

Reward the Child

Review the Session Points and Notes (Therapist Form 5) with the child, and praise the child for the positive behaviors that earned points in the session. Add up the total points earned for this session, and indicate that the child may spend or save the points.

Conclude the Session

Confirm the next session appointment. Give the child and parent the OTMP Checklist for the next session (Handout 30). Remind the parent to bring the Home Behavior Record (Handout 19), and the child to bring the backpack, DAR folder, and binder, with all OTMP papers, to the next session. In addition, tell the child that he will be completing some of his assignments from school in the next session, as part of a practice exercise; thus the child should bring materials for that day's homework to session. If possible, the child should wait to complete at least part of that day's homework until the session time, so that you can work on some assignments in session.

Time Management
Time Tracking for Homework

You will:

- Review the home exercises for time management completed by parent and child.
- Help the child develop a proposed homework schedule.
- Teach the child how to keep track of the time taken to complete homework assignments.
- Make sure the teacher has received the Teacher's Guide to Time Management and the Time Tracker for In-Class Work, to be used in class (Teacher Forms 7 and 8).

The child will:

- Decide when homework can be fitted into the daily schedule.
- Learn how to keep track of the time taken to complete homework assignments, and practice with simulated assignments.

The parent will:

- Describe efforts to prompt, monitor, praise, and reward target behaviors, using the Home Behavior Record from the previous session (Handout 19).
- Agree to work with the child on completing the Time Tracker for Homework (Handout 32).
- Agree to prompt, monitor, praise, and reward specified target behaviors between sessions, using the Home Behavior Record from this session.

MATERIALS NEEDED

For the parent:

- Handout 19, Home Behavior Record

For you:

- Clocks (digital and analog)
- Grade-appropriate worksheets or tasks (two to three)
- Therapist Form 5, Session Points and Notes
- Handout 3, Guide to the Glitches
- Handout 10, Daily Assignment Record

SESSION SUMMARY CHECKLIST FOR SESSION 11

Item	Item Completed
Review implementation of the behavior-monitoring and point program (with parent/child)	
Review the Home Behavior Record	Yes/No
Review home exercises on time management	Yes/No
Conduct skills building with the child alone: Time tracking	
Conduct OST homework review: Tracking Assignments, Managing Materials, and Time Management	Yes/No
Discuss managing the Time Bandit	Yes/No
Help the child develop a Proposed Homework Schedule (Handout 31)	Yes/No
Provide an introduction to the Time Tracker for Homework (Handout 32)	Yes/No
Conduct in-session practice: Time Tracker for Homework	Yes/No
Wrap up the session (with parent/child)	
Support the child in explaining the Proposed Homework Schedule (Handout 31) and Time Tracker for Homework (Handout 32) to the parent	Yes/No
Review the Home Behavior Record (Handout 19)	Yes/No
Add new target behaviors to the DAR folder	Yes/No
Reward the child (Therapist Form 5)	Yes/No
Conclude the session (Handout 33)	Yes/No

For the child:

- Child's DAR folder, binder, and backpack
- Handout 31, Proposed Homework Schedule
- Handout 32, Time Tracker for Homework (two copies)
- Handout 33, OTMP Checklist: Things to Remember for Session 12

ABOUT THIS SESSION

This session extends the work in the previous session by focusing on the ways in which time management skills can prevent the Time Bandit from stealing the child's free time, especially when the child is completing homework. You will work with the child to create a proposed homework schedule, and to decide when homework should be fit into the daily schedule. In addition, the child will learn how to predict and then record how long each homework assignment takes to complete. This time-tracking skill will help the child with time planning, which will be addressed in Sessions 12–13.

You will begin this session by reviewing how effective the child was in working on the Time Detective activity. Based upon this review and your assessment of the child's ability to tell time using clocks, you may want to add a supplemental session devoted to instruction in telling time and calculating the passage of time in the next meeting (see Session 11a).

IN PREPARATION FOR THIS SESSION

In this session, the child will practice using the Time Tracker for Homework (Handout 32). To facilitate this practice, the child will need to complete some sample assignments—first estimating the time each assignment will take, and then noting how long it took to complete each assignment. If the child has remembered to bring in the actual homework that needs to be completed that day, you may select some assignments (or portions thereof) to use for this time-tracking exercise (see below). In case the child forgets the homework at home or the child's assignments are too complex to use for this exercise, you should have some sample assignments prepared for the child to complete. These assignments should be relatively brief (they should take no more than 5 minutes each to complete) and should be appropriate to the child's achievement level (i.e., not too difficult so as to be frustrating, and not too far below the child's ability level). You may obtain assignments by searching the Internet (e.g., *www. tlsbooks.com*, *www.jumpstart.com*), asking the child's teacher for some sample materials, or reviewing the child's typical assignments for ideas.

DETAILED SESSION CONTENT

Review Implementation of the Behavior-Monitoring and Point Program

Review the Home Behavior Record

Review the Home Behavior Record (Handout 19) with the parent, and discuss the child's performance of the OTMP behaviors between sessions.

- Discuss the behaviors that were observed.
- Ask the parent how she prompted the behaviors.
- Review what rewards were used to reinforce the child's performance of the behaviors.
- Help the family manage any problems with implementation (e.g., problems with prompting, recording points, providing rewards, or implementing organizational routines).

Review Home Exercises on Time Management

Ask the child to present the two handouts on time management that were assigned as home exercises: the Personal Calendar (Handout 28) and the Time Detective Worksheet (Handout 29). Praise the child, and provide session points for bringing these completed forms to session.

Ask the parent and child to confirm that the information on the Personal Calendar is accurate, and to indicate whether the schedule of activities listed is a consistent schedule for the child. Tell the parent that you will be working with the child to set a daily homework schedule, and ask whether there is any other information you should know before you do that. Ask the parent how long the child usually takes to complete homework each day. If the parent indicates that the amount of time spent on homework varies daily, ask the parent for a range, and for any information about whether homework takes longer on certain days of the week.

> **HELPFUL HINT:** You should make a copy of the child's completed Personal Calendar and keep it in the child's chart, as you will need to use it in future sessions on time planning.

Next, review the information recorded on the Time Detective Worksheet, asking the child to report how long some of the activities took. Ask the child whether he was surprised by the length of time needed for certain activities: Were there times when he over- or underestimated the amount of time needed to complete a task? Discuss, with the parent and child, whether the child often has an over- or underestimation bias. Does the child frequently think he will have plenty of time to complete homework, but then runs out of time because it takes longer than predicted? Alternatively, does the child often think he will need much more time than he actually does need to complete a task? Tell the parent and child that you will be using time estimation skills at homework time from this session onward, and that you and the child will work on developing those skills in the remainder of this session.

Conduct Skills Building with the Child Alone: Time Tracking

Begin by awarding the child session points (Therapist Form 5) and providing praise for good listening and discussion with the parent present.

Conduct OST Homework Review: Tracking Assignments, Managing Materials, and Time Management

At this point in treatment, the child has learned a number of organizational routines for tracking assignments, managing materials and papers, and getting work areas Ready to Go. You will not have time to review the child's performance of all these routines in detail at each session meeting. However, you should check in briefly at the start of each session with the child, to make note of certain essential signs of follow-through with the skills taught in the first part of treatment. For example, you should look at the DAR folder, note any problems with completion of the DAR or the Assignment and Test Calendar, and check that the teacher is providing daily points for target behaviors. You should also periodically glance into the child's backpack, checking for loose papers and making sure that papers are appropriately filed in the accordion binder. You can also occasionally ask the child whether the Ready to Go steps are still working well, and note whether the backpack checklist is showing any signs of wear.

Troubleshooting Note: Over the course of treatment, the child will learn many organizational skills and routines for the four OST modules (Tracking Assignments, Managing Materials, Time Management, and Planning). You, the parent, and the teacher will prompt, monitor, praise, and reward each skill as it is being acquired, and then move on to attend to new skills as treatment progresses. Although some children will continue to implement previously learned skills as new skills are targeted, others will have some drop-off in implementation of skills over time. For this reason, it is suggested that you check frequently to determine whether all of the organizational skills are being used appropriately. If the parent, teacher, or child reports that organizational problems have recurred in certain areas, the following steps should be taken:

1. Assess further to evaluate when and why these problems are occurring. Determine which skills are being used incompletely or inaccurately to cause the observed problems.
   Example: During the Time Management module, you learn that the child has started to leave homework-related materials in school. This problem could reflect improper use of one or more of the following: the DAR, binder, and backpack checklist. Review the child's use of each one; check the DAR for completeness, look to see whether papers are in the binder, and ask the child and parent whether the backpack checklist is being used.

2. Determine whether the child needs additional in-session practice to increase understanding of how to use the skills properly.
   Example: You discover that the child is checking off the materials needed on the DAR, but is not reviewing this list of materials during pack-up time at school. You decide that additional practice is needed in session, to help the child see how the DAR should be used to make sure that all materials are in the backpack.

3. Alternatively, if it becomes clear that the child knows how to use the skills but is forgetting to do so, or is not motivated to do so, you may decide to modify the Home Behavior Record by adding the problematic skills to the list of skills that the parent should prompt, monitor, praise, and reward. Use clinical judgment in deciding what needs to be reinforced to resolve the observed problems. It is possible that reinforcing performance of a specific skill is warranted (e.g., "Got desk Ready to Go"). Alternatively, you may choose to add a more general target to the Home Behavior Record, to increase the child's use of a set of skills (e.g., "Used skills for tracking assignments"). Finally, it is possible that rewarding an endpoint behavior (e.g., "Brought home all materials for homework") will be most helpful in motivating the child to perform the desired behavior.

Since a thorough review of the time management home exercises assigned at the end of Session 10 was conducted at the beginning of this session with the parent, you do not have to spend more time reviewing those exercises at this point.

Discuss Managing the Time Bandit

Tell the child:

> "Today we will talk more about how time and actions are connected. Everything we do takes time. You noticed this when you were being a Time Detective: Even the smallest activities take time. If you plan your time well, you should be able to get your tasks, like homework, done without wasting time, so you can have enough time left over for other things you like to do. The Time Bandit loves it when you use up your free time by goofing around or daydreaming when you're supposed to be working. Sometimes it seems like more fun to fiddle with a paper clip on your desk than to do your math assignment, or to daydream on the couch instead of cleaning your room. However, these distracting activities use up time, and your parents and teachers will still make you do your work or chores, even if this means that you have to miss watching your favorite TV show or playing outside with your friends."

At this point, show the child the description of the Time Bandit in the Guide to the Glitches (Handout 3), and review the ways in which the Time Bandit steals the child's free time by making sure that the child does not use time or plan a schedule appropriately. Tell the child that this session and the next few sessions will help the child learn to plan a schedule, so that the child can get work done and still have free time left to play and do things that the child enjoys.

Help the Child Develop a Proposed Homework Schedule

Tell the child:

> "Now that we have your Personal Calendar completed, we can see what activities you have each day after school. Let's talk a little about the homework you have to do each day, so we can understand what you need to be spending your time on each afternoon and evening."

Ask the child some questions to get a sense of the time demands of homework on a typical school day:"

> "What is your typical homework each day? We should have a good sense of that now, after reviewing the DAR for all of these weeks."
> "Do you have some assignments that are due each day and some that are due at the end of the week?"
> "Are there certain days of the week when you know you have to spend more time on homework [e.g., on Thursday nights, if there are weekly assignments that are due on Friday]?"
> "How long does your homework usually take to complete?" [You can refer to the parent's response to this question, which you noted at the beginning of the session, and ask the child whether this time estimate makes sense.]

Use Handout 31 (Proposed Homework Schedule) to help the child determine when to complete homework in the daily schedule. Ask the child to look at each day of the week on the Personal Calendar, and see when the child gets home from school, what activities are scheduled on that day and at what time, and when the child must go to bed. Then, with the information you have collected on how long homework should take each day, help the child decide when homework can be fitted into this schedule. For example, if the child gets home from school at 3:00, has karate from 4:30 to 5:30, has to be in bed by 8:00, and needs to spend approximately 45 minutes on homework, you might decide to schedule homework time from 3:15 to 4:00 on that day. Fill in the weekly calendar on Handout 31 to create a proposed homework schedule, which the child will discuss with the parent at the end of the session.

> **HELPFUL HINT:** Fill out the Proposed Homework Schedule in pencil, as it may need to be revised, based on the parent's input. Keep a copy of Handout 31 in the child's chart, as you will review it in Session 12 and may need to modify it further after the child has used it between sessions.

Provide an Introduction to the Time Tracker for Homework

Tell the child:

> "Last time, you learned how to be a Time Detective, using a stopwatch to figure out how long different activities took to complete. You can also use a regular clock to keep track of how much time is passing while you work on something. We just talked about how long your homework usually takes, and we are going to test out a new schedule for fitting homework into your daily schedule. While you are doing your homework each day, I also want you to start paying attention to how long each individual assignment takes to complete. You will use your time detective skills to guess how long each assignment is going to take, and then you will use the clock to see how long it actually takes to complete."

Show the child the Time Tracker for Homework (Handout 32), and highlight the steps that the child should take before starting an assignment. First, the child should think about how long the assignment (e.g., a math worksheet) should take to complete. Then the child will write down when she plans to begin the assignment and when she plans to finish it, using that estimate. When the child actually begins working on the assignment, she should write down the time, and then should write down the time when she has completed the assignment. Finally, the parent will check to see whether the assignment is complete. If it is not, the parent or child should write down how much more time was needed to finish the assignment appropriately.

Tell the child:

> "If you use this Time Tracker, you will be able to gather some important information about how you use your time when you are doing homework. You will learn whether you tend to over- or underestimate how much time you need to do certain assignments. Some children tend to overestimate how much time they need. For example, they might fear that studying for a math test will take an hour, and be surprised when it only takes 30 minutes. Other children tend to underestimate how much time they need. For example,

they might believe that completing a spelling worksheet will only take 10 minutes, and find that they need to spend 25 minutes to complete it appropriately. We want to help you get better at estimating how long your work will take, so you can make sure that you schedule just the right amount of time to do your work. You can ask your parent to help you fill in this Time Tracker at first, especially with using the clock. Let's practice it now in session, so you can get comfortable with using it."

Conduct In-Session Practice: Time Tracker for Homework

If the child has remembered to bring in homework assignments, ask the child to take out the DAR folder and review the assignments for the day. You will only have approximately 15 minutes for this practice exercise, so try to select assignments that can be completed in a shorter period of time. If necessary, you may decide to work with a portion of an assignment (e.g., half a page of math problems, sentences for 5 out of 10 spelling words).

If the child does not have homework assignments for the day, or has forgotten to bring in the relevant materials, you may conduct this practice with sample assignments. Give the child a copy of the DAR (Handout 10), listing three assignments for homework that are similar to the child's typical assignments in three subject areas (e.g., write sentences with six spelling words; complete math worksheet; read a paragraph in the social studies textbook and answer five questions). Once you have selected the assignments that will be used for this practice, take out the materials for each of the assignments, and ask the child to go through the five steps on the Time Tracker for Homework for each of the three subjects:

- *Step 1*: Think about the amount of homework that you have.
- *Step 2*: Think about how much time you think each assignment will take.
- *Step 3*: Write down the time that you think you will start, and then the time that you think you will finish.
- *Step 4*: When you start each assignment, write down the time.
- *Step 5*: When you are finished with each assignment, write down the time.

Guide the child through this process, providing any help necessary with reading the clock and writing down the time. The child should go through this exercise as if he is actually doing homework—completing the first column on the Time Tracker first, while working on the first assignment; then moving on to the second assignment; and finally doing the third. You should act as the parent for this exercise, reviewing the child's completed assignments and noting whether they are complete or need more work. If the child does need to work additionally on any assignments, help her keep track of how much more time she needs to complete the work. Provide praise and session points for engaging in this practice exercise.

HELPFUL HINT: The child will actually need to complete each assignment, in order to complete the Time Tracker fully. Therefore, make sure that the assignments are relatively short and simple, so that this exercise does not take too much time and is not frustrating to the child. If there is not enough time to complete three assignments for this practice, you may use two. The goal of this practice is to have the child understand how to use the Time Tracker by exercising time estimation and calculation skills.

Wrap Up the Session (with Parent/Child)

Support the Child in Explaining the Proposed Homework Schedule and Time Tracker for Homework to the Parent

Ask the child to share the Proposed Homework Schedule (Handout 31) with the parent, and ask the parent whether this schedule makes sense. If the parent has any concerns about the schedule, modify the suggested times for each day as appropriate. Save a copy of the final schedule in the child's chart, and give a copy to the child to keep in the OTMP folder.

Next, show the parent the Time Tracker for Homework (Handout 32) that the child completed in session, and guide the child in explaining how this form will be used at homework time. Give the child a blank Time Tracker for Homework to keep in the OTMP folder and complete at home. Summarize what you would like the parent to do each night, to support the child's time management efforts at homework time:

- The child will review the assignments listed on the DAR with the parent or other responsible adult.
- The child will check the Proposed Homework Schedule and decide whether that schedule makes sense for that day.
- The child will complete the Time Tracker for Homework, with the parent's help, as he works on each homework assignment. The parent will provide feedback on the completeness of each assignment.
- The parent will praise the child for completing each step.

Tell the parent and child that the child will be completing a Time Tracker for In-Class Work (Teacher Form 8) with the teacher, for a selected in-class assignment. You may give the child a copy of the Time Tracker for In-Class Work to keep in the OTMP folder of the binder, so that it is available for use in school. The teacher should also have received a copy of this form.

Review the Home Behavior Record

Show the parent the Home Behavior Record (Handout 19), and review which behaviors the parent will prompt, monitor, praise, and reward. The following is a suggested list of behaviors that might be appropriate for the Home Behavior Record, though variations might make sense for some children.

- *School behavior 1*: Got the desk Ready to Go.
- *School behavior 2*: Completed the Time Tracker for In-Class Work for an in-class assignment.
- *Home behavior 1*: Had all materials for homework.
- *Home behavior 2*: Used the Proposed Homework Schedule.
- *Home behavior 3*: Completed the Time Tracker for Homework.

Add New Target Behaviors to the DAR Folder

The target behaviors for which the teacher will provide school points are these:

1. Got the desk Ready to Go
2. Completed the Time Tracker for In-Class Work for an in-class assignment.

Reward the Child

Review the Session Points and Notes (Therapist Form 5) with the child, and praise the child for the positive behaviors that earned points in the session. Add up the total points earned for this session, and indicate that the child may spend or save the points.

Conclude the Session

Confirm the next session appointment. Give the child and parent the OTMP Checklist for the next session (Handout 33). Remind the parent to bring the Home Behavior Record (Handout 19), and the child to bring the backpack, DAR folder, and binder, with all OTMP papers, to the next session.

Time Management

Instruction in Telling Time
and Calculating the Passage of Time

GOALS FOR THE SESSION

You will:

- Review the home exercises for time management completed by parent and child.
- Teach the child how to tell time on analog and digital clocks.
- Teach the child how to calculate the passage of time.

The child will:

- Practice telling time on analog and digital clocks.
- Practice calculating the passage of time.

The parent will:

- Describe efforts to prompt, monitor, praise, and reward target behaviors, using the Home Behavior Record from the previous session (Handout 19).
- Agree to work with the child on copies of handouts for calculating the passage of time (Handout 33a) and telling time (Handout 33b).
- Agree to prompt, monitor, praise, and reward specified target behaviors between sessions, using the Home Behavior Record from this session.

▬▬▬▬▬▬▬▬▬▬▬▬▬▬ **MATERIALS NEEDED** ▬▬▬▬▬▬▬▬▬▬▬▬▬

For the parent:

- Handout 19, Home Behavior Record

For you:

- Analog clock with movable hands
- Therapist Form 5, Session Points and Notes

For the child:

- Child's DAR folder, binder, and backpack
- Handout 32, Time Tracker for Homework
- Handout 33, OTMP Checklist: Things to Remember for Session 12
- Handout 33a, How Much Time Has Passed? (two copies)
- Handout 33b, Practice with Telling Time

SESSION SUMMARY CHECKLIST FOR SESSION 11A

Item	Item Completed
Review implementation of the behavior-monitoring and point program (with parent/child)	
Review the Home Behavior Record	Yes/No
Review home exercises on time management	Yes/No
Conduct skills building with the child alone: Time telling	
Help the child learn to tell time on an analog clock	Yes/No
Help the child learn to tell time on a digital clock	Yes/No
Help the child learn to calculate the passage of time (Handout 34A)	Yes/No
Wrap up the session (with parent/child)	
Support the child in explaining the lessons learned for telling time	Yes/No
Review homework in time telling (Handouts 33a and 33b) and time management (Handout 32)	Yes/No
Review the Home Behavior Record (Handout 19)	Yes/No
Add new target behaviors to the DAR folder	Yes/No
Reward the child (Therapist Form 5)	Yes/No
Conclude the session	Yes/No

ABOUT THIS SESSION

This session may be conducted with children who need additional instruction in telling time and calculating the passage of time. If you decide, after reviewing the child's performance on the time management exercises in Sessions 10 and 11, that the child needs extra instruction and practice in using clocks, this supplemental session may be inserted between Sessions 11 and 12. The purpose of this session is to help the child become more comfortable with (1) using analog and digital clocks to tell time, and (2) calculating how much time has passed between one time shown on a clock and another time. Improved proficiency in these two skills will help the child benefit more from the skills-building exercises used for time management in the next sessions.

The materials provided in this supplemental session can be used flexibly and adapted to each child's level of understanding. Although this brief instruction in time telling is certainly not comprehensive, it is intended to provide targeted practice with key time-telling skills that the child will need to use for time management taught in future sessions.

IN PREPARATION FOR THIS SESSION

In order to show the child how to tell time on analog clocks, it is best to use an analog clock or model that can be manipulated, with hour and minute hands that move. You may obtain a model clock from a teacher supply store, or use any type of clock that allows you to move the hands to display various times.

DETAILED SESSION CONTENT

Review Implementation of the Behavior-Monitoring and Point Program

Review the Home Behavior Record

Review the Home Behavior Record (Handout 19) with the parent, and discuss the child's performance of the OTMP behaviors between sessions.

- Discuss the behaviors that were observed.
- Ask the parent how he prompted the behaviors.
- Review what rewards were used to reinforce the child's performance of the behaviors.
- Help the family manage any problems with implementation (e.g., problems with prompting, recording points, providing rewards, or implementing organizational routines).

Review Home Exercises on Time Management

Review the child and parent's completion of the Time Tracker for Homework (Handout 32), gathering information on how the child currently uses time for homework. Ask the parent and child whether the Proposed Homework Schedule (Handout 31) worked well, or whether it needs to be modified.

Tell the parent and child that you will be working on time telling in this session, so that the child will be more comfortable with using clocks to tell time and calculate the passage of time. This will help the child complete the Time Tracker for Homework and other time management worksheets that will be used in future sessions.

Conduct Skills Building with the Child Alone: Time Telling

Begin by awarding the child session points (Therapist Form 5) and providing praise for good listening and discussion with the parent present. Tell the child that you will be reviewing how to tell time, focusing on using an analog clock and reading the hours and minutes for different times. The session will combine instruction in different components of time telling and guided practice with each of the components. You may modify the content as appropriate to the child's understanding of the topics covered. If the child knows specific concepts (e.g., what the hour and minute hands on a clock represent), do not got into detailed instruction on those concepts; instead, ask the child to tell you what he knows, and supplement the child's knowledge as necessary.

Help the Child Learn to Tell Time on an Analog Clock

INSTRUCTION: HOUR HAND

Show the child a model analog clock, and point out the short and long hands. Ask the child to tell you what each hand represents, or, if the child does not know or remember this information, point out that the shorter hand indicates the hour and the longer hand indicate the minutes. Show the child how 12 hours are represented on the clock, moving the hour hand from 1 to 12 and telling what time each hour represents (e.g., "When the small hand—the hour hand—is on the 1, it is 1 o'clock," etc.). Tell the child that the 12 hours can indicate a time in the A.M. or P.M., and review what the different times represent (e.g., "12 o'clock noon is the middle of the day, around lunchtime; 6 o'clock P.M. is the evening, when you eat dinner; 12 o'clock midnight is the middle of the night; 6 o'clock A.M. is when the sun comes up," etc.). This will help the child think about time in a more concrete way.

GUIDED PRACTICE: READING THE HOURS

Ask the child to help you tell the time, leaving the minute hand on the 12 and moving the hour hand to five or six different positions (e.g., 12:00, 2:00, 4:00, 5:00, 7:00, 11:00). Remind the child that when the minute hand stays at the 12, the number at the hour hand tells us the time. Praise the child, and provide session points for completing this exercise.

INSTRUCTION: MINUTE HAND

Next, use the model analog clock to show the child how the minute hand works and how to "read" it. Indicate that the minute hand shows how many minutes have passed since the start of an hour. Ask the child how many minutes are in an hour, and point out that there are small marks on the clock for 60 minutes in every hour. When 1 minute passes, it is 1 minute past the hour (and we say the hour, followed by "01"); when 5 minutes pass, it is 5 minutes past hour (and we say the hour, followed by "05"); and so on. Point out that the numbers on the clock show the hours of the day as reviewed above, but they also represent 5-minute segments past each hour. Count by fives with the child, pointing at each of the numbers on the clock, to show how the numbers represent 5, 10, 15 (etc.) minutes past the hour. Tell the child: "When the long hand—the minute hand—is at the 1, it is 5 minutes past the hour. When the long hand, the minute hand, is at the 2, it is 10 minutes past the hour." Continue with 3 through 11, and then indicate that at 12 the time moves to the next hour, and we start over again.

GUIDED PRACTICE: READING THE MINUTES

Select five or six times on the clock, leaving the hour hand in the same position and moving the minute hand around the clock. Ask the child to tell you what time it is, guiding the child to count by 5's if she is not sure how many minutes a given number represents. If the child makes an error, correct it, and repeat that example again, asking the child to tell you the correct time. Praise the child, and provide session points for completing this exercise.

INSTRUCTION: COMBINING HOURS AND MINUTES TO TELL TIME

Now help the child put these pieces together by showing five times on the model clock and describing how the time is told for each example. For example, for 1:15, explain: "The hour hand is on 1, and the minute hand is on 3; the hour is 1, and the minute hand is [count out loud, while pointing to 1, 2, and 3] 5, 10, 15 minutes after the hour. So the time is 1:15, or 15 minutes after 1."

Make sure to show the child times where the minute hand is on both sides of the 6, so you have a variety of times that include small and large numbers after the hour. Include a few examples for times in the 12 o'clock hour, as children often confuse times for this hour.

GUIDED PRACTICE: COMBINING HOURS AND MINUTES TO TELL TIME

Show the child five or six examples of times from both sides of the 6, changing both the hour and minute hands. Ask the child to tell the time on the clock for each example. Help the child correct any errors, using the strategies taught above. Praise the child, and provide session points for completing this exercise.

HELP THE CHILD LEARN TO TELL TIME ON A DIGITAL CLOCK

Children are likely to be more comfortable with telling time on a digital clock, since the process is far simpler, and digital clocks are more widely prevalent nowadays than analog clocks. However, a brief review of how to "read" time on a digital clock can be useful. For this review, you may simply write down different times on a sheet of paper, and discuss the essential elements of telling time in this format. Show the child the numbers to the left of the two dots and to the right of the two dots. Ask the child what each number represents; the numbers on the left show the hours and the numbers on the right show the minutes. Show a few examples of times at the hours (e.g., 12:00, 2:00, 5:00), and ask the child to tell you what times are shown. Then show a few examples of times with different minutes shown, at 5-minute intervals (e.g., 3:05, 3:15, 3:40), and ask the child to read the times shown. Finally, show a few examples of different times in digital format, with hours and minutes varied, and ask the child to read each example. Help the child self-correct any errors. Praise the child, and provide session points for completing this exercise.

Help the Child Learn to Calculate the Passage of Time

The final part of this instruction focuses on teaching the child how to determine how much time has passed between one time on the clock and another time. For this instruction, you will have the child read two times on an analog clock and translate the time into digital format. You will then teach the child how to subtract the start time from the end time, to determine how much time has passed.

Tell the child:

"Now that we've reviewed how to tell time on the clock, we need to think about how we can figure out how much time has passed from one point to another. We need to do this a lot in our daily lives. In the last two sessions, we've been talking about being a Time Detective and estimating how much time different activities should take. You've also started using the Time Tracker to help you keep track of how much time each homework assignment takes you to complete. This is all important information that can help you manage your time, but you can only figure out this information if you know how to calculate how much time has passed. Your parents can help you with this, of course, but I want to help you learn how to do this too, so you'll be more comfortable with calculating the passage of time.

"Let's look at an example together. [Take out Handout 33a.] I'm going to draw the big and small hands in on this first clock, to show when you finished your homework [5:35] and when you started your homework [5:05]. Now let's figure out together, how much time it took you to do your homework. Let's look at the end time: The hour hand is on the 5 and the minute hand is on the 7, so it's 5, 10, 15, 20, 25, 30, 35 minutes past the hour; it's 5:35. For the start time, the hour hand is on the 5, and the minute hand is on the 1, so it's 5 minutes past the hour, or 5:05. Let's write these numbers down on the blank lines in the last column. We'll put the end time on top and the start time underneath, so that we can subtract the start time from the end time. To subtract one time from another, I am going to ignore the hours and subtract the minutes. How much is 35 − 5? Yes, it is 30. So that means that 30 minutes have passed between these two times; homework took 30 minutes to complete.

"We can also figure this out by looking at the clock and counting by 5's. We started at 5:05 [using the model clock, point to the 1] and ended at 5:35 [point to the 7]. Let's count by 5's, from the 1 to the 7. [Point to each number and count out loud: 5, 10, 15, 20, 25, 30]. So it took 30 minutes to do homework."

Ask the child whether she has any questions, and review the example again as needed. Praise the child, and provide session points for listening to this explanation.

Next, guide the child in completing the calculations for six other examples, using Handout 33a. For each example, draw the hour and minute hands for the start and end times. Then ask the child to read the start and end times, write them in on the appropriate lines, and subtract the minutes to find out how much time has passed.

HELPFUL HINT: This brief instruction in calculating the passage of time is certainly not comprehensive, but it is intended to provide the child with some basic skills for calculating how much time has passed. The examples used focus on calculating the passage of time within 1 hour, so that the hour value does not change. Subtracting time with different hours can be more complicated, and may require more instruction than can be provided in one session. However, we hope that the basic instruction provided here will give the child a starting point for calculating the passage of time. The parent can be instructed to help the child extend these basic skills—showing the child, for example, how to count by 5's on the clock to figure out more complicated problems (e.g., determining how much time has passed from 5:45 to 6:10). If a child does not fully grasp even the basic instruction on calculating the passage of time, parents should be encouraged to help the child determine how much time has passed, especially for the purposes of completing the Time Tracker for Homework (Handout 32).

Wrap Up the Session (with Parent/Child)

Support the Child in Explaining the Lessons Learned for Telling Time

Ask the child to tell the parent what he has learned about telling time on an analog and digital clock. Show the parent the model clock; ask the child to tell the parent the name for each of the hands, and to read a few times on the clock, as you move the hour and minute hands to different positions. Then show the parent the time passage calculation problems that the child completed on Handout 33a, and ask the child to describe the steps for figuring out how much time has passed in those examples. Praise the child, and provide session points for this review.

Review Homework in Time Telling and Time Management

Tell the parent that the child will have to keep practicing these time-telling skills at home, in order to become more confident in telling time and calculating the passage of time. Show the child and parent Handouts 33a and 33b, and ask them to spend 10–15 minutes each day completing copies of these handouts on telling time and calculating the passage of time. The child will receive points on the Home Behavior Record for completing this at-home practice.

Indicate that the parent should also continue supporting the child in using the Time Tracker for Homework (Handout 32) each day, using the same procedures that were reviewed in the previous session:

- The child will review the assignments listed on the DAR with the parent or other responsible adult.
- The child will check the homework schedule and decide if that schedule makes sense for that day.
- The child will complete the Time Tracker for Homework, with the parent's help, for each homework assignment. The parent will provide feedback on the completeness of each assignment.
- The parent will praise the child for completing each step.

Review the Home Behavior Record

Show the parent the Home Behavior Record (Handout 19), and review which behaviors the parent will prompt, monitor, praise, and reward. The following is a suggested list of behaviors that might be appropriate for the Home Behavior Record, though variations might make sense for some children.

- *School behavior 1*: Got the desk Ready to Go.
- *School behavior 2*: Completed the Time Tracker for In-Class Work for an in-class assignment.
- *Home behavior 1*: Had all materials for homework.
- *Home behavior 2*: Completed copies of Handouts 33a and 33b.
- *Home behavior 3*: Completed the Time Tracker for Homework.

Add New Target Behaviors to the DAR Folder

The target behaviors for which the teacher will provide school points are these:

1. Got the desk Ready to Go.
2. Completed the Time Tracker for In-Class Work for an in-class assignment.

Reward the Child

Review the Session Points and Notes (Therapist Form 5) with the child, and praise the child for the positive behaviors that earned points in the session. Add up the total points earned for this session, and indicate that the child may spend or save the points.

Conclude the Session

Confirm the next session appointment. Remind the child and parent to review the items on the OTMP Checklist for the next session (Handout 33). Remind the parent to bring the Home Behavior Record (Handout 19), and the child to bring the backpack, DAR folder, and binder, with all OTMP papers, to the next session.

SESSION 12

Time Management
Time-Planning Conferences at Home and School

You will:

- Review the home exercises for time management completed by parent and child.
- Help the child finalize a daily homework schedule.
- Teach the child how to use a Time-Planning Conference to improve time management.

The child will:

- Discuss the time taken to complete homework assignments (using the completed Time Tracker for Homework, Handout 32)
- Practice using the Time-Planning Conference (Handout 34) to manage time spent on homework and activities

The parent will:

- Describe efforts to prompt, monitor, praise and reward target behaviors, using the Home Behavior Record from the previous session (Handout 19).
- Agree to work with the child on completing a daily Time-Planning Conference (Handout 34).
- Agree to prompt, monitor, praise, and reward specified target behaviors between sessions, using the Home Behavior Record from this session.

MATERIALS NEEDED

For the parent:

- Handout 19, Home Behavior Record

162

For you:

- Clock (digital or analog)
- Grade-appropriate worksheets or tasks
- Therapist Form 5, Session Points and Notes
- Handout 10, Daily Assignment Record
- Therapist Form 20, Review of the Time Tracker for Homework
- Therapist Form 21 (Optional), Time Planning for Adventures

For the child:

- Child's DAR folder, binder, and backpack
- Handout 32, Time Tracker for Homework (two copies)
- Handout 34, Time Planning Conference (two copies)
- Handout 35, Guide to the Time-Planning Conference
- Handout 36, OTMP Checklist: Things to Remember for Session 13

SESSION SUMMARY CHECKLIST FOR SESSION 12

Item	Item Completed
Review implementation of the behavior-monitoring and point program (with parent/child)	
Review the Home Behavior Record	Yes/No
Review home exercises on time management	Yes/No
Conduct skills building with the child alone: Time planning	
Conduct OST homework review: Review of the Time Tracker for Homework (Therapist Form 20)	Yes/No
Provide an introduction to the Time-Planning Conference (Handout 34)	Yes/No
Conduct in-session practice: Time-Planning Conference	Yes/No
Optional: Conduct practice in Time Planning for Adventures (Therapist Form 21)	Yes/No
Wrap up the session (with parent/child)	
Support the child in explaining the Time-Planning Conference to the parent	Yes/No
Review the Home Behavior Record (Handout 19)	Yes/No
Add new target behaviors to the DAR folder	Yes/No
Reward the child (Therapist Form 5)	Yes/No
Conclude the session (Handout 36)	Yes/No

ABOUT THIS SESSION

In this session, the child will learn new skills to control the Time Bandit, focusing on the use of the Time-Planning Conference to manage time spent on homework and other activities. A review of the completed Time Tracker for Homework will inform the creation of a finalized homework schedule. You will then introduce the notion of time planning, emphasizing to the child that planning her time can help her maximize "free" time. Numerous in-session practices with time planning will help the child see how this routine can be fitted into the daily schedule.

IN PREPARATION FOR THIS SESSION

You will need to prepare three simulated DARs (Handout 10) with three practice assignments noted on each (e.g., "Science: 'Caring for the Earth' worksheet; Social Studies: Label a map of the 13 colonies; Math: Worksheet on multiplication"). You should also prepare simulated materials to go with each of the practice assignments, so that the child can judge how long each assignment should take to complete. The child will actually have to complete one of the worksheets in session; thus you should make sure that these assignments are appropriate for the child's achievement level.

DETAILED SESSION CONTENT

Review Implementation of the Behavior-Monitoring and Point Program

Review the Home Behavior Record

Review the Home Behavior Record (Handout 19) with the parent, and discuss the child's performance of the OTMP behaviors between sessions.

- Discuss the behaviors that were observed.
- Ask the parent how he prompted the behaviors.
- Review what rewards were used to reinforce the child's performance of the behaviors.
- Help the family manage any problems with implementation (e.g., problems with prompting, recording points, providing rewards, or implementing organizational routines).

Review Home Exercises on Time Management

If this session follows the supplemental session on time-telling instruction (Session 11a), you will review the child's completion of the time-telling home exercises, and will determine to what extent the child will need continued support with the time telling necessary for time management. If the child is still struggling with the time-telling exercises, you may decide, with the parent, that the child should continue practicing with these types of exercises. In addition, you may need to inform the parent that she will have to assist the child in completing the time tracking that will be necessary in the home exercises related to time management. Also indicate that the parent may need to provide reminders when a child is completing tasks (e.g., homework) for which there is a time deadline.

For all children, you will review the child and parent's completion of the Time Tracker for Homework (Handout 32), gathering information on how the child currently uses time for homework. Ask the parent and child whether the Proposed Homework Schedule (Handout 31) worked well, or whether it needs to be modified.

Conduct Skills Building with the Child Alone: Time Planning

Begin by awarding the child session points (Therapist Form 5) and providing praise for good listening and discussion with the parent present.

Conduct OST Homework Review: Review of the Time Tracker for Homework

Ask the child to take out the Time Tracker for Homework, and award session points for bringing this handout to the meeting. Using Therapist Form 20, review the information recorded on the Time Tracker for Homework, noting the average amount of time needed for homework and any factors that caused variations in homework time (e.g., certain assignments were given only on specific days of the week and required more time; the child took longer to complete homework on days when he started homework later and was tired; homework in certain subjects took longer, because the child dislikes those subjects). Discuss whether the child typically under- or overestimates the time needed for homework.

Finally, determine how long homework should take on each day of the week, and decide upon a finalized homework schedule, taking all of the accumulated information into account. You may revise the times recorded on the Proposed Homework Schedule (Handout 31) completed in Session 11, if necessary. Remind the child that using this schedule will help to ensure that homework is completed as efficiently as possible. When the child uses time efficiently, the Time Bandit cannot steal the child's free time as easily. Thus the child will have more time to do what she wants to do each day, if she plans and follows an appropriate homework schedule.

Provide an Introduction to the Time-Planning Conference

Tell the child:

> "Now you have a schedule that should help you get homework done efficiently each day. This is a great first step toward defeating the Time Bandit. I want to teach you another routine that you can do each day with your parents after school, which will help you really keep the Time Bandit under control. This new routine is called a Time-Planning Conference, and it's a way for you and your parent to discuss how you will spend your time each day. Remember that we all have only a limited number of hours in the day, so we need to make sure we use them wisely. If we're not careful, we might not get things like homework finished quickly enough, and we might not have enough time for other activities, like playing. A Time-Planning Conference will help you know what you *need* to spend your time on each day (things like homework, after-school activities, and lessons), so you can figure out when to fit those activities into your schedule. If you use the Time-Planning Conference to make sure you fit in the things you need to do, you will have time left over to do the things you want to do each day. Let me show you how the Time-Planning Conference works. We can practice using time planning with some pretend assignments."

Conduct In-Session Practice: Time-Planning Conference

Show the child Handout 34, the Time-Planning Conference Guide. Use a sample DAR (see "In Preparation for this Session," above) and the child's own Personal Calendar to illustrate how the worksheet is used to guide a time planning discussion. For example, you may engage in the following discussion, as you go through the steps on the form, referring to a sample DAR (Handout 10) and the child's Personal Calendar:

- *Step 1*: "Let's look at the DAR to see what homework you have tonight."
- *Step 2*: [Ask the child to report what needs to be done.] "You have to study for a spelling test, do a math worksheet, and read for 20 minutes."
- *Step 3*: "Let's check your Personal Calendar. Do you have any activities on Monday? Yes, you have a piano lesson from 5:00 to 6:00 tonight."
- *Step 4*: "You have to eat dinner at 6:00, and have to be in bed by 8:30."
- *Step 5*: "What do you want to do for fun tonight? Ok, you want to have 30 minutes to play on your Nintendo DS tonight."
- *Step 6*: [Ask the child for time estimates for each of the assignments. The child will need to see the materials to make these estimations.] "You think that it should take about 15 minutes to study the 15 words on the spelling list, 20 minutes to do your math worksheet, and 20 minutes to read. So you need about 55 minutes to do all of your homework."
- *Step 7*: [Ask the child when to fit in homework, given this information. Take a look at the Homework Schedule and see whether the proposed time period on the schedule makes sense.] "You will do your homework from 4:00 to 5:00. That way, you can take a break and relax when you get home. If you follow this schedule, you should have plenty of time to play on the DS after dinner."

As you go through the steps in this discussion, fill in the appropriate boxes on the Time-Planning Conference handout, so the child sees how to engage in this process. Start in the second column, under Monday, and go down the rows as you complete each step. Put a check mark next to each of the first four steps, to indicate that you and the child have considered each of those sources of information. You do not need to make notes in those boxes, as the information is already written down in the original sources (the DAR, the Assignment and Test Calendar, and the Personal Calendar). In the fifth row, you can jot down the child's desired leisure activity. In the sixth row, you can write in the time estimates for homework, and in the final row, note when the child will fit in homework that day.

> **HELPFUL HINT:** You may decide that it makes most sense for you to write the information on the Time-Planning Conference handout, as the child discusses each point with you, instead of having the child do the writing. You do not want to overwhelm the child with excessive writing demands; the goal of the conference is for the child and adult to have a discussion about how to plan the child's time. The goal of using the Time-Planning Conference is to get the child comfortable with approaching homework carefully and with an understanding of time requirements. Expecting the child to write out responses may interfere with the child's acceptance of this routine.

Practice using the Time-Planning Conference two more times, following the same steps for two more sets of assignments on the sample DARs. Continue filling in Handout 34, selecting different days of the week, and checking the Personal Calendar for each of those days to provide realistic practice. Praise the child for engaging in the time-planning steps, and provide session points for each practice.

At the end of the final practice Time-Planning Conference, tell the child that she will continue to use the Time Tracker for Homework (Handout 32) at home, so that she can keep track of how long each assignment actually takes to complete. Therefore, if time allows, you will practice using the Time Tracker again in this session for one of the assignments on the final practice list of assignments. Select a worksheet or other simple task, and tell the child to write down the estimated start and end time on the Time Tracker, and then to begin working on that task. When the child is done, write down the actual beginning and ending time for the task, and compare to the original estimate.

After the child has concluded these practice rounds, review the Guide to the Time-Planning Conference (Handout 35) together, and summarize the steps in using the Time-Planning Conference. The child should understand, at a conceptual level, that time planning involves (1) looking at the assignment list for the day; (2) looking at the weekly calendar of activities; (3) understanding what needs to be done that day and when; (4) estimating how long homework will take; and (5) deciding how to fit homework into the schedule for the day. Praise the child and provide session points for describing each of these steps.

Optional: Conduct Practice in Time Planning for Adventures

If time permits, you may use the optional materials on Time Planning for Adventures (Therapist Form 21) to engage in extended practice with time planning. You may select one or more of the adventures described in the optional materials, and ask the child to review the description of the adventure(s), discuss what special tasks must be completed today, estimate how long those tasks will take, determine what other activities must be done, and decide when the child would fit in work on the special tasks. This extended practice should be fun for the child, and should reinforce the idea that the steps in time planning can be useful in many situations.

Wrap Up the Session (with Parent/Child)

Support the Child in Explaining the Time-Planning Conference to the Parent

Ask the child to show the parent the Time-Planning Conference (Handout 34) and to review the steps for conducting the conference each day, after school. The child may use the Guide to the Time-Planning Conference (Handout 35) to facilitate this review. Ask the child to show the parent a sample Time-Planning Conference handout that was completed in session, with practice assignments, and to point out how each step was completed.

Tell the parent and child that they should conduct a Time-Planning Conference each day, when the child gets home from school. Point out that, while the child now has the tools to plan her time appropriately, she will only learn to use these tools on a regular basis if she practices them every day, while considering her actual homework assignments and schedule of activities. Thus this at-home practice is a vital part of the child's development of improved time management skills. The parent and child should also continue to use the Time Tracker for Homework (Handout 32) to help the child estimate and track the time needed to complete assignments.

HELPFUL HINT: Some children do not see a parent right after school, as they attend after-school programs or have another person caring for them after school. In this situation, you can instruct the parent and child to use the time-planning routines flexibly, in a way that makes sense with their schedule. For example, the parent and child might discuss how the child will fit in homework with the various after-school activities while driving to school in the morning, anticipating what is usually assigned for daily homework. Alternatively, the parent and child might hold a brief Time-Planning Conference by phone when the child gets home, or another caregiver could be trained in using the Time-Planning Conference with the child.

Review the Home Behavior Record

Show the parent the Home Behavior Record (Handout 19), and review which behaviors the parent will prompt, monitor, praise, and reward. The following is a suggested list of behaviors that might be appropriate for the Home Behavior Record, though variations might make sense for some children.

- *School behavior 1*: Got work area Ready to Go.
- *School behavior 2*: Completed the Time Tracker for In-Class Work for an in-class assignment.
- *Home behavior 1*: Had all materials for homework.
- *Home behavior 2*: Engaged in a Time-Planning Conference.
- *Home behavior 3*: Completed the Time Tracker for Homework.

HELPFUL HINT: You should staple the Time Tracker for Homework (Handout 32) to the Time-Planning Conference (Handout 34), so that the parent and child have both forms in the same place, and remember to use both, as tools for planning and then executing time management skills.

Add New Target Behaviors to the DAR Folder

The target behaviors for which the teacher will provide school points are these:

1. Got the desk Ready to Go.
2. Completed the Time Tracker for In-Class Work for an in-class assignment.

Reward the Child

Review the Session Points and Notes (Therapist Form 5) with the child, and praise the child for the positive behaviors that earned points in the session. Add up the total points earned for this session, and indicate that the child may spend or save the points.

Conclude the Session

Confirm the next session appointment. Give the child and parent the OTMP Checklist for the next session (Handout 36). Remind the parent to bring the Home Behavior Record (Handout 19), and the child to bring the backpack, DAR folder, and binder, with all OTMP papers, to the next session.

Time Management

Time Planning for Longer-Term Assignments and Avoiding Distractions

---

GOALS FOR THE SESSION

You will:

- Review the home exercises for time planning and tracking completed by parent and child.
- Discuss the impact of distractions on free time.
- Teach the child how to use time planning for assignments that are completed over a more extended period of time.

The child will:

- Discuss how the Time-Planning Conference was used at home.
- Learn about the impact of distractions on free time, through a simulated exercise.
- Practice using a Time-Planning Conference to integrate work on longer-term assignments into the daily homework schedule.

The parent will:

- Describe efforts to prompt, monitor, praise, and reward target behaviors, using the Home Behavior Record from the previous session (Handout 19).
- Agree to work with the child on completing a daily Time-Planning Conference, including a consideration of longer-term assignments (Handout 34).
- Agree to use a Time-Planning Conference with the child for a home situation in which the Time Bandit often interferes (Handout 37).
- Agree to prompt, monitor, praise, and reward specified target behaviors between sessions, using the Home Behavior Record from this session.

▄▄▄▄▄▄▄▄▄▄▄▄▄▄ MATERIALS NEEDED ▄▄▄▄▄▄▄▄▄▄▄▄▄▄

For the parent:

- Handout 19, Home Behavior Record

For you:

- Stopwatch and kitchen timer
- Grade-appropriate worksheets or tasks
- Toys/games and a CD player or digital music player
- Therapist Form 5, Session Points and Notes
- Therapist Form 22, Work Observation Sheet
- Therapist Form 23, Practice: Short- and Long-Term Assignments
- Therapist Form 24, Time Planning for Short- and Long-Term Adventure Activities (Optional)

SESSION SUMMARY CHECKLIST FOR SESSION 13

Item	Item Completed
Review implementation of the behavior-monitoring and point program (with parent/child)	
Review the Home Behavior Record	Yes/No
Review home exercises on time management	Yes/No
Conducts skills building with the child alone: Time planning, continued	
Observe work and use of time when distractions are present	Yes/No
Conduct OST homework review: Time-Planning Conference	Yes/No
Discuss time management for longer-term assignments	Yes/No
Conduct in-session practice: Time-Planning Conference for longer-term assignments	Yes/No
Wrap up the session (with parent/child)	
Support the child in explaining the Time-Planning Conference for longer-term assignments to the parent	Yes/No
Obtain information about the Time Bandit	Yes/No
Review the Home Behavior Record (Handout 19)	Yes/No
Add new target behaviors to the DAR folder	Yes/No
Reward the child (Therapist Form 5)	Yes/No
Conclude the session (Handout 39)	Yes/No

For the child:

- Child's DAR folder, binder, and backpack
- Handout 32, Time Tracker for Homework
- Handout 34, Time-Planning Conference (two copies)
- Handout 37, Time-Planning Conference for Problem Situations
- Handout 38, Practice: Time Planning for Longer-Term Assignments
- Handout 39, OTMP Checklist: Things to Remember for Session 14

ABOUT THIS SESSION

This session continues to focus on control of the Time Bandit, through the use of time planning. The child will extend the use of Time-Planning Conferences to include consideration of partial work that should be done on longer-term assignments each day. In addition, the child will understand, through a simulated work situation with distracting items present, how distractions in the work area may result in the child's going off task, which can increase the time required to complete assignments and reduce the amount of free time available.

IN PREPARATION FOR THIS SESSION

You will need to prepare a simulated work situation for the child, with a selection of grade-appropriate reading, math, and writing worksheets that should take a total of approximately 10 minutes to complete. In addition, you will need to set up the work area with a variety of potentially distracting items, such as small toys, markers, bouncing balls, or figurines, and a music player. You will also need to provide toys/games that the child would enjoy using for free time that is earned (e.g., computer or tablet computer games, sticker book, board game).

In addition, you should refer to your notes from earlier contacts with the teacher, to determine what assignments the child regularly has that are completed over the course of a few days (e.g., reading log, studying for a weekly social studies quiz, journal entries). This information will help to make the conversation about time planning for longer-term assignments relevant for the child.

DETAILED SESSION CONTENT

Review Implementation of the Behavior-Monitoring and Point Program

Review the Home Behavior Record

Review the Home Behavior Record (Handout 19) with the parent, and discuss the child's performance of the OTMP behaviors between sessions.

- Discuss the behaviors that were observed.
- Ask the parent how she prompted the behaviors.
- Review what rewards were used to reinforce the child's performance of the behaviors.
- Help the family manage any problems with implementation (e.g., problems with prompting, recording points, providing rewards, or implementing organizational routines).

Review Home Exercises on Time Management

Ask the parent and child how they used the Time-Planning Conference (Handout 34) and Time Tracker for Homework (Handout 32) at home. Provide session points for bringing these forms back to this session. Find out whether the parent and child were able to engage cooperatively in these routines. If they did not complete the conference, ask what interfered with its use (e.g., difficulty finding time to complete it), and provide suggestions for ways to make sure that the conference can be used appropriately. If the parent or child has questions about how to use the forms, provide guidance and examples (if necessary) of how to complete the forms.

If the parent and child did complete the Time-Planning Conference at home, ask whether they noticed any changes in the homework routine as a result of using time-planning skills. Finally, confirm that the parent praised the child for using these new skills, and that the child was rewarded appropriately.

Conduct Skills Building with the Child Alone: Time Planning, Continued

Begin by awarding the child session points (Therapist Form 5) and providing praise for good listening and discussion with the parent present.

Observe Work and Use of Time When Distractions Are Present

Show the child the work area that you have set up, which should contain worksheets and a small collection of potentially distracting toys/games (see "In Preparation for This Session"). Also, point out to the child the toys/games that are set up in a different part of the room, which the child will be able to play with after the work has been completed.

Tell the child:

"Today we're going to do something a little different. I want you to practice working on some reading, math, and writing worksheets for 10 minutes. When you are done, you can play with one of these toys/games for up to 5 minutes. How much time you use the toys/games will depend on your work period. If you stay focused on your work for the whole 10 minutes, you will get to use all 5 minutes of your playtime. I might watch to see whether the Time Bandit takes you off track and costs you any free time.

"Here are the worksheets. Please get your work area Ready to Go, and start working on the worksheets when I start the timer. If you finish one worksheet, you can just go on to the next one and keep working until the timer rings. When the time is up, you will be able to play with the toys/games."

Start the timer. While the child is working, keep track of any off-task behavior, using the Work Observation Sheet (Therapist Form 22). Put a hash mark down on the sheet each time the child is off task (e.g., fiddling with pencil, staring out window, playing with zipper, playing with or starting at one of the toys/games). If the child is off task, start the stopwatch (try to do this so that the child does not notice) and stop it when the child returns to work. Do not reset the time; simply restart the stopwatch if the child gets off task again and stop when the child return to work. This way, you will be able to record the total amount of time the child is off task. The total time spent off task will be subtracted from the 5 minutes of free time allowed to the child.

When the timer sounds at the end of 10 minutes, let the child know that the work period is over, and that he may use the special toys/games now. If the child was on task for the entire work period, praise him for not allowing the Time Bandit to steal any of his free time by distracting him, and tell him that he may play with the toys/games for 5 minutes. If the child was off task at all during the work period, let him know how long he was off task, and tell him that he will be able to play for 5 minutes minus that amount of time. Discuss this reality with the child, emphasizing the impact that the Time Bandit can have on free time.

Tell the child:

"You did great work on these worksheets, and you completed a lot of items. However, I noticed that you stopped working a few times, and [state the amount of time] passed while you were not working. [State what you observed the child doing during the off-task periods—e.g., fiddling with pencil, playing with toys.] Sometimes, it seems like more fun to do these kinds of things instead of working, but these distractions take away from the time you could spend doing things you *really* enjoy, like playing with your iPad or riding your bike. This can happen at home, when you are supposed to be doing your homework but you play with a paper clip on your desk instead. The time you lose on that distraction will come out of your free time that night. Just for practice, we are going to show you how this works, with the free time you can spend now. I am going to subtract [state amount of time] from your 5 minutes of free time. So you have [__ minutes] to play now."

Start the timer, and allow the child to play with the toys/games for up to 5 minutes. While the child is playing, mark down on the Work Observation Sheet (Therapist Form 22) how many items were completed on the worksheets. Save this sheet in the child's chart, as you will refer to it in the next session.

Conduct OST Homework Review: Time-Planning Conference

Tell the child:

"We know that the Time Bandit can steal your free time by convincing you to lose focus on your work. The Time Bandit can also get you in trouble by making sure that you don't get all of your work done, because you haven't set up a good schedule for yourself. Let's talk about the work you did with Time-Planning Conferences since the last session, with your parent. How did that go? Did you find out anything interesting about how you use your time?"

Review the information on the copies of the Time-Planning Conference (Handout 34) that the child completed at home. Note whether the child showed a bias in estimating the time needed to complete homework. Is the child consistently over- or underestimating the time needed? How can the child try to correct this bias and become a more accurate Time Detective?

Discuss Time Management for Longer-Term Assignments

Tell the child:

"We will spend the rest of this session talking about how you can use time planning to make sure that work gets done on longer-term assignments—ones that are usually completed over the course of a few days (such as a book log, weekly journal writing, or research for a small project). We will talk about the steps you should take to make sure those assignments get done, including figuring out how much time each assignment should take and deciding when you can fit the steps for that assignment into your schedule, so you don't have to cram all the work in at once. We will discuss how you can fit in your work on these longer-term assignments with the other activities and homework assignments you have each day."

Briefly, gather some information from the child about the types of longer-term assignments she is given in school. You are not discussing larger long-term projects, like book reports or research papers; rather, these "longer-term" assignments are those that are typically completed over the course of a few days (e.g., studying a spelling list for an end-of-week test, responding to questions about a reading assignment, writing a response to a reading passage). The teacher may have given you some examples of these types of assignments in your initial phone contact, and you may be aware of some examples from your review of the child's DAR and Assignment and Test Calendar in each session. Ask the child whether she has ever had any problems completing these longer-term assignments. For example, has she ever had to cram in work on an assignment, because she did not remember to work on it until the day before it was due?

Conduct In-Session Practice: Time-Planning Conference for Longer-Term Assignments

Discuss how the child can fit these longer-term assignments into the daily Time-Planning Conference. The child will follow the steps for the Time-Planning Conference that were practiced in the previous session and at home; he will pay special attention to any longer-term assignments that are listed on the Assignment and Test Calendar or DAR, making sure to add those assignments to the list of things to work on that day when appropriate. The child will consider the following factors in deciding when to add work on longer-term assignments:

> "How long will it take to complete the steps for this assignment?"
> "What assignments must I complete for tomorrow, and how long will those assignments take me to do?"
> "What other activities do I have tonight?"
> "Based on my answers to these questions, do I have time to fit in some work on my longer-term assignment today?"

Conduct separate Time-Planning Conferences (Handout 34) with two lists of simulated short- and longer-term assignments, which are similar to those that the child usually completes. You may use examples from Therapist Form 23, or create simulated assignment descriptions, based on your knowledge of typical assignments given to the child. If you think it will be useful or interesting to the child, you may also conduct a practice Time-Planning Conference for one of the optional "adventures" in Therapist Form 24. This adventure practice should be conducted only if time permits, but can be a useful way to reinforce the concept that time planning skills can be applied in many different situations. Provide the child with praise and points for completing each of the practice Time-Planning Conferences.

Wrap Up the Session (with Parent/Child)

Support the Child in Explaining the Time-Planning Conference for Longer-Term Assignments to the Parent

Ask the child to explain to the parent how to include consideration of longer-term assignments in the daily Time-Planning Conference (Handout 34). The child may show the parent the notes on the practice Time-Planning Conferences that were conducted in session, and explain the steps for fitting work on longer-term assignments into the daily schedule.

Tell the parent and child that they should conduct a Time-Planning Conference each day, and that they should include a consideration of longer-term assignments in the conference. If the child does not have any longer-term assignments, ask the parent to use one of the assignments described on Handout 38, and ask the child to discuss how she would fit that into the schedule, to allow for practice with this skill. The child should also continue to use the Time Tracker for Homework (Handout 32) to estimate and keep track of the time spent on homework each day.

Obtain Information about the Time Bandit

Tell the parent that you and the child have been talking a lot in session about the Time Bandit and how it can steal time from the child in multiple situations. Ask the parent and child for further information about tasks that the child has difficulty completing on time at home. For example, does the Time Bandit get the child to start certain tasks late or stop doing them in the middle? Does the child get distracted and not get certain tasks done at all because of those distractions?

Ask the parent and child to think about two situations when the Time Bandit interferes at home (e.g., when the child is getting ready for school, taking a shower, or getting ready for bed). Ask them to complete a special Time-Planning Conference for Problem Situations (Handout 37) between now and the next meeting. The child will use Time Detective skills for this activity as well, to determine how long it takes to complete the task that is being planned.

For example, if the parent and child have identified getting dressed in the morning as a task with which the Time Bandit typically interferes, the child will conduct a special Time-Planning Conference regarding how to manage time for this task. The parent might want to prompt the child to think about the following questions in the evening, so that the child is prepared to get dressed quickly in the morning:

"How long should it take me to get dressed?"
"When should I start getting dressed?"
"When should I be finished getting dressed?"

In the morning, the child can use the responses to these three questions to stay on track while getting dressed. Then, after getting dressed, the child can discuss the following questions with the parent:

"What time did I start getting dressed?"
"What time did I finish?"
"Did I get done on time?"
"If I didn't get done on time, how did the Time Bandit get to me? I might have to ask my

parents to help me figure this out. Did I start slowly? Did I get distracted while I was getting dressed? How far behind was I?"

Review the Home Behavior Record

Show the parent the Home Behavior Record (Handout 19), and review which behaviors the parent will prompt, monitor, praise, and reward. The following is a suggested list of behaviors that might be appropriate for the Home Behavior Record, though variations might make sense for some children.

- *School behavior 1*: Got work area Ready to Go.
- *School behavior 2*: Responded to prompt to complete the Time Tracker for In-Class Work for an in-class assignment, and stored it in the accordion binder.
- *Home behavior 1*: Had all materials for homework.
- *Home behavior 2*: Engaged in a Time-Planning Conference for homework *and* longer-term assignments.
- *Home behavior 3*: Completed a Time-Planning Conference for Problem Situations.

Add New Target Behaviors to the DAR Folder

The target behaviors for which the teacher will provide school points are these:

1. Got the desk Ready to Go.
2. Completed the Time Tracker for In-Class Work for an in-class assignment.

Note: At this point in treatment, it is a good idea to check in with the teacher regarding how the child is doing with Managing Materials and Time Management skills in the classroom. Thus, you should contact the teacher and ask her to complete the Skills Check-Up (Teacher Form 9), indicating whether the child hands in homework, has all materials needed for class, and gets in-class work done on time. You may fax/e-mail the form to the teacher, or send it with the child to give to the teacher. The teacher should return the completed form to the child, and the child should bring the form to the next session.

Reward the Child

Review the Session Points and Notes (Therapist Form 5) with the child, and praise the child for the positive behaviors that earned points in the session. Add up the total points earned for this session, and indicate that the child may spend or save the points.

Conclude the Session

Confirm the next session appointment. Give the child and parent the OTMP Checklist for the next session (Handout 39). Remind the parent to bring the Home Behavior Record (Handout 19), and the child to bring the backpack, DAR folder, and binder, with all OTMP papers, to the next session.

Time Management
Time Planning for Regular Routines

You will:

- Review the home exercises on time planning for homework and problem situations completed by parent and child.
- Discuss the child's personal Time Bandit problems.
- Develop strategies for battling the child's personal Time Bandit problems.
- Learn how to use a Time-Planning Conference for Regular Routines.

The parent will:

- Describe efforts to prompt, monitor, praise, and reward target behaviors, using the Home Behavior Record from the previous session (Handout 19).
- Discuss how the Time-Planning Conference was used at home, for both homework and problem situations.
- Agree to work with the child on completing daily Time-Planning Conferences, including a consideration of longer-term assignments and of a problem situation (Handouts 34, 37).
- Agree to work with the child on completing a daily Time-Planning Conference for Regular Routines (Handout 41).
- Agree to prompt, monitor, praise, and reward specified target behaviors between sessions, using the Home Behavior Record from this session.

For the parent:

- Handout 19, Home Behavior Record

For you:

- Therapist Form 5, Session Points and Notes
- Therapist Form 22, Work Observation Sheet (completed in Session 13)
- Therapist Form 25, Time Bandit Record Sheet
- Therapist Form 26, How Might Homework Time Change?

For the child:

- Child's DAR folder, binder, and backpack
- Handout 32, Time Tracker for Homework
- Handout 40, Ideas for Battling the Time Bandit
- Handout 41, Time-Planning Conference for Regular Routines (two copies)
- Handout 42, Time-Planning Conference (Including Review of the Problem Situation)
- Handout 43, OTMP Checklist: Things to Remember for Session 15

SESSION SUMMARY CHECKLIST FOR SESSION 14

Item	Item Completed
Review implementation of the behavior-monitoring and point program (with parent/child)	
Review the Home Behavior Record	Yes/No
Review home exercise: Time-Planning Conferences	Yes/No
Conduct skills building with the child alone: Time planning, continued	
Discuss the Time Bandits	Yes/No
Conduct OST homework review: The Time Bandit in the problem situation (Therapist Form 25)	Yes/No
Discuss the child's personal Time Bandit problems (Therapist Form 26)	Yes/No
Discuss ideas for battling the Time Bandit (Handout 40)	Yes/No
Discuss the Time Bandit's interference in regular routines	Yes/No
Conduct in-session practice: Time-Planning Conference for Regular Routines (Handout 41)	Yes/No
Wrap up the session (with parent/child)	
Support the child in discussing the Time Bandit (Handout 40)	Yes/No
Review the Home Behavior Record (Handout 19)	Yes/No
Add new target behaviors to the DAR folder	Yes/No
Reward the child (Therapist Form 5)	Yes/No
Conclude the session (Handout 43)	Yes/No

ABOUT THIS SESSION

This session is the final one in the Time Management module, and focuses on summarizing what has been learned about how the Time Bandit interferes with the child's completion of homework and other tasks. The child will identify specific, personal ways in which the Time Bandit steals the child's free time by interfering with completion of homework and other routines, and will develop ideas for battling these tactics of the Time Bandit. Finally, the child will learn how to extend the use of Time-Planning Conferences to planning for regular routines (e.g., getting ready in the morning, bedtime routine), and will learn to pay attention to how the Time Bandit might interfere with completion of these routines.

IN PREPARATION FOR THIS SESSION

In this session, you will discuss how the Time Bandit interferes with the child's completion of regular routines at home, like getting ready for school, getting ready for bed, or doing chores. You may want to review the original Parent COSS and your notes from the first session, to gather some information on whether the child has particular difficulty with time management related to any of these regular routines. This will supplement the information you will gather in this session from the child, and will help you focus your discussion.

DETAILED SESSION CONTENT

Review Implementation of the Behavior-Monitoring and Point Program

Review the Home Behavior Record

Review the Home Behavior Record (Handout 19) with the parent, and discuss the child's performance of the OTMP behaviors between sessions.

- Discuss the behaviors that were observed.
- Ask the parent how he prompted the behaviors.
- Review what rewards were used to reinforce the child's performance of the behaviors.
- Help the family manage any problems with implementation (e.g., problems with prompting, recording points, providing rewards, or implementing organizational routines).

Review Home Exercise: Time-Planning Conferences

Ask the parent and child how they used the Time-Planning Conference (Handout 34) for homework and longer-term assignments. Discuss whether the conference helped the child fit work into the daily schedule and complete both short-term and longer-term assignments on time. In addition, review information on the Time Tracker for Homework (Handout 32), and ask the parent and child whether the child is getting better at understanding how long typical assignments take to complete. Ask whether using the Time-Planning Conference for longer-term assignments has helped the child get those assignments done in a timelier manner. If the child is still having difficulty completing longer-term assignments over the course of a few days, determine which tactics of the Time Bandit might be contributing to this difficulty (e.g., the child might be too tired at the end of the day to fit in work on "extra" assignments, or the child insists that the work can be done quickly the day before it is due).

Next, ask the parent and child what they learned about the problem situation they chose to focus on with the Time-Planning Conference for Problem Situations (Handout 37). Did the child estimate time accurately? Which tactics of the Time Bandit interfered with performance in the selected situation? If the child is still having difficulty completing the problem situation (e.g., is still not ready for bed by 8:30), ask the parent and child to think briefly about what needs to be done to make sure this situation is resolved. Discuss this only briefly, as you will spend more time on this question in the session time with the child alone.

Conduct Skills Building with the Child Alone: Time Planning, Continued

Begin by awarding the child session points (Therapist Form 5) and providing praise for good listening and discussion with the parent present.

Discuss the Time Bandit

Tell the child:

> "Today we will talk more about time. We know that time keeps moving, and there is nothing we can do to stop the clock or slow the calendar. However, even though we can't change the passage of time, we *can* change how quickly we work and how we schedule our time. This is sometimes hard to do. Sometimes our minds drift while we are working, and we lose track of time, so it seems like time has stood still—but it keeps on chugging by. This might happen in class, when you're working on an assignment and you start to daydream—and then you realize that you have to hand in your paper in 5 minutes, and you've only completed a small part of it. At other times, you can't move as quickly as you'd like because you are hungry, tired, or not feeling well. Some kids have a really hard time moving quickly in the morning, because they are still sleepy, and then they have to listen to their moms yell at them because they are not ready when the bus arrives. Kids with ADHD often have trouble keeping track of time. The Time Bandit gobbles up their time, because they are daydreaming or getting distracted by other things. Then not only do they get in trouble for not getting the work done; they also lose out on free time that could have been spent doing something fun. Today, we are going to talk about the specific tactics of the Time Bandit that might be bothering you and stealing your free time. We are going to do some detective work, in this session and at home, to learn more about your personal Time Bandit problems. Then we are going to try to figure out some ways to stop these Time Bandits from bothering you."

Remind the child of what happened in the previous session, when the child had to stay focused on the worksheets and not get distracted by the toys and other interesting items in the work area. If the child did get distracted, remind him that he lost out on free-play time with the really interesting toys/games. If the child did not get distracted, talk about what might happen at home or at school when things do distract him, and he is not able to complete his work on time.

Conduct OST Homework Review: The Time Bandit in the Problem Situation

Tell the child:

"Please take out the sheet that you used to discuss time planning for problematic situations [Handout 37, Time-Planning Conference for Problem Situations], which you completed at home. Let's see what you learned when you gathered information on the problem situation. [Specify which problem situation the child used for this exercise.] How long did it take you to complete the activity? What problems did the Time Bandit throw at you? Did it win? Were you able to complete the activity in the time you set aside for it, or did it take you longer?"

Help the child make a list of the problems that interfered with timely completion of the activity in the problem situation. Make a list of these problems on the Time Bandit Record Sheet (Therapist Form 25).

Discuss the Child's Personal Time Bandit Problems

Tell the child:

"Just like the Time Bandit has specific ways of interfering in the problem situation, the Time Bandit uses other tactics to get in the way when you are working on homework or other routines. For example, your surroundings can influence how well and how quickly you get your work done. Do you find that a busy or noisy setting makes it more difficult for you to get your work done? Remember last time, when I had music on while you were working, and there were toys all over your work area? Did those distractions make it harder for you to get the work done in the time given? Different people have different Time Bandit problems that affect them more than others. Some people get very distracted by music, and some people don't. Some people get distracted when there are random materials like paper clips or glue on their desks, and some people get distracted by daydreams. Let's think about the ways the Time Bandit interferes with your work at home."

Using Therapist Form 26 as a guide, ask the child a series of hypothetical questions about how different factors may affect how long a homework assignment would take to complete. Consider each example assignment on the form, like completing 10 math problems in a workbook, and ask the child how long that assignment should take to complete. Then ask how that time estimate would change if the child was tired, was hungry, checked e-mail, and so on. As you complete this exercise, praise the child and give session points (Therapist Form 5), and note which Time Bandit problems the child endorses as being most problematic.

Discuss Ideas for Battling the Time Bandit

Tell the child:

"Now that we have a better idea of the ways the Time Bandit can interfere when you're trying to get things done, let's see if we can think of some strategies for battling the Time Bandit in specific situations."

Show the child Handout 40 (Ideas for Battling the Time Bandit), and begin by discussing how the child can battle the Time Bandit during homework time. Consider the kinds of

Time Bandit problems the child has described to you as being most problematic (e.g., music playing in the background, extraneous items in the work space, a little brother watching TV in the same room), and think of some ideas that might help the child stay focused on work, despite the influence of the Time Bandit. For example, if the child indicates that he often finds himself playing with random items during homework time, like the salt shaker that is on the dining room table where he works, you can suggest that he get Ready to Go before starting homework as a good option for battling the Time Bandit in that situation. If the child indicates that background TV is a problem, you might want to suggest that the child do homework in a different room. Whenever possible, try to have the child think of solutions to the problems posed by the Time Bandit, and praise the child's efforts to manage the Time Bandit.

Next, work with the child to think of some strategies for battling the Time Bandit in the problem situation that was discussed earlier. Consider the issues that the child identified as interfering with completion of the required activity in that situation, and think of some solutions that can address those problems. For example, if the child has difficulty getting ready for school because she continues to press the snooze button on the alarm clock, leaving very little time for her to get dressed and ready to go to school, you may decide that the clock should be moved away from the bed, so that the child must get out of bed to turn it off. Award session points for participating in this discussion.

Discuss the Time Bandit's Interference in Regular Routines

Tell the child:

> "There are lots of routines that you have to get done at home, aside from the routine we talked about as being a 'problem situation.' Just like with your school work, the Time Bandit can get in the way when you're trying to do those routines—like putting your dishes in the sink, taking a shower, getting ready for bed, or getting ready for karate [or other after-school activity]. Are there any routines that take you a lot of time to complete? Does the Time Bandit trick you so that your parents scold you for not finishing on time?"

If the child indicates frequent problems in completing these routines on time, gather some more information about these types of problems, and determine how the Time Bandit interferes with completion of these activities. Does the child have difficulty getting ready for school in the morning, packing the school bag, or doing chores?

Remind the child that when we are distracted by other things when we're supposed to be completing one of these routines, we often lose time that we could have spent doing things that we really enjoy. For example, the child might take too long in the shower because he is playing with a bottle cap instead of washing his hair. Because of this, the child will lose time that could have been spent reading a favorite book before bed.

Tell the child:

> "Remember, the Time Bandit loves to take away time you could have spent on your favorite activities by having you use up all your time on silly or unimportant things. We have to plan our time carefully, so we can spend it on the things we have to do (like homework or important routines) and on things we like to do best (in the time that's left over)."

Take out Handout 40 (Ideas for Battling the Time Bandit), and select one or two regular routines that the child has noted as being problematic. Work with the child to think of some potential solutions for the problems posed by the Time Bandit in these situations (e.g., if the child wastes time in the morning because she can't decide what to wear, a solution might be to leave clothes out the night before).

Conduct In-Session Practice: Time-Planning Conference for Regular Routines

Tell the child that you want him to start thinking about time planning for two to three regular routines that are difficult for the child to complete on time at home. The child will use the Time-Planning Conference for Regular Routines (Handout 41) to estimate the amount of time each routine should take, decide when to fit it into the schedule, record how long it took to complete, and note whether there were any problems getting it done (i.e., which Time Bandit tactics interfered).

Using one copy of Handout 41 for practice, select a simple routine that may be practiced in session (e.g., cleaning up the desk or packing the backpack), to demonstrate how to use this handout. For example, you might make a mess on the desk, scattering pens, pencils, and other office supplies around. Have the child think about how long it should take to clean up this mess, and then have her record this number on Handout 41 in the second row. Tell the child that this task has to be completed by a specific time, because you need to get the parent in just a few minutes, and have her record this time in the third row on the form. Ask the child when she should start working, in order to get done on time. Then have the child clean up the desk and record how long it takes to do this task. Finally, note whether there were any problems completing the task in time. If there were, discuss which Time Bandit tactics interfered. Did the child take a long time putting away the highlighters, choosing to line them up in rainbow order (an unnecessary step)? Did the child stop to talk to you while she was working, and lose focus on what had to be done?

Tell the child that the Time-Planning Conference for Regular Routines will be conducted at home each day, in addition to the Time-Planning Conference for homework. This exercise will help the child be both a Time Detective (identifying the things that might get in the way of completing usual routines) and a Time Planner (thinking more carefully about when things should get done and how long they should take, and trying to stick to those plans).

Wrap Up the Session (with Parent/Child)

Support the Child in Discussing the Time Bandit

Tell the parent that you discussed the Time Bandit in this session, noting that each person has specific Time Bandit problems that interfere with completion of important tasks, like homework or daily routines. Explain that you and the child learned about the impact of the surroundings and other factors on the child's ability to complete tasks on time. Ask the child to show the parent Handout 40, and to discuss some of the ideas for battling the Time Bandit when completing homework, the problem situation, or other regular routines. The child should keep this handout in the OTMP folder in the binder, and should try to implement some of these ideas at home.

Then ask the child to show the parent the Time-Planning Conference for Regular Routines (Handout 41), and to discuss how this handout can be used to help the child learn how to manage time better in getting these routines done. Ask the parent and child to select two to three regular routines that the child must complete at home, and to write those routines down in the first row of this form. Then explain that they will work together to complete the steps in this special Time-Planning Conference, to help the child identify Time Bandit tactics that interfere with these routines and develop strategies for completing these routines in a timelier manner.

Tell the parent and child that they will also continue using the Time-Planning Conference for homework and longer-term assignments (Handout 34) and the Time Tracker for Homework (Handout 32), and will include a discussion each day of the problem situation and when that can fit into the schedule (Handout 42). Ask whether there are any questions about the home exercises, and provide the child with session points for explaining what was covered in session to the parent.

Review the Home Behavior Record

Show the parent the Home Behavior Record (Handout 19), and review which behaviors the parent will prompt, monitor, praise, and reward. The following is a suggested list of behaviors that might be appropriate for the Home Behavior Record, though variations might make sense for some children.

- *School behavior 1*: Completed all in-class assignments on time.
- *School behavior 2*: Completed the Time Tracker for In-Class Work for an in-class assignment.
- *Home behavior 1*: Engaged in a Time-Planning Conference for homework and longer term assignments.
- *Home behavior 2*: Completed the Time-Planning Conference for Regular Routines.
- *Home behavior 3*: Completed the Time Tracker for Homework.

Add New Target Behaviors to the DAR Folder

The target behaviors for which the teacher will provide school points are these:

1. Completed all in-class assignments on time.
2. Completed the Time Tracker for In-Class Work for an in-class assignment.

Reward the Child

Review the Session Points and Notes (Therapist Form 5) with the child, and praise the child for the positive behaviors that earned points in the session. Add up the total points earned for this session, and indicate that the child may spend or save the points.

Conclude the Session

Confirm the next session appointment. Give the child and parent the OTMP Checklist for the next session (Handout 43). Remind the parent to bring the Home Behavior Record (Handout 19), and the child to bring the backpack, DAR folder, and binder, with all OTMP papers, to the next session.

Task Planning
Introduction to Task Planning

━━━━━━━━━━━━ **GOALS FOR THE SESSION** ━━━━━━━━━━━━

You will:

- Review the home exercises on time management completed by parent and child, focusing on the Time Bandit tactics that interfered with the child's task completion.
- Help the parent and child develop a plan to control the Time Bandit.
- Introduce the child to the steps for task planning.
- Contact the teacher before the next session to discuss task planning, and send the teacher materials on Task-Planning Conferences (see Teacher Contact 5).

The child will:

- Discuss the Time Bandit tactics that interfered with task completion at home, and help in developing a plan for controlling the Time Bandit.
- Understand the steps in task planning.
- Practice using the first steps in task planning: describing the activity/goal, and breaking it down into the steps needed to meet the goal.

The parent will:

- Describe efforts to prompt, monitor, praise, and reward target behaviors.
- Discuss the Time Bandit tactics that interfered with task completion at home, and help in developing a plan for controlling the Time Bandit.
- Agree to work with the child on completing a daily Time-Planning Conference, integrating ideas about how to manage the Time Bandit.
- Agree to work with the child on completing practice task-planning exercises.
- Agree to prompt, monitor, praise, and reward specified target behaviors between sessions, using the Home Behavior Record.

MATERIALS NEEDED

For the parent:

- Handout 19, Home Behavior Record

For you:

- Therapist Form 5, Session Points and Notes

For the child:

- Child's DAR folder, binder, and backpack
- Handout 3, Guide to the Glitches
- Handout 32, Time Tracker for Homework
- Handout 42, Time-Planning Conference, Including Review of the Problem Situation
- Handout 44, Steps in Task Planning
- Handout 45, Task-Planning Conference: First Steps (eight copies, collated into two stapled packets)
- Handout 46, Home Exercise Ideas: Task Planning
- Handout 47, OTMP Checklist: Things to Remember for Session 16

SESSION SUMMARY CHECKLIST FOR SESSION 15

Item	Item Completed
Review implementation of the behavior-monitoring and point program (with parent/child)	
Review the Home Behavior Record	Yes/No
Review home exercise: The Time Bandit	Yes/No
Conduct skills building with the child alone: Task planning	
Discuss the Go-Ahead-Don't-Plan Glitch (Handout 3)	Yes/No
Provide an introduction to the steps in task planning (Handout 44)	Yes/No
Conduct in-session practice: First steps in task planning (Handout 45)	Yes/No
Wrap up the session (with parent/child)	
Support the child in discussing task-planning steps (Handout 44)	Yes/No
Review the Home Behavior Record (Handout 19)	Yes/No
Add new target behaviors to the DAR folder	Yes/No
Reward the child (Therapist Form 5)	Yes/No
Conclude the session (Handout 47)	Yes/No

ABOUT THIS SESSION

This session introduces the child to the importance of planning in accomplishing tasks efficiently and effectively. The child will learn about the different steps involved in task planning, and will understand how each of the steps is essential in making sure that tasks are completed efficiently, neatly, and completely. The child will then practice the first of these steps—stating the goal and breaking it down—using an abbreviated Task-Planning Conference. In Sessions 16–19, the child will learn how to add the other steps in planning, and how to complete a Task-Planning Conference with the parent's assistance.

In addition, you will review the information gathered at home about the Time Bandit tactics that hinder the child's completion of tasks, and will help the child and parent develop a plan for controlling those tactics. Although the parent should continue to support the child in using time management tools (i.e., time planning, strategies to control the Time Bandit) at home, the focus in this and subsequent sessions will be on teaching the steps in task planning.

DETAILED SESSION CONTENT

Review Implementation of the Behavior-Monitoring and Point Program

Review the Home Behavior Record

Review the Home Behavior Record (Handout 19) with the parent, and discuss the child's performance of the OTMP behaviors between sessions.

- Discuss the behaviors that were observed.
- Ask the parent how she prompted the behaviors.
- Review what rewards were used to reinforce the child's performance of the behaviors.
- Help the family manage any problems with implementation (e.g., problems with prompting, recording points, providing rewards, or implementing organizational routines).

Review Home Exercise: The Time Bandit

Ask the parent and child what they learned about the specific Time Bandit tactics that interfere with the child's completion of tasks on time. Whenever possible, ask the child to provide information on these tactics and their negative effects, so that the child feels like a constructive member of the discussion and does not feel attacked. Praise the child for noticing problems with getting things done on time, and for describing which tactics of the Time Bandit contributed to those problems. Ask the parent to provide clarification if necessary, and to discuss how the Time Bandit contributes to family conflict and interferes with the child's life.

Use a problem-solving approach to help the child come up with a plan for diminishing the impact of the Time Bandit. For example, if the child reports that she has trouble getting ready for bed on time because she spends too much time in the shower, help the child think of ways to deal with this problem. The child might decide to bring a timer into the bathroom each evening, and to set the timer for 5 minutes, so that she does not spend too much time in the shower. Write down the solutions the child and parent suggest for controlling the

Time Bandit, and tell the child and parent to incorporate these solutions into the daily Time-Planning Conference. When they discuss the problem situation at the end of each conference, they should discuss what steps the child will take to make sure that this task gets done on time, with minimal interference from the Time Bandit.

Conduct Skills Building with the Child Alone: Task Planning

Begin by awarding the child session points (Therapist Form 5) and providing praise for good listening and discussion with the parent present.

Discuss the Go-Ahead-Don't-Plan Glitch

Tell the child:

> "Today we are going to talk about a new skill that can help you get things done and be more organized. You have been doing a good job keeping track of your assignments and managing your materials, so the Go-Ahead-Forget-It and Go-Ahead-Lose-It Glitches haven't been bothering you as much lately. You are also working to control the Time Bandit. The final Glitch that we need to take care of is the Go-Ahead-Don't-Plan Glitch. Let's look again at the Guide to the Glitches [Handout 3] and see how this Glitch gets people in trouble. [Review the narrative with the child, and discuss how the child has gotten into trouble because of a lack of planning.]
>
> "In order to control the Go-Ahead-Don't-Plan Glitch, we are going to learn an important new skill, which we'll call 'task planning.' This skill will help you consider all the steps you need to take to meet a goal. The goal could be just about anything, like making a snack, building a ramp for a skateboard, doing your homework, planning a sleepover with a friend, or finishing a book report for school. Every activity will go more smoothly if you plan ahead."

Provide an Introduction to the Steps in Task Planning

Give the child Handout 44 (Steps in Task Planning), and review these steps:

1. *Think about the goal*: Describe your goal in a short sentence.
2. *Get Ready to Go*:
   a. *Break it down*: What steps do you need to take to reach your goal?
   b. *Stuff you need*: What materials do you need to complete the steps?
3. *Manage your time*:
   a. *Arrange the steps*: In what order will you complete the steps?
   b. *Plan your time*: How much time will you need for each step?
   c. *Fit it in*: How will you fit the steps into your schedule?
4. *Check It Out:* Did you get everything done neatly and completely?

Ask the child whether these steps make sense, and whether the child has any questions. Then conduct a brief, interactive review of the planning steps with an example from your own experience. You may use the example below, or another example that would be interesting to the child, highlighting the planning steps that allowed you to reach your goal.

Tell the child:

"Today I had to get to work by 4:00 [describe your goal]. In order to get to work on time, I had to do a number of smaller things and prepare a lot of stuff [break it down, stuff you need]: get dressed in work clothes, pack my briefcase, write some notes, eat a snack, find my keys, and drive to work. I had to decide what to do first [arrange the steps] and how much time all of this would take [plan your time]. I decided that all of the steps at home would take about 30 minutes, and my drive to work would take 30 minutes, so I started getting ready at 3:00 [fit it in]. First I got dressed; then I prepared a snack; then I ate my snack while I wrote my notes; then I packed my briefcase with my notes and files; then, I found my keys; then, I checked that I had everything I needed [Check It Out]; and finally I drove to work. I got here at 4:00, just as I had planned."

Now briefly review the planning steps again, using an example from the child's experience. For example, you may discuss the steps that were involved in getting to the office for today's session appointment. Ask the child to describe the goal (e.g., getting to the office by 4:00); break it down into steps, with a consideration of the "stuff" that was needed (e.g., eating a snack, packing backpack with OTMP papers, checking that Mom or Dad was ready, getting into the car); arrange the steps (i.e., describe what he did first, second, third, etc.); indicate how long each step took and how he fit it into this schedule (e.g., he got home from school at 3:00 and prepared a snack, etc.); and review how he checked that all the steps were completed. Write down the steps and their order as the child describes them, so the child can see how this task of getting to the session on time can be broken down into distinct, planned steps.

Conduct In-Session Practice: First Steps in Task Planning

Tell the child that you will now practice the first steps in task planning: describing the goal (Step 1 in Handout 44) and breaking the goal down into steps (Step 2a). Guide the child in using these steps for four to five hypothetical practice activities, and record the child's responses on Handout 45 (Task-Planning Conference: First Steps). For each practice activity, help the child complete a copy of Handout 45, by summarizing the goal of the activity and then outlining the steps needed to complete the activity. You may write the child's responses on the handout, so that the child can focus on practicing the planning steps.

The child should practice planning for some activities that are fun and/or interesting (e.g., planning a sleepover) and for some regular chores and school-related projects. You may suggest some activities for which the child must plan, elicit ideas from the child, or use some of the following sample activities:

- Getting packed for school
- Cleaning your room
- Eating a snack after school
- Playing catch with your friend in the backyard
- Getting dressed for school
- Taking a bike ride
- Going to the park
- Writing a paragraph about a U.S. president, using information from the Internet

- Planning a sleepover
- Getting ready for swim practice

Provide praise and session points as the child engages in the first two task-planning steps for each practice activity.

> **HELPFUL HINT:** As children engage in the process of breaking an activity down into steps, they might include very minute or detailed steps (e.g., for eating a snack after school, they might include going into the kitchen, opening the refrigerator, taking out the bread, taking out peanut butter and jelly, walking to the counter, etc.). You should encourage children to list only the *essential* steps in planning for each activity (e.g., getting all the food and utensils needed to make the sandwich; getting bread, peanut butter, and jelly; making sandwich; eating it), so that they do not waste time while engaging in the planning process.

Wrap Up the Session (with Parent/Child)

Support the Child in Discussing the Task-Planning Steps

Have the child explain the steps in task planning to the parent, using the information on Handout 44 as a guide. The child should then show the parent the copies of Task-Planning Conference: First Steps (Handout 45) that were completed in session. Tell the parent that the child should practice using these first steps at home, completing one copy of Handout 45 daily for a practice activity. The parent can use activities from Handout 46 for the task-planning exercise, or think of other activities that are relevant for the child. Explain that the next few sessions will teach the child to use all of the steps in task planning, after the child has mastered the first two steps.

Finally, remind the parent and child that they should also complete a Time-Planning Conference (Handout 42) each day, with a review of short- and longer-term assignments and of a problem situation if this can be included. If the parent believes that the Time Tracker for Homework (Handout 32) helps the child stay on track with timely homework completion, the parent may continue to encourage its use at home; however, use of this form can be presented as optional, at this point in treatment.

Review the Home Behavior Record

Show the parent the Home Behavior Record (Handout 19), and review which behaviors the parent will prompt, monitor, praise, and reward. The following is a suggested list of behaviors that might be appropriate for the Home Behavior Record, though variations might make sense for some children.

- *School behavior 1*: Completed all in-class assignments on time.
- *School behavior 2*: Completed the Time Tracker for In-Class Work for an in-class assignment.
- *Home behavior 1*: Engaged in a Time-Planning Conference for homework, longer-term assignments, and a problem situation.

- *Home behavior 2*: Used strategies for controlling the Time Bandit.
- *Home behavior 3*: Completed practice Task-Planning Conferences.

Add New Target Behaviors to the DAR Folder

The target behaviors for which the teacher will provide school points are these:

1. Completed all in-class assignments on time.
2. Completed the Time Tracker for In-Class Work for an in-class assignment.

Reward the Child

Review the Session Points and Notes (Therapist Form 5) with the child, and praise the child for the positive behaviors that earned points in the session. Add up the total points earned for this session, and indicate that the child may spend or save the points.

Conclude the Session

Confirm the next session appointment. Give the child and parent the OTMP Checklist for the next session (Handout 47). Remind the parent to bring the Home Behavior Record (Handout 19) and the child to bring the backpack, DAR folder and binder, with all OTMP papers, to the next session.

Task Planning
Next Steps—Managing Materials and Time

You will:

- Review the Task-Planning Conferences completed by the parent and child at home.
- Discuss and demonstrate the next steps in task planning with the child: knowing what materials are needed for each step, arranging the steps, and estimating how long each step will take.

The child will:

- Understand how to integrate task planning with management of materials and time.
- Practice using the next steps in task planning: knowing what is needed for each step, ordering the steps, and estimating how long each step will take.

The parent will:

- Describe efforts to prompt, monitor, praise, and reward target behaviors.
- Agree to work with the child on completing two Task-Planning Conferences each day, for homework and another activity.
- Agree to prompt, monitor, praise, and reward specified target behaviors between sessions, using the Home Behavior Record.

For the parent:

- Handout 19, Home Behavior Record

For you:

- Therapist Form 5, Session Points and Notes
- Therapist Form 27, Task-Planning Conference: Example

For the child:

- Child's DAR folder, binder, and backpack
- Handout 44, Steps in Task Planning
- Handout 46, Home Exercise Ideas: Task Planning
- Handout 48, Task-Planning Conference Worksheet (four copies for in-session practice; eight copies for home practice, stapled)
- Handout 49, OTMP Checklist: Things to Remember for Session 17

SESSION SUMMARY CHECKLIST FOR SESSION 16

Item	Item Completed
Review implementation of the behavior-monitoring and point program (with parent/child)	
Review the Home Behavior Record	Yes/No
Review home exercise: Task-Planning Conferences	Yes/No
Conduct skills building with the child alone: Task planning, continued	
Discuss the next steps in task planning (Handout 44)	Yes/No
Provide a demonstration of expanded task planning (Therapist Form 27)	Yes/No
Conduct in-session practice: Task planning with steps fore managing materials and time (Handout 48)	Yes/No
Wrap up the session (with parent/child)	
Support the child in discussing expanded task-planning steps (Handout 44)	Yes/No
Describe home exercise: Task-Planning Conferences (Handout 48)	Yes/No
Review the Home Behavior Record (Handout 19)	Yes/No
Add new target behaviors to the DAR folder	Yes/No
Reward the child (Therapist Form 5)	Yes/No
Conclude the session (Handout 49)	Yes/No

ABOUT THIS SESSION

In this and subsequent sessions, the child will learn the steps in planning sequentially, getting ample opportunity to understand and practice each step and add new steps to the ones learned in Session 15. In this session, the child will learn how to integrate skills for materials and time management with task planning. In addition to stating the goal of an activity and breaking it down into steps, the child will now focus on considering what materials are needed to complete each step (i.e., how to get Ready to Go) and how to sequence the steps in a logical way. Finally, the child will estimate how long each step should take. In the next session, the child will use these time estimates to decide when to fit the planning steps into the schedule.

DETAILED SESSION CONTENT

Review Implementation of the Behavior-Monitoring and Point Program

Review the Home Behavior Record

Review the Home Behavior Record (Handout 19) with the parent, and discuss the child's performance of the OTMP behaviors between sessions.

- Discuss the behaviors that were observed.
- Ask the parent how he prompted the behaviors.
- Review what rewards were used to reinforce the child's performance of the behaviors.
- Help the family manage any problems with implementation (e.g., problems with prompting, recording points, providing rewards, or implementing organizational routines).

Review Home Exercise: Task-Planning Conferences

Ask the parent and child to discuss the Task-Planning Conferences they conducted at home, and review the copies of Handout 45 that they completed. Ask whether they had any difficulty completing these conferences, and problem-solve any issues that may have interfered with completion. Indicate that the handout they will be using after today's session will be expanded slightly, to include the next steps in planning: considering what materials are needed for each step, arranging the steps, and thinking about how long each step will take.

Conduct Skills Building with the Child Alone: Task Planning, Continued

Begin by awarding the child session points (Therapist Form 5) and providing praise for good listening and discussion with the parent present.

Discuss the Next Steps in Task Planning

Begin by reviewing the first steps (1 and 2a) in planning, which were learned and practiced in the previous session and at home: stating the goal and breaking it down into steps. Explain that using these steps to plan our actions can help us control the Go-Ahead-Don't-Plan Glitch, by helping us accomplish our goals. When we break down what needs to be done into smaller steps, we ensure that we don't miss anything in getting that task done. Praise the child for using these first steps with practice activities, and indicate that this session will focus on adding the next few steps in planning to the child's repertoire. Show the child Handout 44, and point out the next steps:

2b. *Stuff you need*: What materials will you need to complete the steps?
3a. *Arrange the steps*: In what order will you complete the steps?
3b. *Plan your time*: How much time will you need for each step?

Tell the child:

"The first steps in planning—knowing your goal and breaking down your goal into smaller steps—are important actions for controlling the Go-Ahead-Don't-Plan Glitch. In order for your plan to run really smoothly, though, you also need to control the Go-Ahead-Forget-It Glitch and the Time Bandit. To make sure the Go-Ahead-Forget-It Glitch doesn't get in the way of your plan, you'll need to figure out what supplies or materials you need to complete each of the steps you have listed. You can plan a visit to the park to shoot hoops with your friends and list all of the steps well, but if you forget to take the basketball, you won't be able to play ball when you get there.

"Don't forget that the Time Bandit loves it when you waste time, so you have to watch out for that Glitch, too, when you plan. You want to make sure the steps are put in a logical order, so that you don't waste your time doing things in a way that doesn't make sense. For example, if you want to bake brownies, and decide to mix the eggs with the flour, cocoa, and sugar before you break the eggs, the shell will be mixed in with the other ingredients. You don't want to have crunchy brownies, so you'll have to spend a lot of time picking out the tiny pieces of shell from your batter. If you consider the order of your steps first, you won't run into these problems; you'll know to crack the eggs before you add them to the rest of the batter. Finally, to really keep the Time Bandit under control, you need to think about how long each step will take, so you can make sure to leave enough time to get all of the steps done."

Provide a Demonstration of the Next Steps in Task Planning

To further clarify how to use the next steps in task planning, use a brief example of an activity that requires planning, and describe how each of the planning steps must be used to make sure the activity gets done. For example, describe how you planned a surprise party with a special meal for a family member, how you planned for a race or other sport, or how you prepared for an important presentation or report, highlighting the importance of considering what you need for each step and managing your time. You may use Therapist Form 27 to illustrate the steps in planning, as you describe how you planned for one of these activities (planning a surprise party). Or you can use another example activity, and fill in the appropriate columns on a blank copy of Handout 48 as you go through the steps.

Conduct In-Session Practice: Task Planning with Steps for Managing Materials and Time

Guide the child through at least four practice Task-Planning Conferences, using two activities related to school projects and two activities that are interesting to the child. Using Handout 48, prompt the child to describe how to answer the questions under "Getting Ready to Go" and the first two steps under "Time Management" (ordering the steps and determining how long each step should take), taking notes as the child describes the plan. As you discuss the "Time Management" steps, point out how these steps are similar to the steps in a Time-Planning Conference: The child must consider what needs to be done and estimate how long each step will take. The child will then be able to determine how to fit each of the steps into the schedule (this last step will be practiced extensively in Session 17).

For the practice Task-Planning Conferences, you may select an example from the following list or create your own, using information about the child's typical school projects or activities that the child enjoys.

1. *Sleepover.* You want to have a friend sleep over at your house, and you want to plan your night, so you make sure to have as much fun as possible.
2. *Getting ready for the game.* You are the equipment manager for the [insert name of regional baseball, basketball, hockey, football, or soccer team]. You have to make sure that the players' equipment is ready for their game. Consider things like uniforms (which must be laundered), play equipment, playbooks, and so on.
3. *Book report.* You have to write a book report about a novel, including a summary of the plot, a description of the main character, and a description of your favorite part of the book. You also have to draw a picture of a scene from the book.
4. *Homework.* You have to study for a social studies quiz on a chapter in your textbook, and complete math worksheets (one sheet with 6 word problems and one sheet with 10 calculations). The social studies chapter is about 15 pages long, and you have a set of 10 study questions you must complete.
5. *Fashion show.* You are the producer for a major designer's fashion show. To be ready for the show, you must make sure that all the models' outfits are ready, prepare the music list for the show, and arrange for hairdressing and makeup for the models.
6. *Lemonade stand.* You want to earn some money by setting up a lemonade and cookie stand in front of your house.
7. *Science project.* You have to complete a science project, exploring how flowers attract bees. You must conduct research on the topic, do one observation outside, and create a poster that describes your findings.

Provide praise and session points as the child engages in the task-planning steps for each practice activity.

HELPFUL HINT: You may provide suggestions if the child has difficulty with any of the steps (e.g., determining how long a given step might take), but should attempt to elicit most of the ideas from the child. Task-Planning Conferences are meant to be collaborative experiences; it is not expected that the child will be able to complete an entire plan for an activity independently, especially when this skill is still being learned. An adult will need to work with the child to encourage a thoughtful and appropriate consideration of each of the planning steps, and may need to write in the responses on Handout 48 to prevent this task from seeming too tedious to the child. This handout is meant to shape an understanding of how to consider all relevant steps in planning; ultimately, the parent and child should be able to engage in a brief planning "conference" without the use of this handout, in an informal manner, once these steps are internalized.

Wrap Up the Session (with Parent/Child)

Support the Child in Discussing Expanded Task-Planning Steps

Have the child review Steps 1–3b in task planning, with their more detailed components, for the parent; the information on Handout 44 should be used as a guide. The child should also show the parent the sample copies of Handout 48 that were completed in session, pointing out how she stated the goal for each activity and then broke it down into steps, considered what was needed for each step, arranged the steps, and determined how long each step would take.

Describe Home Exercise: Task-Planning Conferences

Ask the parent to work with the child each day to complete two Task-Planning Conferences (Handout 48), using the steps practiced in this session. Explain that one Task-Planning Conference should be used daily to replace the Time-Planning Conference in planning homework completion. The child should use Handout 44 to plan for homework, answering each of the planning questions:

1. *Think about the goal*: Complete homework.
2. *Get Ready to Go*;
   a. *Break it down*: List the homework assignments for the day.
   b. *Stuff you need*: Consider what materials are needed for each assignment.
3. *Manage your time*:
   a. *Arrange the steps*: Decide which assignment to do first, second, third, and so forth.
   b. *Plan your time*: Estimate how long it will take to do each assignment.
   c. *Fit it in*: Look at the Personal Calendar and daily schedule, and then decide when to complete homework. (*Note*: "Fitting it in" has not been emphasized in this session's task-planning practice; however, the child should be familiar with fitting homework into the daily schedule, since this has been practiced extensively in Time-Planning Conferences.)
4. *Check It Out*: The child can put a check mark in this column on Handout 48 when each assignment is completed appropriately.

In addition to the Task-Planning Conference to be completed for homework each day, the parent should support the child in completing a Task-Planning Conference for another activity—either an imaginary activity (see Handout 46 for ideas), or a chore or other task that the child must complete (e.g., cleaning a room, setting the table, going to an extracurricular activity). For this activity, the child only needs to focus on the planning steps that were practiced in this session; the child does not have to determine how to fit it into the schedule or check it out.

Review the Home Behavior Record

Show the parent the Home Behavior Record (Handout 19), and review which behaviors the parent will prompt, monitor, praise, and reward. The following is a suggested list of behaviors that might be appropriate for the Home Behavior Record, though variations might make sense for some children.

- *School behavior 1*: Completed all in-class assignments on time.
- *School behavior 2*: Completed the Time Tracker for In-Class Work for an in-class assignment, *or* completed a Task-Planning Conference for an in-class assignment.
- *Home behavior 1*: Completed a Task-Planning Conference for homework.
- *Home behavior 2*: Completed a Task-Planning Conference for another activity.
- *Home behavior 3*: Completed a home task (selected by parent) on time.

Add New Target Behaviors to the DAR Folder

The target behaviors for which the teacher will provide school points are these:

1. Completed all in-class assignments on time.
2. Completed the Time Tracker for In-Class Work for an in-class assignment, *or* completed a Task-Planning Conference for an in-class assignment.

HELPFUL HINT: The completion of an in-class Task Planning Conference may not be realistic or necessary for some children and teachers. Thus you may use your discretion in selecting target behaviors for the DAR at this point in treatment. If you have spoken with the teacher and determined that the child must use planning skills at school, multiple times each week (e.g., planning time for independent work time; working on a long-term independent research project), you may suggest that the teacher use the Task-Planning Conference as a useful tool for helping the child plan his time at school. If the teacher does not believe that task planning will be relevant to the child for in-class work, you may continue to suggest that the teacher praise and award points for the use of time management skills. Alternatively, you may decide, with the teacher, that the child could use additional reinforcement for skills that were learned earlier in treatment (e.g., getting Ready to Go or keeping track of assignments), and you may add those skills to the list of target behaviors for the DAR. Keep in mind that target behaviors should be those that have a good probability of occurring on a given day; the child should not be returning home more days than not with a DAR that has "N/A" noted in the column for the teacher points. This will decrease the child's motivation for earning those points, and will make it difficult for the parent to award points and rewards at home.

Reward the Child

Review the Session Points and Notes (Therapist Form 5) with the child, and praise the child for the positive behaviors that earned points in the session. Add up the total points earned for this session, and indicate that the child may spend or save the points.

Conclude the Session

Confirm the next session appointment. Give the child and parent the OTMP Checklist for the next session (Handout 49). Remind the parent to bring the Home Behavior Record (Handout 19), and the child to bring the backpack, DAR folder, and binder, with all OTMP papers, to the next session.

SESSION 17

Task Planning
Fitting the Steps into the Schedule

━━━━━━━━━━━━━━━ **GOALS FOR THE SESSION** ━━━━━━━━━━━━━━━

You will:

- Review the Task-Planning Conferences completed by the parent and child at home.
- Confirm the child's understanding of the task-planning steps practiced thus far.
- Teach the child how to use time management skills to fit task-planning steps into the daily schedule.
- Contact the teacher, before Session 18, to check on progress and ask about any long-term, multistep assignments that the child must complete in the near future.

The child will:

- Understand how to use Steps 1–3 of task planning (think about the goal, get Ready to Go, and manage your time) in their entirety.
- Learn how to coordinate time management with task planning by fitting steps into the schedule.
- Practice fitting in the steps for imaginary and school-related activities.

The parent will:

- Describe efforts to prompt, monitor, praise, and reward target behaviors.
- Agree to work with the child on completing two Task-Planning Conferences daily, for homework and another activity.
- Agree to prompt, monitor, praise, and reward specified target behaviors between sessions, using the Home Behavior Record.
- Think about an upcoming family activity or project that will require planning.

200

MATERIALS NEEDED

For the parent:

- Handout 19, Home Behavior Record

For you:

- Therapist Form 5, Session Points and Notes
- Therapist Form 28, Sample Projects for In-Session Practice

For the child:

- Child's DAR folder, binder, and backpack
- Handout 44, Steps in Task Planning
- Handout 46, Home Exercise Ideas: Task Planning
- Handout 48, Task-Planning Conference (four copies for in-session practice; eight copies for home practice, stapled)
- Handout 50, OTMP Checklist: Things to Remember for Session 18

SESSION SUMMARY CHECKLIST FOR SESSION 17

Item	Item Completed
Review implementation of the behavior-monitoring and point program (with parent/child)	
Review the Home Behavior Record	Yes/No
Review home exercise: Task Planning Conferences	Yes/No
Conduct skills building with the child alone: Task planning, continued	
Review task-planning steps (Handout 44)	Yes/No
Discuss time management and planning: Fitting it in	Yes/No
Conduct in-session practice: Task planning with a focus on fitting it in (Handout 48)	Yes/No
Wrap up the session (with parent/child)	
Support the child in discussing "Fitting It In"	Yes/No
Describe home exercise: Task-Planning Conferences (Handout 48)	Yes/No
Review the Home Behavior Record (Handout 19)	Yes/No
Add new target behaviors to the DAR folder	Yes/No
Reward the child (Therapist Form 5)	Yes/No
Conclude the session	Yes/No

ABOUT THIS SESSION

In this session, the child will focus on how to integrate time management skills with task planning by fitting the steps for task completion into the usual schedule. This is an important component of task planning for long-term projects, as well as for projects that must be completed over a shorter period of time. The child will practice this skill with a number of imaginary projects and one actual school-related project, by going through all of the steps in planning covered thus far (thinking about the goal, breaking it down, and managing your time) and then focusing on how to fit the planned steps into the schedule, which is the final part of Step 3.

DETAILED SESSION CONTENT

Review Implementation of the Behavior-Monitoring and Point Program

Review the Home Behavior Record

Review the Home Behavior Record (Handout 19) with the parent, and discuss the child's performance of the OTMP behaviors between sessions.

- Discuss the behaviors that were observed.
- Ask the parent how she prompted the behaviors.
- Review what rewards were used to reinforce the child's performance of the behaviors.
- Help the family manage any problems with implementation (e.g., problems with prompting, recording points, providing rewards, or implementing organizational routines).

Review Home Exercise: Task-Planning Conferences

Ask the parent and child to discuss the planning conferences they conducted at home, and review the copies of Task-Planning Conference handout (Handout 48) that they completed. Ask whether they had any difficulty completing these conferences, and problem-solve any issues that may have interfered with completion. Indicate that the child will be focusing on fitting in the steps for completing an activity or project (Step 3c in Handout 44) in today's session.

Conduct Skills Building with the Child Alone: Task Planning, Continued

Begin by awarding the child session points (Therapist Form 5) and providing praise for good listening and discussion with the parent present.

Review Task-Planning Steps

Review the task-planning steps, asking the child to summarize what must be done for each of the steps (Handout 44). Look at the Task-Planning Conferences that were completed at home in more detail, focusing on how effectively the child broke down homework and other activities into steps, considered what was needed for each step, arranged the steps, and estimated how long each step would take. If the child seems confused about how to use any of the planning steps, clarify how to use the steps, reviewing their appropriate use for the activities that were considered for the home exercise.

Discuss Time Management and Planning: Fitting It In

Tell the child:

> "In the previous session, we talked about the importance of thinking about time when you are planning an activity or project. You learned how to arrange the steps in your plan so that you use your time well, and you also practiced estimating how long each step in your plan would take. At home, you also practiced using the last important time management skill that's related to planning, when you thought about how to fit your completion of homework assignments into your daily schedule. Today we're going to practice fitting the planned steps for an activity or project into your schedule, by using some imaginary examples of projects that have to be completed over a few days. We will also practice fitting it in by thinking about how you could fit a typical long-term school assignment into your schedule. We will use your Personal Calendar to decide when you could fit in the steps for completing all of these activities."

Conduct In-Session Practice: Task Planning with a Focus on Fitting It In

Guide the child through two or three practice Task-Planning Conferences, using activities that the child selects from the Sample Projects for In-Session Practice (Therapist Form 28). Show the child the description for each sample project, to make it easier to break each task down into steps. Using the complete Task-Planning Conference handout (Handout 48) to record the child's responses, prompt the child to consider the questions under "Getting Ready to Go" and "Time Management." In order to decide when each step should be fitted into the schedule, instruct the child to consult the Personal Calendar. (This should be part of the child's file; the child should also have a copy in the OTMP folder.) The child should use the current day of the week as the starting point for each of the projects. You can prompt the child with targeted questions such as these:

> "Do you have any time to work on [insert the child's suggested first step for the selected project] tomorrow?"
> "Look at your homework assignments for today. Will you have any time left over to start working on one of the steps for this project?"
> "What about the weekend? Could you get one of the bigger steps done on Saturday or Sunday?"

Provide praise and session points as the child engages in the task-planning steps for each practice activity. Then ask the child to think about long-term school projects (e.g., book reports, science fair projects, research projects, biographies) that have been assigned during this school year. Or, if the child already knows of an upcoming school project, you can begin to engage in planning for that assignment. (If the child is not aware of such a project, you will be consulting with the teacher to determine whether there is such a project, in preparation for Session 18.) Choose one of the assignments and practice planning for completion of that assignment, as if it were due in the next week or two (depending on the nature of the project).

Record the child's responses to each of the planning prompts on Handout 48. Then help the child determine when to fit in each of the steps toward completing the project, by considering the Personal Calendar and other assignments that are due. Provide praise and session points for this practice.

Wrap Up the Session (with Parent/Child)

Support the Child in Discussing Fitting It In

Guide the child in explaining the process of fitting in the steps for task completion, considering the Personal Calendar and other assignments that are due. Show the parent the copies of the Task-Planning Conference (Handout 48) that were completed in session for the sample projects and school assignment, and describe how the child determined when to fit in each of the steps for the projects.

Describe Home Exercise: Task-Planning Conferences

Ask the parent to work with the child each day to complete two Task-Planning Conferences (Handout 48), using all of the steps practiced in this session (Steps 1–3 on Handout 44). One Task-Planning Conference should be used to plan for homework completion (during the week) or a leisure activity (for the weekend). Another one should be used to practice planning for another activity or project; if there are no relevant activities/projects, the parent and child may select an imaginary activity from Home Exercise Ideas: Task Planning (Handout 46). For both of the daily Time-Planning Conferences, the parent should guide the child to consider when to fit in each of the steps for completion of the activity/project.

Finally, ask the parent to think about any upcoming family projects, activities, or events for which the child may need to plan (e.g., a holiday meal, a family member's birthday party, a family vacation). The parent should be prepared to describe this activity/event/project in detail during the next session, as it will be used for in-session planning practice.

Review the Home Behavior Record

Show the parent the Home Behavior Record (Handout 19), and review which behaviors the parent will prompt, monitor, praise, and reward. The following is a suggested list of behaviors that might be appropriate for the Home Behavior Record, though variations might make sense for some children.

- *School behavior 1*: Completed all in-class assignments on time.
- *School behavior 2*: Completed the Time Tracker for In-Class Work for an in-class assignment, *or* completed a Task-Planning Conference for an in-class assignment.
- *Home behavior 1*: Completed a Task-Planning Conference for homework.
- *Home behavior 2*: Completed a Task-Planning Conference for another activity.
- *Home behavior 3*: Completed a home task (selected by parent) on time.

Add New Target Behaviors to the DAR Folder

The target behaviors for which the teacher will provide school points are these:

1. Completed all in-class assignments on time.
2. Completed the Time Tracker for In-Class Work for an in-class assignment, *or* completed a Task-Planning Conference for an in-class assignment.

Reward the Child

Review the Session Points and Notes (Therapist Form 5) with the child, and praise the child for the positive behaviors that earned points in the session. Add up the total points earned for this session, and indicate that the child may spend or save the points.

Conclude the Session

Confirm the next session appointment. Give the child and parent the OTMP Checklist for the next session (Handout 50). Remind the parent to bring the Home Behavior Record (Handout 19), and the child to bring the backpack, DAR folder, and binder, with all OTMP papers, to the next session.

SESSION 18

Task Planning
Planning for Long-Term Projects

━━━━━━━ **GOALS FOR THE SESSION** ━━━━━━━

You will:

- Review the Task-Planning Conferences completed by the parent and child at home.
- Work with the child on planning for an upcoming school project (based on information gathered from the teacher, if applicable).
- Help the child apply all of the task-planning steps to planning for long-term projects at home and for school.

The child will:

- Practice using task-planning steps to plan for long-term projects at home and for school.

The parent will:

- Describe efforts to prompt, monitor, praise, and reward target behaviors.
- Share information about long-term activities/projects that the child could plan at home.
- Agree to conduct two Task-Planning Conferences daily with the child.
- Agree to prompt, monitor, praise, and reward specified target behaviors between sessions, using the Home Behavior Record.

━━━━━━━ **MATERIALS NEEDED** ━━━━━━━

For the parent:

- Handout 19, Home Behavior Record

For you:

■ Therapist Form 5, Session Points and Notes

For the child:

■ Child's DAR folder, binder, and backpack
■ Handout 48, Task-Planning Conference (four copies for in-session practice; eight copies for home practice, stapled)
■ Handout 51, OTMP Checklist: Things to Remember for Session 19

ABOUT THIS SESSION

This session is intended to consolidate the child's use of task-planning skills, by helping the child apply the planning steps to planning for long-term projects that must be completed over the course of a few days or weeks. The child will not learn any new steps in this session; instead, the child will practice the use of the steps learned thus far, in planning for upcoming

SESSION SUMMARY CHECKLIST FOR SESSION 18	
Item	Item Completed
Review implementation of the behavior-monitoring and point program (with parent/child)	
Review the Home Behavior Record	Yes/No
Review home exercise: Task-Planning Conferences	Yes/No
Discuss home activities that require planning	Yes/No
Conduct skills building with the child alone: Task Planning, continued	
Conduct OST homework review: Task-Planning Conferences	Yes/No
Discuss applying task-planning steps to long-term projects	Yes/No
Conduct in-session practice: Task planning for long-term projects (Handout 48)	Yes/No
Wrap up the session (with parent/child)	
Support the child in discussing planning for long-term projects	Yes/No
Describe home exercise: Task-Planning Conferences (Handout 48)	Yes/No
Review the Home Behavior Record (Handout 19)	Yes/No
Add new target behaviors to the DAR folder	Yes/No
Reward the child (Therapist Form 5)	Yes/No
Conclude the session (Handout 51)	Yes/No

projects that must be completed at home (e.g., planning a party, sleepover, or vacation) or for school (e.g., book report, research project, or diorama). This practice will help the child integrate the skills of tracking assignments (i.e., listing the steps necessary for completion of the project), managing materials (i.e., determining what is needed for each step), time management (i.e., estimating the time needed for each step and fitting it into the schedule), and task planning (i.e., putting all of these steps together into a coherent, reasonable plan). The real-life application of task planning to a project that must be completed in the near future will also help the child see how this skill can be useful in daily life.

DETAILED SESSION CONTENT

Review Implementation of the Behavior-Monitoring and Point Program

Review the Home Behavior Record

Review the Home Behavior Record (Handout 19) with the parent, and discuss the child's performance of the OTMP behaviors between sessions.

- Discuss the behaviors that were observed.
- Ask the parent how he prompted the behaviors.
- Review what rewards were used to reinforce the child's performance of the behaviors.
- Help the family manage any problems with implementation (e.g., problems with prompting, recording points, providing rewards, or implementing organizational routines).

Review Home Exercise: Task-Planning Conferences

Ask the parent and child to discuss the Task-Planning Conferences they conducted at home, and review the copies of the Task-Planning Conference handout (Handout 48) that they completed. Ask whether they had any difficulty completing these conferences, and problem-solve any issues that may have interfered with completion. Check to make sure that the child remains motivated to use the Task-Planning Conferences at home, and that the parent is providing enough support (e.g., taking notes for the child during the discussion, praising the child for any efforts to discuss planning) to keep the child engaged in this process.

Discuss Home Activities That Require Planning

Ask the parent to help you make a list of family activities that are likely to happen in the next few weeks (e.g., a family trip or vacation, a party, an important outing, a family project). Focus on activities that the child could realistically help plan. Indicate that you will work with the child in this session to apply the planning steps to preparations for one of these family activities.

Conduct Skills Building with the Child Alone: Task Planning, Continued

Begin by awarding the child session points (Therapist Form 5) and providing praise for good listening and discussion with the parent present.

Conduct OST Homework Review: Task-Planning Conferences

Review the copies of Handout 48 that the child completed at home with the parent between sessions. Ask the child to describe how he came up with the planning steps listed, and praise the child for engaging in this process. Reinforce the importance of developing and following a plan to get things done appropriately, and indicate that as the child gets better at using these planning steps, these Task-Planning Conferences will become brief discussions.

Discuss Applying Task-Planning Steps to Long-Term Projects

Tell the child:

> "So far, we have practiced the task-planning steps with homework, imaginary assignments and projects, and daily activities. You've gotten more comfortable with the steps: thinking about the goal; getting Ready to Go by breaking it down and considering the stuff you need; and managing your time by arranging the steps, planning your time, and fitting the steps into your schedule. Today we will practice using these steps for real school and home projects that have to be completed over the course of a few days or weeks."

Ask the child to describe any long-term assignments that have been completed over the course of the school year (e.g., book reports, research projects, biographies). You may already know about these assignments from prior discussions with the child or teacher; if that is the case, review the information you already have, instead of asking the child to describe the details again. Then ask whether there are any long-term assignments that are due in the next few weeks (referring to your conversation with the teacher, if applicable). Tell the child that you will practice using Task-Planning Conferences to plan for a past and a future school assignment, and for one or more of the family activities that the parent mentioned at the start of the session.

Conduct In-Session Practice: Task Planning for Long-Term Projects

Take out a blank copy of Time-Planning Conference handout (Handout 48), and ask the child to think about a recent long-term project that was completed for school—going through the planning steps in reconstructing the goal, the steps that had to be completed, and the materials that were needed. Then ask the child to pretend that this project is due in the next week. After consulting the Personal Calendar, ask the child to arrange the steps, estimate how long each step would take, and then fit the steps into the schedule for the next week. Provide praise and session points for this mock planning practice. Alternatively, continue the process with the assignment that was discussed in the previous session. Redundant review and reconsideration of these steps are not considered detrimental, as planning is a complex process that is enhanced through extensive practice.

Next, if it has not been done already, ask the child to consider one of the upcoming long-term assignments that are due in the near future. Use another blank copy of Handout 48 to help the child develop a plan for completing this assignment by the due date. Tell the child to file this copy in the binder, and to use it as a guide for completing this long-term assignment.

HELPFUL HINT: If there are no upcoming long-term assignments due in school, create an assignment description that is similar to the types of assignments the child has had in the past, and ask the child to practice planning for this assignment.

Finally, consider one of the family activities that will occur in the next few weeks. Ask the child to develop a plan for completing this activity, using another blank copy of Handout 48. Praise the child and provide session points for cooperative engagement in this process.

Wrap Up the Session (with Parent/Child)

Support the Child in Discussing Planning for Long-Term Projects

Ask the child to explain which school projects and family activities were used to practice planning in session. Have the child show the parent the copies of the Task-Planning Conference handout that were completed for the upcoming school and home projects, and to describe the steps that she will take in completing the projects, the materials she will need, and the plan for fitting these steps into the schedule. Ask the parent to provide feedback on the proposed plans, and encourage the parent and child to discuss any modifications that should be made to the plans, to make sure they can be realistically completed. Provide the child with praise and points for reviewing these plans with the parent.

Describe Home Exercise: Task-Planning Conferences

Ask the parent to continue using task planning daily, aiming to complete at least one Task-Planning Conference (Handout 48) each day for a school or home task. Explain that by continuing to use these planning skills, the child and parent will begin to see planning as a normal part of the daily routine.

Review the Home Behavior Record

Show the parent the Home Behavior Record (Handout 19), and review which behaviors the parent will prompt, monitor, praise, and reward. The following is a suggested list of behaviors that might be appropriate for the Home Behavior Record, though variations might make sense for some children.

- *School behavior 1*: Completed all in-class assignments on time.
- *School behavior 2*: Completed the Time Tracker for In-Class Work for an in-class assignment, *or* completed a Task-Planning Conference for an in-class assignment.
- *Home behavior 1*: Completed a Task-Planning Conference for homework.
- *Home behavior 2*: Completed a Task-Planning Conference for another activity.
- *Home behavior 3*: Completed a home task (selected by parent) on time.

Add New Target Behaviors to the DAR Folder

The target behaviors for which the teacher will provide school points are these:

1. Completed all in-class assignments on time.
2. Completed the Time Tracker for In-Class Work for an in-class assignment, *or* completed a Task-Planning Conference for an in-class assignment.

Reward the Child

Review the Session Points and Notes (Therapist Form 5) with the child, and praise the child for the positive behaviors that earned points in the session. Add up the total points earned for this session, and indicate that the child may spend or save the points.

Conclude the Session

Confirm the next session appointment. Give the child and parent the OTMP Checklist for the next session (Handout 51). Remind the parent to bring the Home Behavior Record (Handout 19), and the child to bring the backpack, DAR folder, and binder, with all OTMP papers, to the next session.

SESSION 19

Task Planning
Checking It Out and Planning for Graduation

═══════════ **GOALS FOR THE SESSION** ═══════════

You will:

- Review the Task-Planning Conferences completed by the parent and child at home.
- Introduce the final step in task planning—Check It Out, which requires a check of the final product for neatness and completeness.
- Help the child plan a script for a personalized commercial, presenting a testimonial about the skills learned in the OST treatment.
- Contact the teacher to indicate that the child should check classwork for neatness and completeness.

The child will:

- Understand how to check work to make sure it is neat and complete.
- Practice the final task-planning skill, Check It Out, with simulated materials.
- Plan a script for a personalized commercial, presenting a testimonial about the skills learned in OST.

The parent will:

- Describe efforts to prompt, monitor, praise, and reward target behaviors.
- Understand how to guide the child in considering whether work is neat and complete.
- Agree to conduct a daily Task-Planning Conference with the child for homework.
- Agree to guide the child in practicing the personalized commercial script between sessions.

MATERIALS NEEDED

For the parent:

- Handout 19, Home Behavior Record
- Handout 53, Helping Your Child Maintain Good Organizational Skills

For you:

- Computer with printer (optional)
- Therapist Form 5, Session Points and Notes
- Therapist Form 29, Materials for Practicing Checking It Out

For the child:

- Child's DAR Folder, binder, and backpack
- Handout 48, Task-Planning Conference (one copy for in-session practice; four copies for home practice, stapled)

SESSION SUMMARY CHECKLIST FOR SESSION 19

Item	Item Completed
Review implementation of the behavior-monitoring and point program (with parent/child)	
Review the Home Behavior Record	Yes/No
Review home exercise: Task-Planning Conferences	Yes/No
Conduct skills building with the child alone: Checking It Out and planning a commercial	
Introduce the last step in task planning: Check It Out	Yes/No
Conduct in-session practice: Check It Out (Therapist Form 29)	Yes/No
Discuss planning a personalized commercial (Handout 52)	Yes/No
Wrap up the session (with parent/child)	
Support the child in discussing how to Check It Out	Yes/No
Describe home exercise: Task-Planning Conferences and practicing the personalized commercial (Handouts 48, 52)	Yes/No
Review the Home Behavior Record (Handout 19)	Yes/No
Add new target behaviors to the DAR folder	Yes/No
Reward the child (Therapist Form 5)	Yes/No
Introduce the concepts of fading and thinning to the parent (Handout 53)	Yes/No
Conclude the session (Handout 54)	Yes/No

■ Handout 52, Personalized Commercial Script Outline
■ Handout 54, OTMP Checklist: Things to Remember for Session 20

ABOUT THIS SESSION

In this session, the child learns the final step in task planning—Check It Out, which involves checking work for neatness and completeness—and practices its use with simulated work products. In addition, the child will use planning skills to develop the script for a personalized commercial, providing a testimonial about the skills learned in the OST treatment. The child must plan for the recording of this commercial, which will occur in the next session. The process of planning for the commercial and reviewing the script with the parent for neatness and completeness reinforces the application of planning to any project. In addition, the task of creating an organized script detailing how OST has been helpful is a useful activity for the child and therapist to complete prior to the final session. This organized review helps the child focus on the skills learned and on the tools that should be used in the future, even after formal treatment has ended.

DETAILED SESSION CONTENT

Review Implementation of the Behavior-Monitoring and Point Program

Review the Home Behavior Record

Review the Home Behavior Record (Handout 19) with the parent, and discuss the child's performance of the OTMP behaviors between sessions.

- Discuss the behaviors that were observed.
- Ask the parent how she prompted the behaviors.
- Review what rewards were used to reinforce the child's performance of the behaviors.
- Help the family manage any problems with implementation (e.g., problems with prompting, recording points, providing rewards, or implementing organizational routines).

HELPFUL HINT: As this is the penultimate session, the parent's use of behavior modification procedures should (ideally) be well established by this point. If so, then you will follow the suggestions at the end of this session regarding parental use of fading and thinning procedures after treatment has ended. However, if implementation remains problematic, you should take some time in this session to identify the lingering issues that have made it difficult for the parent to follow through on these procedures at home. You should then consider developing a simplified behavior modification system and presenting it to the parent in the final session, as an alternative approach to be used when treatment ends. Some suggestions for developing this simplified system are presented in Session 20.

Review Home Exercise: Task-Planning Conferences

Ask the parent and child to discuss the Task-Planning Conferences they conducted at home, and review the copies of the Task-Planning Conference handout (Handout 48) that they completed. Ask whether they had any difficulty completing these conferences, and problem-solve any issues that may have interfered with completion. Check to make sure that the child remains motivated to use the Task-Planning Conferences at home, and that the parent is providing enough support (e.g., taking notes for the child during the discussion, praising the child for any efforts to discuss planning) to keep the child engaged in this process.

Tell the child and parent that the child will learn the final step in task planning in this session: checking work for neatness and completeness. The child will then plan a special, personalized commercial, to be recorded in the next session, describing what the child has learned in OST.

Conduct Skills Building with the Child Alone: Checking It Out and Planning a Commercial

Begin by awarding the child session points (Therapist Form 5) and providing praise for good listening and discussion with the parent present.

Introduce the Last Step in Task Planning: Check It Out

Tell the child:

"Now that you know how to use all components of the first three steps in task planning, let's talk about the final step, which we call 'Check It Out.' In this step, you have to ask yourself the questions 'Did I meet my goal, and is the work correct, neat, and complete?' You must look at your plan and at the work you did, and check whether they are done well and whether your work is neat and complete. So, for example, if you are planning to write a book report, you will first spell out the steps that have to be done; then, as you complete each step, you'll check to see that you have done what you needed to do. When you complete the book report, you'll Check It Out by making sure it is neat (for instance, typed neatly, spelled correctly) and complete (that is, all the necessary parts are included). You can also check your work for neatness and completeness when you are doing a smaller task or assignment. For example, when you complete a school assignment, you might rush through it and hand in a messy paper, or forget to complete some of the items. Your teacher won't like that, and your parents won't be happy, either. If you check your work before you hand it in, and correct any mistakes, you will be able to make sure that the Go-Ahead-Don't-Plan Glitch doesn't get you in trouble.

"So today we're going to practice checking out your work to make sure it is neat and complete. First, let's think a little more about what you should check for when you're looking at some different assignments or projects."

Conduct a brief discussion with the child, giving examples of some assignments and projects, and asking the child to describe what could be checked in each. Below are some examples of assignments to consider, and some elements that could be checked:

1. Written book report (spelling, handwriting, use of full sentences, appropriate capitalization, illustrated cover page, etc.)
2. Diagram of a volcano, with labeled parts (spelling of words, neatness of drawing, labeled parts)
3. Math worksheet (neatness of writing, no missed problems, numbered answers, accuracy of answers, etc.)
4. Packing for a beach vacation (remembering all clothes/shoes needed, including beach toys, making sure all items fit into the suitcase, etc.)

Praise the child and provide session points for thoughtfully considering these examples.

Conduct In-Session Practice: Check It Out

Show the child a set of materials (Therapist Form 29) that are either samples of school work or planning steps for projects. The materials have obvious mistakes in them; the child's job is to critique the materials by checking them for neatness and completeness, and identifying what needs to be fixed. Introduce the materials to the child by saying, "Let's look at some examples of results for school assignments and other projects, and see if we can check the results to see if they are neat and complete." For each sample assignment/project, guide the child in checking the results by asking directed questions:

- Spelling list: "Is this spelling homework neat and complete? If not, why not?"
- Picture of a desk that was supposed to be Ready to Go for homework: "Is this desk Ready to Go for homework time? If not, why not?"
- Picture of an incomplete puzzle: "Is this puzzle complete? If not, why not?"
- Task-Planning Conference handout for soccer practice and picture of soccer bag: "This child wrote out a plan to make sure she had everything she needed for soccer practice. Look at this picture of her packed soccer bag. Did she forget anything? If yes, what did she forget? Is her work neat and complete? If not, why not?"
- Task-Planning Conference handout for sleepover: "Is this plan for a sleepover neat and complete? If not, why not? Did this child forget anything? If yes, what did the child forget?"

As the child responds to prompts to check out the results of these activities and assignments, praise the child for appropriate responses. Remind the child that with this final step in task planning, the child should be able to control the Go-Ahead-Don't-Plan Glitch by making sure that all projects, tasks and assignments are completed correctly, neatly, and completely.

Discuss Planning a Personalized Commercial

Tell the child:

"Since the next session is our last one together, I want to work with you on a special project that will help us think about all the things you have learned in OST. In our final session, we will record a short commercial (about 4–5 minutes long), using a video camera, which would tell other kids about the OST program. We won't actually be putting the commercial on TV; it will just be for you and your parents to keep, to remind you of what you've learned here. Today we're going to work on writing a script, so you will know what to say when we record the commercial next time. We will think about all the parts of the program, and about all the skills you have learned here for controlling the Glitches and becoming more organized. Let's start by planning what needs to be done, so we can record this commercial and do a good job with it."

HELPFUL HINT: Some children may indicate that they do not wish to make a video recording for the commercial. If the child expresses an worries or concerns, you can offer to make an audio recording.

Take out a blank copy of the Task-Planning Conference handout (Handout 48), and help the child consider what steps to take to complete this project (e.g., writing a script, getting a digital recorder, creating cue cards, etc.) and what will be needed for each step (e.g., pencil, paper, digital recorder, index cards). Then help the child decide what to do first, second, third, and so forth, and consult the Personal Calendar to see when the child can fit in practice time with the script at home. Finally, discuss how the child will review the script with the parent to make sure it is neat and complete.

Tell the child that you will work together in this session to create the script, and that the child will review and practice it at home, with the parent. Using Handout 52 (Personalized Commercial Script Outline), guide the child to consider and answer each of the listed questions. Use this outline to create a script that the child can use during the commercial recording. The child is not expected to memorize the script, and can read from the notes while being recorded.

HELPFUL HINT: There are many ways that you can help the child organize and write the script. You may use Handout 52 to write in the child's responses, and allow the child to read directly from that handout, when recording the commercial. Alternatively, you may find that it is simpler to use a computer to type the child's responses and integrate them into a seamless script, which the child can follow. You may also decide to use index cards to record each of the child's responses, and instruct the child to read from the cards. Select a method that is simple for you to implement and for the child to understand and use. You will give the child a copy of the script to take home and practice, and you should retain a copy in the child's file, in case the child forgets the script at home for the next session.

Wrap Up the Session (with Parent/Child)

Support the Child in Discussing How to Check It Out

Ask the child to tell the parent about the final step in task planning, Check It Out, and to explain why it is important to check that assignments or projects are done correctly, neatly, and completely. The child may share some of the examples discussed in session, to show the parent how different types of assignments/projects can be checked for neatness and completeness. Indicate that this final step should be included from now on in all Task-Planning Conferences at home.

Describe Home Exercise: Task-Planning Conferences and Practicing the Personalized Commercial

Ask the parent to continue using task planning daily, aiming to complete at least one Task-Planning Conference each day for homework (using Handout 48), including the final step of Checking It Out. Explain that by continuing to use these planning skills, the child and parent will begin to see planning as a normal part of the daily routine.

In addition, ask the child to show the parent the personalized commercial script, and explain that this commercial will be recorded in the next session. Ask the parent and child to review the script at home and make sure it is neat and complete. If the parent believes that the child has left out any aspect of the program that was helpful, the parent can work with the child to integrate more information into the script. In addition, the parent should prompt the child to practice the script at home before the next session.

Review the Home Behavior Record

Show the parent the Home Behavior Record (Handout 19), and review which behaviors the parent will prompt, monitor, praise, and reward. The following is a suggested list of behaviors that might be appropriate for the Home Behavior Record, though variations might make sense for some children.

- *School behavior 1*: Completed all in-class assignments on time.
- *School behavior 2*: Showed evidence of Checking It Out by handing in a selected assignment that was neat and complete.
- *Home behavior 1*: Completed a Task-Planning Conference for homework, and included checking it out.
- *Home behavior 2*: Practiced the personalized commercial script.
- *Home behavior 3*: Completed tasks at home on time.

Add New Target Behaviors to the DAR Folder

The target behaviors for which the teacher will provide school points are these:

1. Completed all in-class assignments on time.
2. Checked all in-class assignments for neatness and completeness.

Reward the Child

Review the Session Points and Notes (Therapist Form 5) with the child, and praise the child for the positive behaviors that earned points in the session. Add up the total points earned for this session, and indicate that the child may spend or save the points.

Introduce the Concepts of Fading and Thinning to the Parent

When the parent has been consistently using the behavior modification system at home, say that he can make some changes to the prompting and reward procedures after treatment has ended. These changes are intended to help the child become more self-reliant in using the OTMP skills learned during the OST program. Give the parent Handout 53 (Helping Your Child Maintain Good Organizational Skills), and ask the parent to read it before the next session. Tell the parent that there will be an opportunity to review and answer any questions about the information in the handout during the next session.

Conclude the Session

Confirm the next session appointment. Give the child and parent the OTMP Checklist for the final session (Handout 54). Remind the parent to bring the Home Behavior Record (Handout 19), and the child to bring the backpack, DAR folder, and binder, with all OTMP papers, to the next session.

SESSION 20

Program Summary
Personalized Commercial and Graduation

GOALS FOR THE SESSION

You will:

- Provide the child with an interactive overview of the basic concepts and skills learned over the course of the program.
- Record the child's personalized commercial.
- Review with the parent and child how they can continue to implement the OTMP skills and praise–point–reward systems at home and in school.

The child will:

- Understand why it is important to keep working on organization: To keep the Glitches under control.
- Demonstrate understanding of the different OTMP skills (keeping track of assignments, managing materials, managing time, and planning tasks).
- Present a personalized commercial, and view the recording with you and the parent.

The parent will:

- Describe efforts to prompt, monitor, praise, and reward target behaviors.
- Demonstrate understanding of how to continue to motivate the child to use the OTMP skills at home and in school, using an appropriate praise–point–reward system.

MATERIALS NEEDED

For you:

- Video recorder with playback feature
- Therapist Form 5, Session Points and Notes

For the child:

- Child's DAR folder, binder, and backpack
- Personalized commercial script (completed in Session 19, with Handout 52 as a guide)
- Handout 55, Owner's Manual for Organizational Skills
- Handout 56, OST Graduation Certificate

IN PREPARATION FOR THIS SESSION

You should set up a digital video recorder to record the child's personalized commercial. The recorder should contain a playback feature, so that the child and parent can view the commercial at the end of the session (even if it is only viewed on the small recorder screen). It is suggested that you burn a CD of the commercial after the session and mail it to the parent and child, or e-mail them a copy of the video file

At the end of this session, you must be prepared to discuss how the parent can continue to motivate the child to use organizational skills at home and school. You should consider how effectively the parent has implemented the behavior modification system throughout treatment. If the parent has been able to use the full behavior modification system with ease, consistently recording points and giving rewards, she can be advised to begin using the fading and thinning procedures (which are described in Handout 53) to modify the way in

---

SESSION SUMMARY CHECKLIST FOR SESSION 20

Item	Item Completed
Review implementation of the behavior-monitoring and point program (with parent/child)	
Review the Home Behavior Record	Yes/No
Review home exercise: Task-Planning Conference and commercial	Yes/No
Conduct skills building with the child alone: Program summary	
Review basic OST concepts	Yes/No
Discuss how to keep controlling the Glitches (Handout 55)	Yes/No
Review and record the personalized commercial	Yes/No
Wrap up the session (with parent/child)	
Show the commercial to the child and parent	Yes/No
Present the OST Graduation certificate (Handout 56) and Owner's Manual for Organizational Skills (Handout 55)	Yes/No
Review behavior modification techniques	Yes/No
Reward the child (Therapist Form 5)	Yes/No

which she prompts and rewards the child's use of organizational skills. However, if the parent has been inconsistent in implementation, or does not believe that this full system can be realistically used after treatment ends, you should help the parent develop a simplified system for prompting, praising, and rewarding the use of organizational skills. See the "Review Behavior Modification Techniques" section near the end of this session for guidelines and suggestions.

ABOUT THIS SESSION

This session provides an opportunity to summarize the main concepts, principles, and skills learned throughout treatment, and to praise the child for successful completion of the program. You will review why the child must work to control the Glitches, as well as the organizational skills that the child can use to keep the Mastermind in charge. The child will also recognize which Glitches are most problematic, and will develop a plan for keeping those Glitches in check. You and the parent will praise the child's accomplishments, noting the ways in which the child has learned to improve OTMP skills. Finally, the parent will work with you to develop an appropriate reinforcement system that will motivate continued use of these skills. By the end of this session, the child and parent should feel confident about their ability to continue working on managing the Glitches.

DETAILED SESSION CONTENT

Review Implementation of the Behavior-Monitoring and Point Program

Review the Home Behavior Record

Review the Home Behavior Record (Handout 19) with the parent, and discuss the child's performance of the OTMP behaviors between sessions and the rewards that were earned for the most recently acquired skills. Indicate that at the end of this session you will discuss ways to continue reinforcing the child's use of OTMP skills.

Review Home Exercise: Task-Planning Conferences and Commercial

Ask the parent and child to discuss the Task-Planning Conferences they conducted at home, and review the copies of the Task-Planning Conference handout (Handout 48) that they completed. Ask if they had any difficulty completing these conferences, and problem-solve any issues that may have interfered with completion. Check to make sure that the child remains motivated to use the Task-Planning Conferences at home, and that the parent is providing enough support (e.g., taking notes for the child during the discussion, praising the child for any efforts to discuss planning) to keep the child engaged in this process.

Next, ask the parent and child whether they reviewed the script for the personalized commercial at home, and (if so) whether they made any modifications to the script. Indicate that the child will record the commercial in this session, and that they will be able to view the commercial together at the end of the session.

Conduct Skills Building with the Child Alone: Program Summary

Begin by awarding the child session points (Therapist Form 5) and providing praise for good listening and discussion with the parent present, and for bringing in all appropriate materials.

Review Basic OST Concepts

The following list summarizes the basic concepts underlying the OST program:

- Children with ADHD have difficulty with organizational tasks like tracking assignments, managing materials, managing time, and planning.
- There are different Glitches that lurk in everyone's brain. These Glitches can get children in trouble, by making them forget important events or assignments, lose things they need, get things done on time, and plan appropriately for important projects or assignments.
- If children ignore the Glitches and pretend that there are no problems, the Glitches will cause a lot of trouble.
- The child can fight the Glitches and stay more organized by using the organizational tools and skills that have been learned in this program and practiced repeatedly.
- Parents and teachers can help the child control the Glitches by reminding the child to use organizational tools and skills.

Present a brief review of these fundamental concepts, checking to confirm the child's understanding and encouraging the child to ask questions. You may present this information as a brief monologue, or use questions and answers to involve the child. The following is one way to lead this discussion; however, the review should be personalized for the child, focusing on the particular difficulties that the child has had and the issues that have been most relevant in your work together.

Tell the child:

"Today is our last session, and I want to take some time to review the things we've learned together. Do you remember the very first session, when we talked about ADHD and what children with ADHD experience? We talked about the fact that children with ADHD sometimes have difficulty paying attention, sitting in one place, and making careful decisions. We also learned that children with ADHD have a harder time staying organized—keeping track of assignments, managing materials (like papers, books, and backpacks), getting things done on time, and planning for important assignments and tasks. We've also talked about Glitches: those annoying little creatures that steal our free time, make us forget assignments and lose things we need, and convince us that planning ahead is not really important.

"Now that we've worked together for all these weeks, we know a lot more about how to deal with the Glitches. For example, what will happen if you pretend the Glitches aren't there and you say you have no problems with getting things done at home or school? The Glitches will be thrilled, because they can keep getting you in trouble, convincing you that you don't have to do anything special to stay organized and get things done. Your parents will be angry when you forget things at school and get poor grades for work that is incomplete. Your teachers will be angry when you forget to study for a test or leave your homework at home. You and your parents and teachers will not be working together; instead, it will feel like everyone is ganging up on you.

"In our time working together, we've worked to make sure that everyone is on the same team. You, your parents, and your teacher are all working together to fight the Glitches. You now know all about the Glitches, and you know how they cause problems for you. You've also learned how to use special tools for keeping these Glitches under control. You've learned to keep your papers and books in special places, so they don't get lost; you've learned to keep your workspaces organized, so you are ready to work; you use written reminders, like the backpack checklist, to make sure you don't forget anything; you've learned to use clocks and calendars to organize your schedule and get work done on time; and you've learned to plan your actions. You've also learned to accept help and reminders from the adults who care about you, and you've earned rewards for learning new organizational skills and for continuing to use them.

"If you keep using the skills you've learned here, and working with your parents and teachers to keep an eye on the Glitches, you will be able to keep your Mastermind in control and stay organized. You will have to remember that the Glitches can always get you if you're not careful. But if you use simple steps that you practice all the time, you will be able to keep these Glitches under control in your life."

Discuss How to Keep Controlling the Glitches

Ask the child which Glitches are the trickiest and the most likely to cause problems for her. Emphasize that the child should be extra careful about looking out for situations when those Glitches can cause problems, and then using OTMP skills to keep them under control. Remind the child about the skills learned in each of the following areas, and tell the child that tips for using these skills can be found in the Owner's Manual for Organizational Skills (Handout 55), which the child and parent will take home today. Conduct an interactive review, asking the child to tell you which skills can help with the different areas, and filling in the skills that the child does not mention.

Tracking Assignments
- DAR
- Assignment and Test Calendar

Managing Materials
- Accordion binder
- Backpack checklist
- Other checklists for activity bags
- Ready to Go

Time Management
- Personal Calendar
- Time Trackers for Homework and In-Class Assignments

- Time-Planning Conferences for homework and regular routines
- Strategies for battling personal problems with the Time Bandit

Task Planning

- Task-Planning Conferences, including these steps:
  - Think about the Goal
  - Get Ready to Go
  - Manage your time
  - Check It Out

Review and Record the Personalized Commercial

Ask the child to take out the commercial script and practice reading through it once. If the child wants to use any props, make sure those are set up. Then tell the child that you will record the commercial, and remind the child to speak clearly and slowly. After recording, show the child the video; if the child would like to make any changes, you may record the commercial again until the child is pleased with the result.

Wrap Up the Session (with Parent/Child)

Show the Commercial to the Child and Parent

Play the commercial for the child and parent, and praise the child for completing the commercial and thinking about the ways that OST has been helpful. Tell the child and parent that you will create a copy of the commercial and send it to them, by U.S. mail or e-mail.

Present the OST Graduation Certificate and Owner's Manual

Support the child in telling the parent what you discussed in this session—that is, reviewing how the child must continue using the OTMP skills and tools to battle the Glitches. Present the child and parent with the Owner's Manual for Organizational Skills (Handout 55), and show them the major features. Point out that many forms and guidelines for using the various organizational skills can be found in the manual. Encourage the parent and child to use the Owner's Manual as a resource, to help the child continue using these skills in school and at home. Finally, present the child with the OST Graduation Certificate (Handout 56), and congratulate the child and parent for completing the program successfully.

Review Behavior Modification Techniques

Remind the parent that adult encouragement and support will be essential in helping the child continue to use the organizational skills learned in the program. If the parent and child have been using the points and rewards system appropriately and it has been useful, the parent should continue prompting, monitoring, praising, and rewarding the child for using these skills at home and school. However, to help the child become less dependent on the parent and more self-reliant in using the skills, the parent can begin to cut back on the frequency of prompts and rewards. Reducing prompts is called "fading," and reducing rewards is called "thinning," as described in Handout 53. Ask whether the parent has any questions about why and how to fade prompts and thin rewards. Inform the parent that the information about fading and thinning is also included in the Owner's Manual (Handout 55), which the parent should refer to as needed to implement the behavior modification system at home after treatment has ended.

If the family has had difficulty implementing the behavior modification system throughout treatment, you may present a simplified system that you believe will work for the family. For example, if the parent does not have the time to keep a daily chart, the parent can give the child a certain number of points and a reward at the end of the week for meeting organizational demands throughout the week. Whatever point–reward system the parent decides to use, it is important to emphasize that the parent must continue to give the child frequent reminders to use organizational skills, and must follow up with consistent praise when the child demonstrates positive performance.

Reward the Child

Review the Session Points and Notes (Therapist Form 5) with the child and praise the child for the positive behaviors that earned points in the session. Add up the total points earned for this session, along with any points saved from previous sessions, and indicate that the child may spend the points on a final reward.

PART III

OST Forms and Handouts

THERAPIST FORMS

Form number	Form title	Applicable sessions
Therapist Form 1	Session Points and Notes—Session 1	1
Therapist Form 2	Interview Record of Problems in Organization, Time Management, and Planning	1
Therapist Form 3	Interference and Conflict Rating Scales	1
Therapist Form 4	Interview Form for Family's Schedule and Activities	1
Therapist Form 5	Session Points and Notes	Multiple sessions (introduced in Session 3)
Therapist Form 6	Interview Form for Tracking Assignments	3
Therapist Form 7	Sample Assignments for DAR and Assignment and Test Calendar Practice	4
Therapist Form 8	Interview Record for School Materials	4
Therapist Forms 9 (Optional)	Trekking Adventure: Instructions for a Special Instrument	4 (Optional)
Therapist Form 10 (Optional)	Trekking Adventure: Instructions to your destination— The Adventurers' General Store	4 (Optional)
Therapist Form 11 (Optional)	Trekking Adventure: Supply List—Use this at the Adventurers' General Store	4 (Optional)
Therapist Form 12 (Optional)	Trekking Adventure: The Special Code	4 (Optional)
Therapist Form 13	Interview on School Materials	7
Therapist Form 14	Photos of Backpacks	8
Therapist Form 15	Ready to Go: What's Up with That Desk?	9

Therapist Form 16 (Optional)	Ready to Go: Materials for Adventure Practice	9 (Optional)
Therapist Form 17	My Personal Calendar: Crystal	10
Therapist Form 18	My Personal Calendar: Carl	10
Therapist Form 19	Time Detective Worksheet: In-Session Activities	10
Therapist Form 20	Review of the Time Tracker for Homework	12
Therapist Form 21 (Optional)	Time Planning for Adventures	12 (Optional)
Therapist Form 22	Work Observation Sheet	13
Therapist Form 23	Practice for Short- and Long-Term Assignments	13
Therapist Form 24 (Optional)	Time Planning for Short- and Long-Term Adventure Activities	13 (Optional)
Therapist Form 25	Time Bandit Record Sheet	14
Therapist Form 26	How Might Homework Time Change?	14
Therapist Form 27	Task-Planning Conference: Example	15
Therapist Form 28	Sample Projects for In-Session Practice	17
Therapist Form 29	Materials for Practicing Checking It Out	19

PARENT AND CHILD HANDOUTS

Handout number	Handout title	Applicable sessions
Handout 1	Overview of Session Content	1
Handout 2	Treatment Expectations	1
Handout 3	Guide to the Glitches	Multiple sessions (introduced in Session 1)
Handout 4	Helping Your Child Use Organizational Skills	2
Handout 5	Interview for Developing a Reward Menu	2
Handout 6	Homework: Let's Consider Possible Rewards	2, 3
Handout 7	Home Behavior Record: Behaviors to Prompt, Monitor, and Praise	2
Handout 8	OTMP Checklist: Things to Remember for Session 3	2
Handout 9	Reward Menu	3
Handout 10	Daily Assignment Record	Multiple sessions (introduced in Session 3)
Handout 11	Assignment and Test Calendar	Multiple sessions (introduced in Session 3)
Handout 12	Reminder for the Daily Assignment Record	3
Handout 13	Home Behavior Record: Behaviors to Prompt, Monitor, and Praise	3
Handout 14	OTMP Checklist: Things to Remember for Session 4	3

Handout 45	Task-Planning Conference: First Steps	15
Handout 46	Home Exercise Ideas: Task Planning	Multiple (introduced in Session 15)
Handout 47	OTMP Checklist: Things to Remember for Session 16	15
Handout 48	Task-Planning Conference	Multiple (introduced in Session 16)
Handout 49	OTMP Checklist: Things to Remember for Session 17	16
Handout 50	OTMP Checklist: Things to Remember for Session 18	17
Handout 51	OTMP Checklist: Things to Remember for Session 19	18
Handout 52	Personalized Commercial Script Outline	19
Handout 53	Helping Your Child Maintain Good Organizational Skills	19
Handout 54	OTMP Checklist: Things to Remember for Session 20	19
Handout 55	Owner's Manual for Organizational Skills	20
Handout 56	OST Graduation Certificate	20

TEACHER FORMS

Form number	Form title	Applicable contact/time
Teacher Form 1	Teacher's Guide to Organizational Skills Training	Contact 1 Beginning of Week 1
Teacher Form 2	Detailed OST Schedule	
Teacher Form 3	Guide to the Daily Assignment Record	
Teacher Form 4	Sample Daily Assignment Record	
Teacher Form 5	Guide to the Accordion Binder	Contact 2 End of Week 2
Teacher Form 6	Getting Ready To Go: Teacher Guidelines	Contact 3 End of Week 4
Teacher Form 7	Introduction to Time Management	Contact 4 End of Week 5
Teacher Form 8	Time Tracker for In-Class Work	
Teacher Form 9	Skills Check-Up	
Teacher Form 10	Introduction to Task Planning	Contact 5 Beginning of Week 8
Teacher Form 11	Sample Task-Planning Conference	

THERAPIST FORMS

Session Points and Notes—Session 1

Talking about how you might become better organized	
Listening carefully to a short story about the Glitches	
Staying calm while hearing about some problems that happen	
Answering questions about activities at home and at school	
Taking home a folder of new materials	
Total points earned today	

Session notes. _____

_____

_____

_____

Interview Record of Problems in Organization, Time Management, and Planning

LAPSES IN MEMORY AND MATERIALS MANAGEMENT

Lapses in memory and materials management—Forgetting about assignments and losing track of materials, including papers, books, and other needed materials.	
What concerns do you have about your child's remembering assignments and keeping track of supplies and papers? Could you tell me more about that? When and in what situations do you notice those problems? What has the child's teacher said about those kinds of problems in school?	Notes:
What specific problems do you notice with keeping track of supplies?	
How much do those problems interfere with your child's functioning?	Interference score → 1 to 4
How much do those problems result in conflict at home?	Conflict score → 1 to 4

(continued)

What specific problems do you notice with keeping track of papers?	
How much do those problems interfere with your child's functioning?	Interference score → 1 to 4
How much do those problems result in conflict at home?	Conflict score → 1 to 4
What specific problems do you notice with keeping track of assignments? With knowing what to do for homework and what to bring home in order to do homework?	
How much do those problems interfere with your child's functioning?	Interference score → 1 to 4
How much do those problems result in conflict at home?	Conflict score → 1 to 4

(continued)

Can you think of any other problems in remembering information or items, or losing track of items?	
How much do those problems interfere with your child's functioning?	Interference score → 1 to 4
How much do those problems result in conflict at home?	Conflict score → 1 to 4

PROBLEMS IN TIME MANAGEMENT AND TASK PLANNING

Problems in time management and task planning—Problems in completing tasks on time, problems in knowing what to do to complete tasks, problems in thinking about actions that are required to complete tasks, and problems in executing a plan carefully.	
What concerns do you have with your child completing work and other activities on time and doing things carefully? Could you tell me more about that? When and in what situations do you notice those problems? What has the child's teacher said about those kinds of problems in school?	Notes:

(continued)

Does your child have problems with starting work on time?	
How much do those problems interfere with your child's functioning?	Interference score → 1 to 4
How much do those problems result in conflict at home and at school?	Conflict score → 1 to 4
Does your child have specific problems with completing work on time?	
How much do those problems interfere with your child's functioning?	Interference score → 1 to 4
How much do those problems result in conflict at home and at school?	Conflict score → 1 to 4

(continued)

Does your child have specific problems with doing other activities on time? If yes, what kinds of activities are most problematic?	
How much do those problems interfere with your child's functioning?	Interference score → 1 to 4
How much do those problems result in conflict at home and at school?	Conflict score → 1 to 4
Does your child have specific problems with doing work carefully?	
How much do those problems interfere with your child's functioning?	Interference score → 1 to 4
How much do those problems result in conflict at home and at school?	Conflict score → 1 to 4

(continued)

Does your child have specific problems with planning ahead for assignments, projects, or activities (e.g., play dates, afterschool activities)?	

How much do those problems interfere with your child's functioning?	Interference score → 1 to 4

How much do those problems result in conflict at home and at school?	Conflict score → 1 to 4

Can you think of any other problems in managing time or planning tasks?	

How much do those problems interfere with your child's functioning?	Interference score → 1 to 4

How much do those problems result in conflict at home?	Conflict score → 1 to 4

(continued)

Special Questions on Telling Time	Yes	No
Does your child know how to tell time?		
Does your child know how to read a digital clock?		
To the hour?		
To the half hour?		
To the quarter hour?		
Does your child know how to read an analog clock?		
To the hour?		
To the half hour?		
To the quarter hour?		
Can your child tell how much time has passed from one time on the clock to another time on the clock?		

PROBLEMS WITH ORGANIZED ACTIONS

Problems with organized actions—Insufficient use of proactive behaviors/tools, such as using calendars, making outlines, and using folders or other storage items.	
What concerns do you have with your child's use of organized actions and tools, like planners, calendars, folders, and other storage or organizing tools. Could you tell me more about that? When and in what situations do you notice those problems? What has the child's teacher said about those kinds of problems in school?	Notes:
Does your child have specific problems with using a planner and/or calendar properly to keep track of due dates?	

(continued)

240

How much do those problems interfere with your child's functioning?	Interference score → 1 to 4
How much do those problems result in conflict at home and at school?	Conflict score → 1 to 4
Does your child have specific problems with folders/binders appropriately to manage school papers?	
How much do those problems interfere with your child's functioning?	Interference score → 1 to 4
How much do those problems result in conflict at home and at school?	Conflict score → 1 to 4
Does your child have specific problems with using appropriate storage tools at home to store stuff (e.g., bins for toys, boxes for smaller items, closets and drawers for clothes)?	

(continued)

How much do those problems interfere with your child's functioning?	Interference score → 1 to 4
How much do those problems result in conflict at home and at school?	Conflict score → 1 to 4
Does your child have any other problems with organization, time management, and task planning that we haven't covered?	
How much do those problems interfere with your child's functioning?	Interference score → 1 to 4
How much do those problems result in conflict at home and at school?	Conflict score → 1 to 4

Interference and Conflict Rating Scale

INTERFERENCE RATING SCALE

1. Not at all.

2. Slightly.

3. Pretty much.

4. Very much.

CONFLICT RATING SCALE

1. None.

2. A small amount.

3. Pretty much.

4. Very much.

Interview Form for Family's Schedule and Activities

TYPICAL WEEKDAY

Morning Routine
What time does your child have to get up?
Who is around in the morning while your child is getting ready?
Does anyone help your child get ready?
Who stays with your child until the child gets ready to leave?
What tasks does your child have to take care of before leaving for school?
What time does your child have to leave the house?
How would you say the morning routine goes?

(continued)

After-School Routine
Does your child go to an after-school program? If so, please describe it.
What time does your child arrive home?
When your child arrives home, who else is at home?
When does your child do homework?
How long does it take for your child to do homework?
Does your child have any chores or other regular activities after school (music practice, etc.)?
When do other people arrive home?
When does the family eat dinner?
How would you say the after-school time goes?

(continued)

Evening Routine
What does your child do after dinner?
Who is around after dinner?
What time does your child go to bed?
Who helps your child with the bedtime routine?
How would you say the evening routine goes?

TYPICAL WEEKEND DAY

With what activities is your child involved on the weekend?

(continued)

Does your child have any chores or responsibilities on the weekend?

What does the family do together on the weekends?

Who is usually home on the weekends?

Does your child spend time in different households on the weekend?

Does your child usually have schoolwork to do on the weekends?

Does your child have any other regular activities on the weekend?

How would you describe the weekend time that you have together with your child?

Session Points and Notes

Listening	
Giving examples	
Practicing	
Explaining the new skill	
Packing what you need to take home	
Total points earned today	
Point bank (if saving)	

Session notes: _____

_____

_____

_____

_____

_____

_____

_____

_____

_____

_____

_____

_____

_____

_____

_____

_____

_____

_____

_____

_____

Interview Form for Tracking Assignments

Ask the child the following questions, to guide a discussion on how the child keeps track of assignments for school.

How often do you have homework?

How does your teacher inform the class about assignments?

Have you ever forgotten about assignments, so that you have to call friends? Have you ever gone to school without assignments? Have you ever remembered your assignments too late (e.g., late in the evening or just before school starts)?

(continued)

What are your typical homework assignments?

Do you write down your homework assignments? If so, where do you write them down?

Does the teacher check that the assignments written down are correct?

Do you ever forget the paper/planner/pad that you use for writing down assignments?

(continued)

Does someone at home check your assignment list and then make sure that you have completed the list?

How do you make sure that you have the materials you need to go along with the assignments?

What materials do you typically need at home to complete homework?

(continued)

251

Do you have special items for different subjects, like textbooks, workbooks, notepads, or special notebooks? If so, can you tell me what some of those are?

Do you sometimes get worksheets or special readings for homework? If so, can you give me some examples?

Sample Assignments for DAR and Assignment and Test Calendar Practice

PRACTICE ASSIGNMENT LIST 1

Math—Read pages 23–25 in your math textbook. Do page 19 in your workbook.

Social Studies—You will be writing a report on one tribe of Native Americans, describing the types of homes they used, what foods they ate, and how they interacted with the Europeans. Read about the different tribes, and choose which tribe you want to study by next Friday.

PRACTICE ASSIGNMENT LIST 2

Reading—Read for 20 minutes in your "Reader's Choice" book. Complete a reading response in your reading log.

Math—Complete a worksheet. Begin studying for the math test, which will be next Tuesday.

Science—Read the handout about earthquakes and answer the questions.

PRACTICE ASSIGNMENT LIST 3

Spelling—Do the exercises on page 57 of your workbook (copy the word list three times, and make sentences using the words).

Social Studies—Fill in the state capitals on the map of the United States that was handed out in class. A completed map is due on Monday.

Science—The science fair is coming up. You have to pick a project by Friday. The science fair is on [give a date next month].

PRACTICE ASSIGNMENT LIST 4

Science—Take your mystery powder home. Complete the experiments on the worksheet, and write down your observations. What happens to the powder when you mix it with water? What happens when you mix it with salt?

Math—Complete the problems on pages 16 and 18 in your math workbook. Play the dice game listed on your worksheet with one of your parents or siblings.

Language Arts—Select a new book. A book report is due in 3 weeks, on [give date].

Interview Record Form for School Materials

Let's review your school day and materials.

1. What subjects do you have in school?

2. What materials do you need for each subject, and where do you put these materials?

Subject	Books	Papers	Other supplies	Where do you put these materials?

(continued)

3. Do you get any other papers (e.g., announcements, permission slips, notes from the teacher)?

4. Where do you put your books during the school day?

5. Where do books go when it's time to pack up and go home?

6. Where do you put handouts that your teacher gives you to work on in class?

7. Where do you put homework sheets?

8. Where do you put announcements, permission slips, or other papers that have to go home?

Trekking Adventure: Instructions for a Special Instrument

A "trek" is a long journey. Your "trekking adventure" is one in which you are walking and riding camels through a flat desert with long stretches of sand and rock. On your adventure, you are going to need to find food and water. When you leave on the adventure, you will only have enough food and water for 1 day. At the end of each day, you will need to find hidden treasures of food and drink. These hidden treasures are all over the landscape, but they are buried or hidden from the hot sun.

To help find the supplies, you will need a special tool. It is called the Supply Finder.

To use the Supply Finder, follow these directions:

1. Hold it in your hand.

2. Point the arrow on the top front at the ground in front of you.

3. Wave it back and forth.

4. When it makes a loud "beeping" sound, and the light on the front flashes bright green, that means you have it pointed in the direction of the supplies.

5. Walk in that direction, still holding the finder.

6. The "beeping" gets louder as you get closer and starts letting out a strong, steady siren noise when you are on top of the supplies.

7. Dig a little under the sand, and take out your supplies.

Trekking Adventure: Directions to Your Destination— The Adventurers' General Store

Use your compass and go west for 3 miles. At the first set of rocks, turn 20° to the north, and walk for another 2 miles. Turn to the left, and the Adventurers' General Store is straight in front of you.

Trekking Adventure:
Supply List—Use This at the Adventurers' General Store

1. Map for your next destination

2. Sunglasses

3. Hats

4. A new tent

5. A flashlight

6. Camel treats for the camels

7. A portable fan

8. A portable video game

9. Extra batteries

10. Soda

11. Candy bars

12. A pocket knife

13. Your code paper

14. The directions for the next leg of the trek

Trekking Adventure: The Special Code

Use this code to determine what message has been sent to you while you are on your trek. On many occasions, you will be approached by messengers who will provide you with a warning, a change in plans, or special clues for completing your mission. The messages will include a list of numbers. You must be ready to add every two numbers and use the result to decide what letter should be in the message.

Number	1	2	3	4	5	6	7	8	9	10	11	12	13
Letter	Z	Y	X	W	V	U	T	S	R	Q	P	O	N
Number	14	15	16	17	18	19	20	21	22	23	24	25	26
Letter	M	L	K	J	I	H	G	F	E	D	C	B	A

Example: 11 9 5 7 6 6 13 10 8 7 2 4 18 6 9 7

11 + 9 = 20/G

5 + 7 = 12/O

6 + 6 = 12/O

13 + 10 = 23/D

8 + 7 = 15/L

2 + 4 = 6/U

18 + 6 = 24/C

9 + 7 = 16/K or GOOD LUCK

Interview on School Materials

Questions	Child's Responses
1. How do you figure out what to put in your backpack when you're packing up at the end of the school day or at home? (*Note:* The child may not have an organized method. In this case, ask what the child would probably do or has done in the past to be sure of remembering items to take home or take to school.)	
2. How well has that method worked? Have you had any problems with forgetting to pack certain things that you need in your backpack?	

(continued)

3. What do you almost always have to take back and forth between school and home?	Every day:	On a regular basis (e.g., every Wednesday):
4. What do you have to take back and forth sometimes, but not every day (e.g., project materials, reports, Show and Tell items)?		

Photos of Backpacks

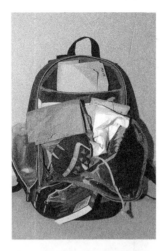
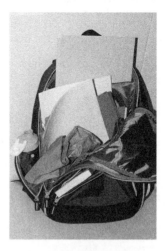
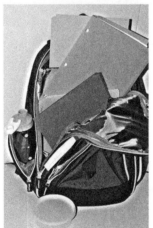
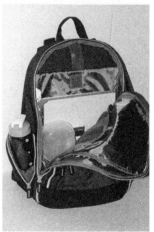
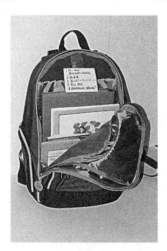

Ready to Go: What's Up with That Desk?

FOR HOME

Where do you usually do homework?	
What supplies or items do you have in that area?	
What supplies or items do you sometimes have to find and bring to that area?	
Do you ever have to stop working to get something?	
Is the space big enough so you can work carefully and neatly?	
When you are done with your homework, do you put things away? By yourself?	

(continued)

Do any Glitches get you when you work in that area or do your homework?	
Are there any other things I should know?	

FOR SCHOOL

Tell me about your workspace at school. Do you have a desk or a table?	
Where do you keep your papers and books in class?	
What about supplies, like pencils, markers, and paper?	
Are you able to find the things you need easily?	
Are there any times when you have trouble finding the things you need?	

(continued)

If there are, why/when does that happen?	
Does your teacher ever tell you that your desk should be neater?	
Does your teacher ever tell you to clear off your desk or put things away while you are working?	
Do you sometimes have to stop work to get supplies?	
Do you sometimes have to stop to put things away because they interfere with your work?	
Is your work area usually clear, and is it large enough for you to do your work?	
Do you have problems with any Glitches when you work at your desk?	
Is there anything else that you can tell me about your desk at school?	

Ready to Go: Materials for Adventure Practice

Note: In preparation for this optional practice, you will need to obtain the following items:

For Activity 1: Adventure to Mars
1. Items that are relevant to the task:
   a. A map of Mars (go to this webpage NASA: *http://mars.jpl.nasa.gov/gallery/atlas/index.html*; use the rectangular map at the top of this page)
   b. A ruler
   c. A pencil or pen
2. Items that are irrelevant to the task:
   a. A compass
   b. A blank DVD in a case, with a label that reads: "SpongeBob on Mars"
   c. Any other distracter items (toys, balls, snacks)

For Activity 2: Superstar Concert Adventure
1. Items that are relevant to the task:
   a. A list of made-up songs (see below)
   b. A list of musicians needed for each song (see below)
   c. Blank paper and pen/pencil
2. Items that are irrelevant to the task:
   a. A *Teen People* (or other) magazine
   b. A music CD and appropriate player or an MP3 player
   c. Some school workbooks or notebooks

For Activity 3: Fashion Show Adventure
1. Items that are relevant to the task:
   a. A listing of models and contact numbers (see below)
   b. A blank calendar (see below)
   c. Writing materials and paper
   d. A telephone (simulated, if necessary)
2. Items that are irrelevant to the task:
   a. A fashion magazine
   b. Art supplies
   c. Toys, games, homework materials, etc.

Activity 1: Adventure to Mars

Directions for the task:

1. You need to map out a route for an exploration team. Your ship has landed on Mars in the Elysium Planitia. You have to describe the route that the group will use to travel to the Olympus Mons.
2. Get the materials Ready to Go: Consider everything you need for this task, put away things you don't need, check that your work area is clear, and make sure there are no things out that could distract you.

(continued)

Activity 2: Superstar Concert Adventure

Directions for the task:

1. A pop star is depending on you to plan her next concert. The star is not feeling well, and is not able to prepare the order of the show for the next concert. You have to make a list of the songs and the order in which they are to be performed. You also have to make a list of the musicians needed for the show.
2. Get the materials for this task Ready to Go: Consider everything you need for this task, put away things you don't need, check that your work area is clear, and make sure there are no things out that could distract you.

Activity 3: Fashion Show Adventure

Directions for the task:

1. You have to arrange to find models for a show that is happening in two weeks. In order to do this, you have to call the models' agents, and then make a list of models who are available to present to the designers.
2. Get the materials that you need Ready to Go: Consider everything you need for this task, put away things you don't need, check that your work area is clear, and make sure there are no things out that could distract you.

SUPERSTAR CONCERT ADVENTURE MATERIALS
Song List

Hits from the '90s

A
"All about Me"
"Always in Love"
"Adventures of the Heart"

B
"Beyond Belief"
"Back Off"
"Blues Rap"

C
"Calling All Dancers"
"Class Trip Cha-Cha"

D
"Dance till You Drop"

E
"Every One Loves Me"
"Endless Dancing"
"Errors of the Heart"

F
"Falling All over Myself"
"Friends Forever"

Recent Songs

"End of the Line"
"Fever for You"
"A Harsh Wind"
"New Century"
"Ride the Waves"
"Show Me the Truth"

(continued)

List of Instruments Needed

Hits from the '90s

A

"All about Me"	Guitars, bass, drums, horns
"Always in Love"	Guitars, bass, drums, flute
"Adventures of the Heart"	Guitars, bass, drums, piano

B

"Beyond Belief"	Guitars, bass, drums, electric organ, chorus
"Back Off"	Guitars, bass, cymbals, drum machine
"Blues Rap"	Beat box, scratching tables, guitars, bass, drums

C

"Calling All Dancers"	Guitars, horns, bass, drums
"Class Trip Cha-Cha"	Orchestra

D

"Dance till You Drop"	Funk band

E

"Every One Loves Me"	Guitars, bass, drums
"Endless Dancing"	Funk band and drum machine
"Errors of the Heart"	Acoustic guitar, bass, piano

F

"Falling All over Myself"	Orchestra
"Friends Forever"	Guitars, bass, drums, horns

Recent Songs

"End of the Line"	Guitars, bass, drums
"Fever for You"	Country band
"A Harsh Wind"	Orchestra
"New Century"	Recorded tape
"Ride the Waves"	Violins, guitars, bass, drums
"Show Me the Truth"	Guitars

FASHION SHOW ADVENTURE MATERIALS
List of Models, Agencies, and Agency Phone Numbers

Model's Name	Agency	Agency Phone Number
Angie Ardslie	We Are Fashion	555-1234
Rob Ringold	Top Models	555-4321
Julie Jones	A to Z Models	555-2314
Samantha Barnes	Miller Agency	555-7895
Christie Brinks	Beautiful People	555-5678
Jon Reynolds	Models 'R' Us	555-8765

(continued)

Charyse	A1 Agency	555-9876
Sonya Reyes	Models of Distinction	555-4567
Tyler Watson	Only the Best	555-6987
Lucy Diamond	Model Citizens	555-6789

SHOW CALENDAR
Next Month

M	T	W	Th	F	Sa	Su
1	2	3	4	5	6	7
8	9	10	11	12	13	14
15	16	17	18	19	20	21
22 Practice	23 Practice	24 Practice	25 4 P.M. Outer- wear	26 3 P.M. Dresses and suits	27 3 P.M. Resort Wear— Women 4:30 P.M. Resort Wear— Men	28 3 P.M. Formal Wear— Women 4 P.M. Formal Wear— Men
29	30					

269

Personal Calendar: Crystal

Fill in your schedule for the week:

1. When do I get home?
2. What time do I have to go to bed?
3. Do I have any special activities after school? If so, what are they, and what times are they scheduled?

	Su	M	Tu	W	Th	F	Sa
Get home	—	3:15	3:15	3:45	4:00	3:45	—
Go to bed	9:00	9:00	9:00	9:00	9:00	10:00	10:00
Any special activities	Help at nursing home 4:00–5:00	—	Dance class 6:00–7:00	Science Club after school 3:15–4:00	Reading to after-school kids 3:15–4:00 Sports practice 6–7	Girl Scouts after school 3:45–4:30	Sports game—variable times

Personal Calendar: Carl

Fill in your schedule for the week:

1. When do I get home?
2. What time do I have to go to bed?
3. Do I have any special activities after school? If so, what are they, and what times are they scheduled?

	Su	M	Tu	W	Th	F	Sa
Get home	—	4:00	3:10	3:10	3:10	3:10	—
Go to bed	9:00	9:00	9:00	9:00	9:00	10:00	10:00
Any special activities	Religion school 10:00– 11:00	Chess after school 3:15– 4:00	Music lesson 5:30– 6:15	Sports practice 4:30– 5:30	—	—	Tennis with Dad 3:00– 4:00

Time Detective Worksheet: In-Session Activities

Activity	Estimated time	Actual time
To blink	_____	_____
To walk across the room	_____	_____
To write an assignment list	_____	_____
To complete a set of math problems	_____	_____
To read a handout or a page in *TIME for Kids*	_____	_____
To throw a ball 10 times	_____	_____
To pack a backpack	_____	_____
To complete a set of puzzles or "brain teasers"	_____	_____
To get the computer running	_____	_____
To find something on the Internet	_____	_____
To write a paragraph	_____	_____
To make a list for a trip or a specific event	_____	_____
To pack a camp bag	_____	_____

Review of the Time Tracker for Homework

	M	Tu	W	Th	F	Sa or Su
How long did homework take to complete?						
Did anything special change the time needed for homework?						
What is the range of time needed for homework?						
Any over- or underestimations?						
Reconsider: When should you schedule homework each day?						

Time Planning for Adventures

ACTIVITY 1: ADVENTURE TO MARS

You have a few assignments to complete for the crew today, Monday.

Special assignment for the day: You have to collect rock samples from the area around the ship. You have to collect a red rock and two blue rocks. When you return to the ship, you have to weigh the rocks and measure their length.

Your **regular assignments for today** are these:
1. Clean the five spacesuits for the crew at 9:30 A.M.
2. Prepare lunch for the crew at 1:00 P.M.

Discuss how much time you think you will need for the activities. Think about when you will start the tasks and when you will finish them.

ACTIVITY 2: SUPERSTAR CONCERT ADVENTURE

You are in Dallas, on the day before a concert.

Special assignment for the day: You have to get batteries for the eight wireless microphones. You have to go to the store, 2 miles away, to buy the batteries.

Your **regular assignments for today** are these:
1. Pick up the dry cleaning for the band at 1:00 P.M.
2. Prepare snacks and get drinks for the concert at 7:00 P.M.

Discuss how much time you think you will need for the activities. Think about when you will start the tasks and when you will finish them.

ACTIVITY 3: FASHION SHOW ADVENTURE

It is the day of the two Formal Wear shows. On the morning before the show, you have a special assignment and some regular activities.

Special assignment for the day: Five pairs of women's shoes have to be polished.
Also, one of the dresses needs new buttons sewn onto the back.

Your **regular assignments for today** are these:
1. You have to check in with the models' agencies at 10:00 A.M.
2. You have to prepare the makeup stand and mirror for the models by 1:00 P.M.

Discuss how much time you think you will need for the activities. Think about when you will start the tasks and when you will finish them.

(continued)

TIME-PLANNING CONFERENCE FOR ALL ADVENTURES

Check your adventure's activity list.	
Discuss what special tasks need to be completed today.	
How long will these special tasks take? (Write down your estimate.)	
When do your regular assignments need to be done?	
What time will you start your special assignment?	
What time will you finish your special assignment?	

Work Observation Sheet

How many times were off-task behaviors noted? (Use tally marks.)
What total amount of time was spent off task?
How much time is available to spend with special materials? (This should be 5 minutes minus the amount of time off task.)
What tactics of the Time Bandit seemed to hinder quick and easy work? (Describe what the child did—e.g., fiddled with pencil, stared out window, played with shirt button.)
How many items were completed?

Practice for Short- and Long-Term Assignments

PRACTICE ROUND 1

Homework assigned:

Math—Complete the worksheet of 40 problems on fractions.

Social Studies—You are studying the countries of South America. Read the textbook content on the climates in the different parts of South America. Answer the questions at the end of the readings.

Reading—Read for 20 minutes, and complete your reading log.

Longer-term assignments:

Science—You have to complete a report on the atmospheres of the planets. You have to find information from two books and one Internet site. Complete the chart that summarizes the average temperature on each planet. This is due in 3 days.

PRACTICE ROUND 2

Homework assigned:

Math—Do pages 34–35 in your math workbook.

Reading—Read for 20 minutes and complete your reading log.

Language Arts—Complete the worksheet on punctuation.

Longer-term assignments:

Vocabulary words—We are adding 15 words to your vocabulary. Write them down three times each. Write a definition for each one. Write a sentence for each one. This is due in 5 days.

PRACTICE ROUND 3

Homework assigned:

Math—Complete the worksheet on probability. You will need two coins and a die from a game.

Reading—Read for 20 minutes, and complete your reading log.

Social Studies—Read the article from *Time for Kids* on global warming. Write a paragraph telling what you think should be done about this problem.

Longer assignments:

Social Studies—You have a test on the materials that you have been studying about your state. You will have to know the capital, the two main economic activities in your state, and the way the government is organized. The test will be in 4 days. Plan on studying several times between now and the test.

Time Planning for Short- and Long-Term
Adventure Activities

ACTIVITY 1: ADVENTURE TO MARS

Regular tasks (done every day):
Check the water supply.
Dispose of the trash.
Clean the spacesuits in the contamination room.
Prepare breakfast for you and the other crew members (they do lunch and dinner).

Special tasks, due in 3 days:
You have to prepare a report on the composition of the rocks on Mars and provide photographs of them. You have to provide reports and photos on the rocks from 4 different locations – you have to go 500 yards from the ship to the North, to the South, to the East, and to the West. You have to send the report and the photos to NASA in 3 days.

ACTIVITY 2: SUPERSTAR CONCERT ADVENTURE

Regular tasks (done every day):
Check the microphones.
Arrange the snacks for the performers.
Tune the guitars.

Special tasks, due in 3 days:
The group needs materials to add smoke to the show. You are told that you need to get large electric fans, 10-gallon metal containers to hold water, and a source of dry ice that smokes when put in water. You have to test the method and have it ready to cover the stage for the show in 3 days.

ACTIVITY 3: FASHION SHOW ADVENTURE

Regular tasks (done every day):
Check on the models to make sure no one is sick.
Find a back-up model for anyone who is sick.
Write out the list of clothes and the model for each outfit.
Write out the order of the show.
Arrange for drinks (water, juice, soda) for the crew and models.

Special tasks, due in 3 days:
The show needs extra accessories. You need to find a collection of costume jewelry from the 20th century, and you need to find vintage clothes for three models. The models will be showing a collection of hats, and they need to wear the vintage clothes and costume jewelry as their outfits. The hats are the focus of the show, so the vintage jewelry and clothing will not be the center of attention. You need to find five outfits in local stores and thrift shops.

(continued)

TIME-PLANNING CONFERENCE FOR ALL ADVENTURES

What are your regular assignments?
How long will they take to do?
When can you start them?
When will you finish them?
What special tasks do you have to do?
How long will they take to complete?
How much time can you work on them each day?
When can you start that work?
When will you finish?

Time Bandit Record Sheet

What problems kept you from completing the problem situation activity on time?

Started too late?	
Got involved in other activities in the middle of completing it?	
Moved too slowly?	
Did not have the right materials or supplies when you started?	
Thought the activity would take less time to complete than it did?	
Did not put it into your schedule?	

How Might Homework Time Change?

Activity: Complete 10 math problems in a workbook.			
Amount of time it should take to complete:	What happens if you are tired?	What happens if you are hungry?	What happens if you notice a text or e-mail from a friend?

Activity: Write sentences for 10 spelling words.			
Amount to time it should take to complete:	What happens if you take a break after each question?	What happens if it is late in the day?	What happens if you feel sick?

Activity: Read a chapter in social studies book.			
Amount to time it should take to complete:	What happens if you take a break to play on your Nintendo DS?	What happens if you draw on a piece of paper on your desk?	What happens if you eat a snack while working?

Task-Planning Conference: Example

1. The Goal	2. Getting Ready to Go		3. Time Management			4. Checking It Out
	a. Breaking it down into steps	b. What stuff is needed?	a. Ordering the steps	b. How long?	c. When to fit it in?	(All done—neat and complete)
Throwing a surprise party for my mother's birthday	Create and send out invitations	Card stock paper, computer, stamps, envelopes	1	1 hour		
	Order food	Lasagna, ziti, salad, garlic bread, veggie/fruit platters	2	30 minutes		
	Order decorations	Flowers, balloons, sign for the door	3	30 minutes		
	Load music onto my iPod	List of songs my mom likes, iPod	6	30 minutes		
	Bake a cake	Cake mix, eggs, oil, frosting, decorating tools	5	1½ hours		
	Figure out how to get my mom to the house at the right time		4	20 minutes		

Sample Projects for In-Session Practice

1. As the manager for a fashion show, you realize that the clothes for the show all have to be fitted to the models who will be wearing them. The clothes will be delivered to your house. You have to arrange for five models to come over and be fitted by a tailor. After that is done, you have to make sure the clothes are pressed neatly, so that there are no wrinkles. The person who will do the ironing is going to come to your house and complete that. You have to supervise all of the steps and watch them happen. Tell how you would complete the tasks and when you would put them into your schedule.

2. The crew for a Mars landing has to come to your house to plan an exploratory hike of the Valles Marineris (the Mariner Valley). You are looking for special rocks and any signs of water. There are three other crew members and you. You have to plan the hike and check the compasses, shovels, and collection boxes to make sure they work. The crew is coming over to your house every day after school for the next week. How can you fit in the time necessary to map out your route, assign tasks to people, and check the equipment?

3. At school, you and three other students are given a group assignment to put on a skit to show how people lived when they traveled on the Oregon Trail. In your skit, you must explain how people packed for the trip and how they dressed, and you have to show the route that they traveled. How can you fit in the steps needed to complete this assignment during the next week?

4. The road crew for a band tour has to bring the sound equipment (e.g., microphones and speakers) and lighting equipment to your house to make sure that they work correctly for a show next week. Each piece of equipment has to be plugged in and tested individually. There are 50 pieces of equipment. Describe your plan for testing the equipment over the next few days.

> **HELPFUL HINT:** Projects 1, 2, and 4 are pretty complicated. They are designed to capture the interest of older children and may not be easily understood by younger children (in third grade or below). However, you can feel free to simplify the tasks by selecting one element for the child to address. For example, in Project 1, have the child describe the plan for models to come to try on the clothes. For Project 2, you could have the child develop the plan for gathering the needed equipment and storing it for the hike. You may also find that you can create other ideas that fit the child's particular interests.

Materials for Practicing Checking It Out

SAMPLE SPELLING LIST

Whear

Shirt

Found

Science

Courtesy

Blose

Notebook

Growl

Finish

Helpful

Thraot

Powr

Birds

(continued)

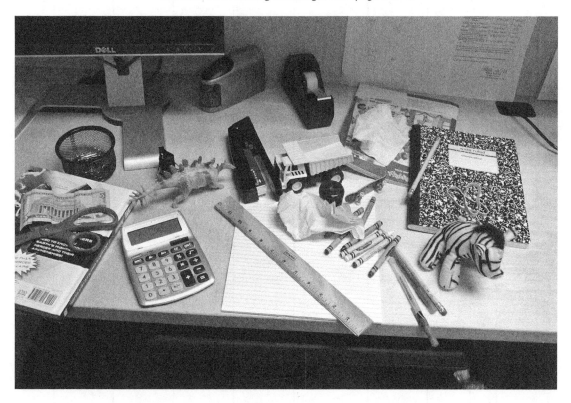

(continued)

TASK-PLANNING CONFERENCE: SAMPLE

1. The Goal	2. Getting Ready to Go		3. Time Management			4. Checking It Out
	a. Breaking it down into steps	b. What stuff is needed?	a. Ordering the steps	b. How long?	c. When to fit it in?	(All done—neat and complete)
Get my equipment and clothes ready for the soccer game	Get clean soccer uniform from laundry	Clean soccer clothes, cleats, shin guards, and goalie gloves	2	5 mins.	Night before the game	
	Check bag for shorts, shirt, cleats, socks, shin guards, and goalie gloves	Soccer bag checklist	6	1 min.	8 A.M., morning of game	
	Fill water bottle	Water bottle	4	2 mins.	8 A.M., morning of game	
	Pack bag	Bag and all the stuff for it	5	5 mins.	8 A.M., morning of game	
	Call friend for a ride to game	Phone and phone number	1	10 mins.	Night before the game	
	Get practice soccer ball	Soccer ball	3	5 mins.	Night before the game	

(continued)

TASK-PLANNING CONFERENCE: SAMPLE

1. The Goal	2. Getting Ready to Go		3. Time Management			4. Checking It Out
	a. Breaking it down into steps	b. What stuff is needed?	a. Ordering the steps	b. How long?	c. When to fit it in?	(All done—neat and complete)
Fun sleepover with a friend	Check calendar to make sure I am free	My Personal Calendar	1	5 mins.	After homework	
	Call to invite friend	Phone and phone number	2	10 mins.	After school Wednesday	
	Get room and beds ready	Clean sheets or sleeping bags, duster, vacuum	3			
	Buy snacks	Ride to store, money, snacks	4	30 mins.	Thursday evening	
	Take friend home	Car	5	30 mins.	Saturday at noon	

287

PARENT AND CHILD HANDOUTS

Overview of Session Content

Session 1. Introduction: Parent and Child Orientation

Session 2. Introduction: Using Social Learning Strategies to Motivate Skills Building (for Parents Only)

Session 3. Tracking Assignments: Implementing Behavior Management Procedures and Getting It All Down

Session 4. Tracking Assignments: The Daily Assignment Record and the Assignment and Test Calendar

Session 5. Managing Materials: Managing Papers for School

Session 6. Managing Materials: Review of Routines for Tracking Assignments and Managing Papers

Session 7. Managing Materials: Introducing a Backpack Checklist

Session 8. Managing Materials: "Other Stuff" and Other Bags

Session 9. Managing Materials: Getting Work Areas Ready to Go

Session 10. Time Management: Understanding Time and Calendars

Session 11. Time Management: Time Tracking for Homework

Session 11a (Optional). Time Management: Instruction in Telling Time and Calculating the Passage of Time

Session 12. Time Management: Time-Planning Conferences at Home and School

Session 13. Time Management: Time Planning for Longer-Term Assignments and Avoiding Distractions

Session 14. Time Management: Time Planning for Regular Routines

Session 15. Task Planning: Introduction to Task Planning

Session 16. Task Planning: Next Steps-Managing Materials and Time

Session 17. Task Planning: Fitting the Steps into the Schedule

Session 18. Task Planning: Planning for Long-Term Projects

Session 19. Task Planning: Checking It Out and Planning for Graduation

Session 20. Program Summary: Personalized Commercial and Graduation

---

Treatment Expectations

This handout highlights what is expected of children and parents in this treatment program. These expectations include the following:

- There will be two meetings a week for most weeks for 10 weeks, for a total of 20 contacts.

- The meetings each week need to be scheduled at least 2 days apart.

- As the child's parent or guardian, you need to come to all meetings. For most meetings, you will be involved at the beginning and the end. The child will meet individually with me, the therapist, for the majority of the time.

- If you are not able to keep to the schedule, I would like you to notify me and arrange for alternative meeting times with at least 24 hours' notice, if possible.

- There are home exercises that you and your child are expected to complete between sessions.

- Of course, all participation and continuation of participation are voluntary. However, we may decide together that the treatment will not be effective if there are many missed sessions.

Guide to the Glitches

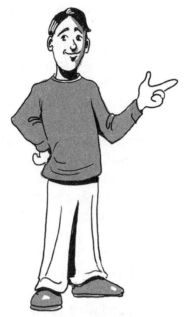

The Mastermind.

"Glitches" are like little creatures that live inside our brains and get in the way when we least expect it. We all have Glitches creeping around in our brains. They get in the way by telling us silly things or by making us forget to use skills that keep us organized and help us get things done, like writing down our assignments or checking that we have the things we need before we leave the house. Have you ever forgotten a book or paper that you needed to take to school? If you have, that was the Glitches' work. Have you ever lost an important paper, like your homework or a special permission slip? That was also caused by Glitches. Every time we slip up and make mistakes—forgetting to hand in assignments, leaving important materials at school, taking too much time to finish homework, forgetting to plan ahead for a big project that is due—the Glitches throw a party. They love when we are not in control of our actions.

The brain also has a "Mastermind" that keeps the Glitches and us in control, most of the time. The Mastermind helps us control our actions, making sure that we do important things like writing down what needs to be done so we don't forget, keeping track of our stuff, using time well, and planning ahead for important tasks. But sometimes the Mastermind is not active enough, and the Glitches take over. When we are tired, nervous, or rushed, the Mastermind has a hard time staying in control. When the Mastermind takes a nap, the Glitches take over, and we get in trouble.

Some people have a lot of trouble keeping the Mastermind in control. Kids with attention-deficit/hyperactivity disorder (ADHD) often find that even when they want to do their best, they can't keep the Mastermind active enough to stop the Glitches from popping through. People sometimes say that kids with ADHD are lazy or careless, but most kids with ADHD want to work hard and do things carefully. They just can't do it all of the time, because the Mastermind is struggling to keep the Glitches under control. This causes a lot of problems for these kids, especially with their parents and teachers.

"Organizational Skills Training," or OST, is a special program that can help you train the Mastermind to be more active, so you can control the Glitches. This program will teach you some new habits, so you know which steps to use to keep the Mastermind in control and stop the Glitches from making mischief. There are several important Glitches that we are going to watch out for, and we will learn about different ways to prevent these Glitches from getting in your way. Let's find out who they are and what they do.

First, there is the "Go-Ahead-Forget-It Glitch." This Glitch doesn't want you to remember important things, like homework assignments, important books that you need to bring home to study for a test, or the chore that your mom asked you to do. This Glitch tricks you and tells you that you don't have to write down your homework or check to see if you have everything with you when you leave school. This Glitch tells you that you will remember what you are supposed to do and what you are supposed to take with you. This Glitch *wants* you to forget things and get into trouble. When it wins, you look silly, because you don't have the right things with you or you don't know what you need to do, and you will probably get into trouble with your parents or teachers.

There is also the "Go-Ahead-Lose-It Glitch." This Glitch takes your mind off your things, so you misplace them or lose them. This Glitch tells you that you will find important papers, no matter where you put them, convincing you to just stuff papers into your backpack or desk, instead of using a folder. When you can't find your homework even though you did it, or you can't find your iPod, because you leave it in a different place each time you use it, the Go-Ahead-Lose-It Glitch has gotten you.

The "Time Bandit" is another Glitch. The Time Bandit makes you lose track of time and forget when things are due. If you ever forgot about a big school project until the night before it was due, this Glitch was around. This Glitch convinces you that you can do things later, without planning out a schedule. The Time Bandit is also around when you find that you did not get your homework done, even though you had several hours to do it. It confuses you, so that you don't estimate how long things will take. It also distracts you while you're working, so that you don't use your time well.

Finally, the last Glitch, the "Go-Ahead-Don't-Plan Glitch," takes away your good thinking skills. This Glitch tells you that you don't have to plan, which means that you don't have to think ahead and consider what steps need to be done to complete important tasks or projects. If you've ever handed in a big school assignment that was missing important parts, or found that you don't enjoy a play date as much because you forgot to plan which toys and games you wanted to bring, you've had trouble with the Go-Ahead-Don't-Plan Glitch.

So let's get ready to beat the Glitches. First, we'll take a closer look at the opponents.

THE GO-AHEAD-FORGET-IT GLITCH

The Go-Ahead-Forget-It Glitch lurks in your memory and wipes out things you should remember or prevents you from remembering things. This Glitch convinces you not to do things (like writing things down or keeping track of important dates on a calendar) that could help you remember important dates, assignments, and tasks.

Some Things the Go-Ahead-Forget-It Glitch Might Say

"Don't worry; you won't forget to take home your math book. You can pack it later, after you go to recess."
"You'll remember what the homework is, without writing it down."
"You don't have to use a calendar to keep track of tests or projects. Your teacher will remind you when those are due."

When Is the Go-Ahead-Forget-It Glitch Around?

This Glitch often shows up when your teacher tells you what the homework assignments are for the day. It also shows up when you are packing up your things, and keeps you from being careful about remembering what things to take with you. Then, when you get home and don't have the materials you need to complete your homework, this Glitch throws a party.

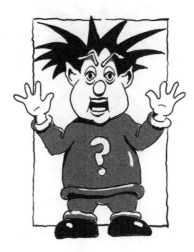

The Go-Ahead-Forget-It Glitch.

THE GO-AHEAD-LOSE-IT GLITCH

The Go-Ahead-Lose-It Glitch gets into the parts of your brain that control what you do and convinces you to put things away in the wrong place or in a place you will forget. It tricks you into misplacing your things, so that you come to school without your homework or get home without your books or papers. This Glitch makes you lose parts of your toys and makes it hard for you to find things when you need them. It also makes your backpack and desk really messy, because you don't take the time to put things away carefully.

What the Go-Ahead-Lose-It Glitch Might Say

"Hurry up; we have to do something else. Just drop that toy over there, and you can put it away later."

"Let's go watch TV. You can put your homework in your backpack when you're done."

"Just put that homework worksheet into your desk. You will find it later."

"Even if you lose your iPod, Mom or Dad will help you find it."

"You're just a kid; you don't have to put your stuff away."

When Is the Go-Ahead-Lose-It Glitch Around?

This Glitch shows up whenever you are given a paper at school, and when you are packing up at the end of the school day. It hangs out whenever you open your backpack, especially when you take things out; it might distract you, so that you forget to put things back in the right spots. When you finish your homework each night, this Glitch lurks in the shadows and might pull you away before you have a chance to put your completed homework in your backpack.

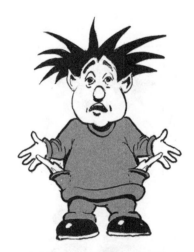

The Go-Ahead-Lose-It Glitch.

THE TIME BANDIT

The Time Bandit gets into the parts of your brain that keep track of time. This Glitch convinces you not to worry about clocks or calendars, or how your behavior has to be linked to the passage of time. It confuses you, so you don't keep track of how much time you have left before you need to do something or how much time has passed while you're working. These tricks often get you into trouble; you might end up being late to school or activities and have trouble fitting in the work you have to do each evening. You also might lose out on free time because of this Glitch. When the Time Bandit slows you down while you are working, you have less time to do the things you really want to do in a day. This Glitch can get you into trouble with your parents and teachers, who might constantly ask, "What is taking you so long?"

What the Time Bandit Might Say

"Take it easy. We can take all the time we want to do this work."
"Don't worry about what time it is; Mom or Dad will make sure you get to school on time."
"Just relax and don't worry about time passing. You'll get everything done eventually."
"It's OK to take a little break from your homework and make a paper clip chain. You have
    plenty of time to get this done."
"Don't worry about how much time you need to finish your homework. You can do each
    assignment in only 10 minutes."

When Is the Time Bandit Around?

It's OK if the Time Bandit takes over when you are on vacation or relaxing on weekends. Everyone needs a break from worrying about schedules, as long as there isn't anything important that needs to get done. But the Time Bandit can also show up during homework time or other times when you have to meet a deadline (like getting to soccer practice by 5 P.M.). That's when the Time Bandit causes problems, because it slows you down and keeps you from being ready on time. The Time Bandit may also try to trick you into thinking that you can wait to start bigger projects, like book reports. The Time Bandit may convince you that you can get a big project done in just a few hours, when you actually need a few days to do the project the right way. This Glitch takes the Mastermind's eyes away from the clock and the calendar, and gets you into trouble.

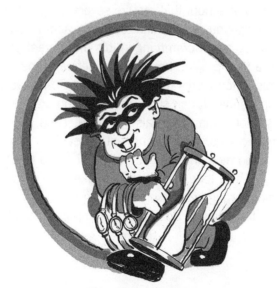

The Time Bandit.

THE GO-AHEAD-DON'T-PLAN GLITCH

The Go-Ahead-Don't-Plan Glitch gets into the parts of your brain that control your thinking. This Glitch convinces you not to think ahead or think too much about the different steps you have to get done in order to complete a task the best way. It may trick you into believing that a project is easy and does not require planning. This Glitch might suggest that you wait until the last minute to start working on a complicated project, convincing you that you can get the work done easily. Or it may suggest that other people (like your parents) will solve your problems for you, so you don't have to think or plan ahead.

What the Go-Ahead-Don't-Plan Glitch Might Say

"This project will be easy. You can get it done in no time, without thinking too much about it."

"Why bother planning how you will do this science project? Mom and Dad always do the planning for you."

"You don't need to think about what materials you need for this project. I'm sure you already have everything you need."

"You don't have to tell your parents about this big test that your teacher just told you about. You can just study the day before the test."

"When your friend comes over, you can just play; you don't need to plan any fun activities."

When Is the Go-Ahead-Don't-Plan Glitch Around?

This is another Glitch that can be great on vacations, when you have lots of free time to do whatever you want. Sometimes it is great just to relax and not decide how you will spend your time. But when you want to get something done that requires planning (like a school assignment or even a fun activity with a friend), this Glitch gets you in trouble. It shows up when you are given projects at school that require several steps (like a research project or book report), and it convinces you not to think too much about how to complete each of those steps. When you find yourself cramming in lots of different pieces of a project at the last minute, and hand in a final project that is incomplete and messy, this Glitch has been in control. Sometimes this Glitch works together with the Go-Ahead-Forget-It Glitch and the Time Bandit to get you in trouble. It can show up when you are starting your homework and tell you not to worry about what materials you need. Then, when you keep jumping up from your desk to get more things, your parents get upset. This Glitch might also be around when you wake up in the morning and tell you not to think too much about the steps you have to take to get ready or how long each step will take. This Glitch is really happy when you get scolded for rushing through your work, handing in assignments that don't meet the teacher's expectations, or forgetting to do something important until the last minute.

298

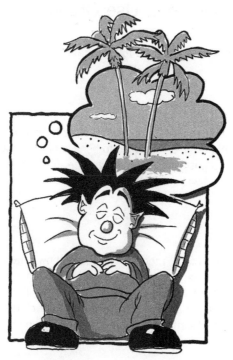

The Go-Ahead-Don't-Plan Glitch.

So let's work on beating the Glitches. We are going to learn how to use special skills to fight the Glitches. We will keep score, so we can find out who wins each day—the Mastermind or the Glitches. We can make you the Mastermind, by giving you the tools to keep the Glitches under control.

Helping Your Child Use Organizational Skills

When children are just learning a new skill, the following parent behaviors are keys for success.

PROMPT

Children with ADHD need frequent, specific reminders in order to behave in new ways. "Prompts" are clear, direct, specific requests that remind your child to behave in a new way. Your child is most likely to listen to your prompts if you use a positive, encouraging voice. A negative or accusatory tone is likely to get your child to stop listening. Kids will ignore harsh messages.

MONITOR

It is important for you to keep track of, or "monitor," when and how often your child uses a skill. Once you have prompted your child in a clear, specific, and positive way, monitor whether or not your child follows through in practicing the behavior, by recording the child's skill use on a chart. When you monitor behaviors, it sends a message that you are invested in helping your child learn new skills and that you will regularly keep track of your child's efforts. This helps you keep an accurate record of your child's success and areas that need further work. Finally, monitoring helps you provide rewards appropriately.

PRAISE

Use "labeled praise" when your child performs a desired behavior or skill. This means praising the child for a specific action, such as looking at you when you make a request. Frequent use of labeled praise during an activity motivates the child to continue performing the desired action. This form of praise helps children with ADHD stay focused on what is important. Remember to describe exactly what you are praising (e.g., "I liked the way you picked up your clothes"). Praising in a sincere, specific, and enthusiastic manner will increase your child's motivation to continue practicing. You don't have to be sugary-sweet or fake; just use your own style and your own words to thank your child and indicate what you like about what the child has done. When a new behavior is first being learned, it is important to praise that behavior very often.

Please use these guidelines:

- Notice and praise small behaviors that lead to a goal.
- Provide labeled praise often.
- Use your style. You do not have to be a cheerleader. Show some excitement, but don't act like a completely different person.
- Sometimes a simple thank you is helpful.
- Use a pleasant voice.
- Do not pay attention to small misbehaviors in the middle of praising your child.
- Remember the examples from your work in treatment sessions.

(continued)

REWARD

Provide a "reward" for desired behaviors. Praise is valuable, but to encourage consistent use of new skills, it helps to provide small rewards for effective use of the skills. We suggest that you provide small rewards at the end of each day if the child practices specific organizational skills, and a larger reward at the end of each week for cumulative use of the skills. Daily rewards keep a child interested in performing specific behaviors each day; this is especially important for children with ADHD, who respond best to immediate rewards. Weekly rewards help children stay interested in showing the behaviors consistently, and teach them about the advantages of consistent effort.

Interview for Developing a Reward Menu

1. What does your child like to do during free time?

Activity	How often does your child engage in this activity?	Does your child get to engage in this activity for free (i.e., without needing to "earn" the privilege)?	Rate how highly valued this activity is (1 = minimally valued; 5 = highly valued)

2. What items or toys does your child like to use?

Toy or item	How often does your child use this toy/item?	Does your child get to use this toy/item for free?	Rate how highly valued this toy/item is (1 → 5)

(continued)

3. What outings does your child enjoy?

Outing	How often does your child go on this outing?	Does your child get to go on this outing for free?	Rate how highly valued this outing is (1 → 5)

4. With whom does your child like to play?

Person	How often does your child play with this person?	Does your child get to play with this person for free?	Rate how highly valued playing with this person is (1 → 5)

(continued)

5. Does your child collect any items or show interest in collecting items?

Item	How often does your child collect this item?	Does your child get to collect this item for free?	Rate how highly valued this item is (1 → 5)

6. Does your child have any favorite snacks or restaurants?

Food or restaurant	How often does your child eat this food or go to this restaurant?	Does your child get to have this type of food or eat at this restaurant for free?	Rate how highly valued this food or restaurant is (1 → 5)

(continued)

7. What does your child like to do on weekends?

Activity/outing/play with friend/ have sleepover with friend	How often does your child engage in this activity?	Does your child get to engage in this activity for free?	Rate how highly valued this activity is (1 → 5)

Homework: Let's Consider Possible Rewards

Directions: Based on your responses to the Interview for Developing a Reward Menu (Handout 5), select some possible rewards that you can use to reinforce your child's performance of selected target behaviors at home and in school. Consider rewards from each of the categories discussed in the interview (activities, toys/items, outings, friends, collectibles, and food/restaurant).

Possible Daily Rewards (i.e., rewards that could be realistically given on a daily basis)

Level One (moderately valued) rewards
Level Two (highly valued) rewards

Possible Weekly Rewards

Level One (moderately valued) rewards
Level Two (highly valued) rewards

Home Behavior Record:
Behaviors to Prompt, Monitor, and Praise

	Day 1	Day 2	Day 3	Day 4	Day 5	Day 6	Day 7
Behavior 1 _____ _____							
Did I **prompt** this behavior? (Y/N)							
Please **monitor** your child's performance of this behavior. (Mark Y if it was done, N if not.)							
Did I **praise** my child for this behavior? (Y/N)							
Behavior 2 _____ _____							
Did I **prompt** this behavior? (Y/N)							
Please **monitor** your child's performance of this behavior. (Mark Y if it was done, N if not.)							
Did I **praise** my child for this behavior? (Y/N)							

OTMP Checklist: Things to Remember for Session 3

Please bring with you:

- ☐ Your Child

- ☐ Your OTMP parent's folder

- ☐ Handout 6, Homework: Let's Consider Possible Rewards (with choices for daily and weekly rewards filled in)

- ☐ Handout 7, Home Behavior Record: Behaviors to Prompt, Monitor, and Praise

- ☐ Any questions or ideas that you want to discuss

Therapist's name: _____

Therapist's phone number: _____

Appointment date and time: _____

Reward Menu

Daily Rewards

Level One rewards
Level Two rewards

For a Home Behavior Record with two target behaviors:

Level One: Use if the child earns 1 out of 2 points for the day.

Level Two: Use if the child earns 2 out of 2 points for the day.

For a Home Behavior Record with five target behaviors:

Level One: Use if the child earns 60% (e.g., 3 out of 5) of the points for the day.

Level Two: Use if the child earns at least 80% (e.g., 4 or 5 out of 5) of the points for the day.

(continued)

Weekly Rewards

Level One rewards

Level Two rewards

Note: Weekly points = the sum of all the points earned over the course of the week.

For a Home Behavior Record with two target behaviors:

Level One: Use if the child earns 6 out of 10 possible points.

Level Two: Use if the child earns 8 out of 10 possible points.

For a Home Behavior Record with five target behaviors:

Level One: Use if the child earns at least 60% (i.e., 15 out of 25) of the points accumulated over the course of the week.

Level Two: Use if the child earns 80% (i.e., 20 out of 25) or more of the points accumulated over the course of the week.

Daily Assignment Record

Date: _____

Subject	What Is for Homework?	What Do I Need to Take?	Other Assignments and Due Dates	Teacher: Check for School Points— Did the child use the skill? If yes, provide a point.
Language Arts		___ Workbook ___ Handouts ___ Textbook ___ Other		**Target Skills:** 1.
Social Studies		___ Workbook ___ Handouts ___ Textbook ___ Other		
Science		___ Workbook ___ Handouts ___ Textbook ___ Other		**Check/Initials** _____
Math		___ Workbook ___ Handouts ___ Textbook ___ Other		

(continued)

Daily Assignment Record (page 2 of 2)

Subject	What Is for Homework?	What Do I Need to Take?	Other Assignments and Due Dates	Teacher: Check for School Points—Did the child use the skill? If yes, provide a point.
Spelling		___ Workbook ___ Handouts . ___ Textbook ___ Other		**Target Skills:** 2.
Second Language		___ Workbook ___ Handouts ___ Textbook ___ Other		
Announcements or Special Papers		___ Handouts ___ Other ___ Permission slip		**Check/Initials** _____
Anything Else?				

Assignment and Test Calendar

Month _____

What Is Due?:
Look at Your Daily Assignment Record

Monday	Tuesday	Wednesday	Thursday	Friday

Reminder for the Daily Assignment Record

Let's Control the Go-Ahead-Forget-It Glitch

How to use the Daily Assignment Record (DAR):

1. Write down the homework for each subject in the "What Is for Homework?" column.

2. Put a check next to any item you need to complete the homework in the "What Do I Need to Take?" column.

3. Write down any tests or assignments that are not due the next day, with their due dates, in the "Other Assignments and Due Dates" column.

4. Show your teacher the completed DAR to get your school praise and points.

Home Behavior Record:
Behaviors to Prompt, Monitor, and Praise

	Day 1	Day 2	Day 3	Day 4	Day 5	Day 6	Day 7
Behavior 1 _____ _____							
Prompt: Did I prompt the behavior?							
Monitor: Did the behavior occur?							
Praise: Did I praise the behavior?							
Put 1 **point** here if the child performed the behavior							
Behavior 2 _____ _____							
Prompt?							
Monitor?							
Praise?							
Put 1 **point** here if the child performed the behavior							
Total Points							
Did your child earn a reward?							
Did your child get the reward?							
Daily Assignment Record: Did the child complete this at school? (Y/N)							

OTMP Checklist: Things to Remember for Session 4

Please bring with you:

☐ Your OTMP parent's folder

☐ Handout 13, Home Behavior Record: Behaviors to Prompt, Monitor, and Praise

☐ The child's DAR folder

☐ The child's school bag

☐ Any questions or ideas that you want to discuss

Therapist's name: _____

Therapist's phone number: _____

Appointment date and time: _____

Home Behavior Record:
Behaviors to Prompt, Monitor, Praise, and Reward

Directions: Give your child 1 point for each behavior that is performed on a given day. There are 5 possible points to be earned each day.

	Day 1	Day 2	Day 3	Day 4	Day 5	Day 6	Day 7
Non-OTMP Behavior 1 _____ _____							
Non-OTMP Behavior 2 _____ _____							
Completed Daily Assignment Record							
Completed Assignment and Test Calendar							
Wrote down papers received at school							
Total points (out of 5)							
Points for the week							

Home Behavior Record:
Behaviors to Prompt, Monitor, Praise, and Reward

Directions: Give your child 1 point for each non-OTMP behavior that is performed on a given day. There are 2 possible points to be earned each day. In addition, indicate whether you prompted, monitored, and praised the three OTMP behaviors below.

	Day 1	Day 2	Day 3	Day 4	Day 5	Day 6	Day 7
Non-OTMP Behavior 1 _____ _____							
Non-OTMP Behavior 2 _____ _____							
Completed Daily Assignment Record							
Completed Assignment and Test Calendar							
Wrote down papers received at school							
Total points (out of 2)							
Points for the week							

Keeping Track of School Papers

	Homework Papers	Announcements	Other Papers
Monday			
Tuesday			
Wednesday			
Thursday			
Friday			

OTMP Checklist: Things to Remember for Session 5

Please bring with you:

☐ Your OTMP parent's folder

☐ Handout 15 and 15a, Home Behavior Record: Behaviors to Prompt, Monitor, Praise, and Reward

☐ The DAR child's folder with completed DARs and Assignment and Test Calendars

☐ The child's school bag

☐ List of papers received at school

☐ Any questions or ideas that you want to discuss

Home Point Bank

Points Earned

Sa	Su	M	Tu	W	Th	F
Total for the Week:						
Sa	Su	M	Tu	W	Th	F
Total for the Week:						
Sa	Su	M	Tu	W	Th	F
Total for the Week:						
Sa	Su	M	Tu	W	Th	F
Total for the Week:						
Sa	Su	M	Tu	W	Th	F
Total for the Week:						

Home Behavior Record

Directions: Give your child 1 point for each behavior that is performed on a given day. There are 5 possible points to be earned each day.

Behaviors	Day 1	Day 2	Day 3	Day 4	Day 5	Day 6	Day 7
School Behavior 1:							
School Behavior 2:							
Home Behavior 1:							
Home Behavior 2:							
Home Behavior 3:							
Total points (out of 5)							
Points for the week							

Accordion Binder Instructions

1. Fill in the Daily Assignment Record (DAR) with homework assignments.

2. Put all papers in the accordion binder, *including* the DAR.

3. Put papers in the right section of the binder.

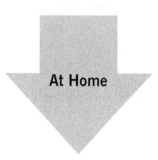

At Home

4. Check the DAR for homework.

5. Fill in the Assignment and Test Calendar with any long-term assignments/tests.

6. Take out and complete homework papers.

7. Put papers back in the right section of the binder.

OTMP Checklist: Things to Remember for Session 6

Please bring with you:

- ☐ Your OTMP parent's folder with:

  - ☐ Handout 19, Home Behavior Record

- ☐ The accordion binder with:

  - ☐ The child's DAR folder with completed DARs and Assignment and Test Calendars

  - ☐ All school papers

- ☐ The child's school bag

- ☐ Any questions or ideas that you want to discuss

OTMP Checklist: Things to Remember for Session 7

Please bring with you:

- ☐ Your OTMP parent's folder with:

    - ☐ Handout 19, Home Behavior Record

- ☐ The accordion binder with:

    - ☐ The child's DAR folder with completed DARs and Assignment and Test Calendars

    - ☐ All school papers

- ☐ The child's school bag

- ☐ Any questions or ideas that you want to discuss

Check It Out: Steps

1. Write down all assignments and items needed on your Daily Assignment Record (DAR).

2. Put all papers in your accordion binder.

3. Put away your DAR in the binder.

4. Put all of your books and your accordion binder in your bag.

5. Check It Out on your backpack checklist.

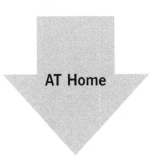

AT Home

6. Take out the DAR, and put information on your Assignment and Test Calendar.

7. Take out papers for homework.

8. Put the papers back, put the DAR back in the binder, and put the binder back in the bag.

9. Check It Out on your backpack checklist.

OTMP Checklist: Things to Remember for Session 8

Please bring with you:

- ☐ Your OTMP parent's folder with:
    - ☐ Handout 19, Home Behavior Record
- ☐ The accordion binder with:
    - ☐ The child's DAR folder with completed DARs and Assignment and Test Calendars
    - ☐ The child's OTMP folder
    - ☐ All school papers
- ☐ The child's school bag with backpack checklist and luggage tag attached
- ☐ Other bags and items used for other activities
- ☐ Any questions or ideas that you want to discuss

OTMP Checklist: Things to Remember for Session 9

Please bring with you:

- ☐ Your OTMP parent's folder with:

    - ☐ Handout 19, Home Behavior Record

- ☐ The accordion binder with:

    - ☐ The child's DAR folder with completed DARs and Assignment and Test Calendars

    - ☐ The child's OTMP folder

    - ☐ All school papers

- ☐ The child's school bag with backpack checklist and luggage tag attached

- ☐ Any questions or ideas that you want to discuss

Getting Ready to Go

1. Before starting homework, decide where you will work.

2. Then consider these questions:

   • Do you have everything you need? (Consider everything, including the kitchen sink!)

   • What should you put away?

   • Is your work area clear?

   • Are there any things that could distract you?

3. You are now *Ready to Go!*

OTMP Checklist: Things to Remember for Session 10

Please bring with you:

- ☐ Your OTMP parent's folder with:

  - ☐ Handout 19, Home Behavior Record

- ☐ The accordion binder with:

  - ☐ The child's DAR folder with completed DARs and Assignment and Test Calendars

  - ☐ The child's OTMP folder

  - ☐ All school papers

- ☐ The child's school bag with backpack checklist and luggage tag attached

- ☐ Any questions or ideas that you want to discuss

Personal Calendar

Fill in your schedule for the week:

1. When do I get home?

2. What time do I have to go to bed?

3. Do I have any special activities after school? If so, what are they, and what times are they scheduled?

	Su	M	Tu	W	Th	F	Sa
Get home							
Go to bed							
Any special activities							

Time Detective Worksheet

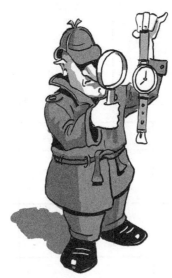

To control the Time Bandit, it is important to plan your time well. The first step in gaining control over the Time Bandit is to gather information. The Mastermind needs to know how long it takes to do many things. You can help the Mastermind by being a Time Detective and finding out some information. How long does it take to do each of the activities below? You can do each activity yourself or observe someone else doing the activity. You can also try some of your own activities (just write them in the last few rows).

Activity	Estimated time (How long do you think it will take?)	Actual time (How long did it take?)
Turn on a computer (press "Power" and see when the welcome screen shows up)		
Print a page on a printer		
Read a page in a book		
Read a school handout		
Travel to school		

(continued)

Travel home from school		
Make a sandwich		
Take a shower		
Put on socks		
Run around the block		
Write three sentences		
Complete a sheet of math problems		

OTMP Checklist: Things to Remember for Session 11

Please bring with you:

☐ Your OTMP parent's folder with:

☐ Handout 19, Home Behavior Record

☐ The accordion binder with:

☐ The child's DAR folder with completed DARs and Assignment and Test Calendars

☐ All school papers

☐ The child's OTMP folder in the accordion binder with completed copies of:

☐ Handout 28, Personal Calendar

☐ Handout 29, Time Detective Worksheet

☐ The child's school bag with backpack checklist and luggage tag attached

☐ Materials for homework assignments (please wait to complete some of your homework until our meeting, if you can)

☐ Any questions or ideas that you want to discuss

Proposed Homework Schedule

Let's Keep the Time Bandit Locked Up

	M	Tu	W	Th	F	Sa or Su
Look at your Personal Calendar. What is on your schedule?						
How much time do you need to complete your homework?						
When should you start your homework?						
When should you finish your homework?						

Time Tracker for Homework

Step 1: Think about the amount of homework that you have.

Step 2: Think about how much time you think each assignment will take.

Step 3: Write down the time that you think you will start, and then the time that you think you will finish.

Step 4: When you start each assignment, write down the time.

Step 5: When you finish each assignment, write down the time.

DAY 1

	Subject 1	Subject 2	Subject 3
I plan to start at:			
I plan to finish at:			
I actually started at:			
I actually finished at:			
Is my work complete?			
How much more time did I spend to complete it?			

DAY 2

	Subject 1	Subject 2	Subject 3
I plan to start at:			
I plan to finish at:			
I actually started at:			
I actually finished at:			
Is my work complete?			
How much more time did I spend to complete it?			

(continued)

DAY 3

	Subject 1	Subject 2	Subject 3
I plan to start at:			
I plan to finish at:			
I actually started at:			
I actually finished at:			
Is my work complete?			
How much more time did I spend to complete it?			

DAY 4

	Subject 1	Subject 2	Subject 3
I plan to start at:			
I plan to finish at:			
I actually started at:			
I actually finished at:			
Is my work complete?			
How much more time did I spend to complete it?			

DAY 5

	Subject 1	Subject 2	Subject 3
I plan to start at:			
I plan to finish at:			
I actually started at:			
I actually finished at:			
Is my work complete?			
How much more time did I spend to complete it?			

OTMP Checklist: Things to Remember for Session 12

Please bring with you:

☐ Your OTMP parent's folder with:

    ☐ Handout 19, Home Behavior Record

☐ The accordion binder with:

    ☐ The DAR folder with completed DARs and Assignment and Test Calendars

    ☐ All school papers

    ☐ The child's OTMP folder in the binder with completed copies of:

        ☐ Handout 28, Personal Calendar

        ☐ Handout 31, Proposed Homework Schedule

        ☐ Handout 32, Time Tracker for Homework

☐ The child's school bag with backpack checklist and luggage tag attached

☐ Any questions or ideas that you want to discuss

How Much Time Has Passed?

End time	Start time	End time: _____
12 11　1 10　2 9　3 8　4 7　5 6	12 11　1 10　2 9　3 8　4 7　5 6	Start time: _____ How much time passed? _____
End time 12 11　1 10　2 9　3 8　4 7　5 6	Start time 12 11　1 10　2 9　3 8　4 7　5 6	End time: _____ Start time: _____ How much time passed? _____
End time 12 11　1 10　2 9　3 8　4 7　5 6	Start time 12 11　1 10　2 9　3 8　4 7　5 6	End time: _____ Start time: _____ How much time passed? _____

(continued)

End time	Start time	End time: _____
12 11 1 10 2 9 3 8 4 7 5 6	12 11 1 10 2 9 3 8 4 7 5 6	Start time: _____ How much time passed? _____
End time	Start time	End time: _____
12 11 1 10 2 9 3 8 4 7 5 6	12 11 1 10 2 9 3 8 4 7 5 6	Start time: _____ How much time passed? _____
End time	Start time	End time: _____
12 11 1 10 2 9 3 8 4 7 5 6	12 11 1 10 2 9 3 8 4 7 5 6	Start time: _____ How much time passed? _____

Practice with Telling Time

12 11 1 10 2 9 3 8 4 7 5 6 **What time is it?**	12 11 1 10 2 9 3 8 4 7 5 6 **What time is it?**	12 11 1 10 2 9 3 8 4 7 5 6 **What time is it?**
12 11 1 10 2 9 3 8 4 7 5 6 **What time is it?**	12 11 1 10 2 9 3 8 4 7 5 6 **What time is it?**	12 11 1 10 2 9 3 8 4 7 5 6 **What time is it?**
12 11 1 10 2 9 3 8 4 7 5 6 **What time is it?**	12 11 1 10 2 9 3 8 4 7 5 6 **What time is it?**	12 11 1 10 2 9 3 8 4 7 5 6 **What time is it?**

Time-Planning Conference

Step 1: Get out the Daily Assignment Record (DAR) and Assignment and Test Calendar.

Step 2: Discuss assignments (short-term and long-term) that must be worked on today.

Step 3: Look at the Personal Calendar. What other activities are occurring tonight?

Step 4: Discuss what you want to do for leisure time today.

Step 5: Don't forget eating and getting ready for bed.

Step 6: Discuss how long each part of homework will take and how long all of homework will take.

Step 7: Decide when you will complete homework today.

Step 8: Fill in the Time Tracker for Homework as you complete each assignment.

Time-Planning Steps	Mon.	Tues.	Wed.	Thurs.	Fri.
Check the DAR for assignments.					
Check the Assignment and Test Calendar for other things to work on.					
Decide what schoolwork has to be worked on today.					
Check the Personal Calendar. Do you have any other activities?					
What do you want to do for leisure time today, and for how long?					
How long will your homework take?					

(continued)

Subject 1:					
Subject 2:					
Subject 3:					
Total time:					
When should you fit in this homework?					

Guide to the Time-Planning Conference

I. Review your DAR and your Assignment and Test Calendars.

What homework do you have?

II. Look at your Personal Calendar find out what other activities you have scheduled.

What activities do I have tonight?

What time are the activities?

How long does each activity take?

What do I want to do for fun tonight?

III. Decide when to do your homework.

How long should each assignment take? How long will all the work take to complete?

When can you fit in your homework?

Record when you plan to start and when you plan to finish homework.

IV. Write down when you actually started and actually finished each assignment on the Time Tracker for Homework.

OTMP Checklist: Things to Remember for Session 13

Please bring with you:

- ☐ Your OTMP parent's folder with:

  - ☐ Handout 19, Home Behavior Record

- ☐ The accordion binder with:

  - ☐ The child's DAR folder with completed DARs and Assignment and Test Calendars

  - ☐ All school papers

  - ☐ The child's OTMP folder with completed copies of:

    - ☐ Handout 28, Personal Calendar

    - ☐ Handout 31, Proposed Homework Schedule

    - ☐ Handout 34, Time-Planning Conference (with Handout 32, Time Tracker for Homework, attached)

- ☐ The child's school bag with backpack checklist and luggage tag attached

- ☐ Any questions or ideas that you want to discuss

Time-Planning Conference for Problem Situations

What do I have trouble finishing on time?
How long should this activity take?
When should I start the activity?
When should I be finished?
What time did I start? Write down the time on the clock.
What time did I finish?
Did I get done on time?   If not . . . I need to use my Time Detective Skills.
How did the **Time Bandit** get to me? I might need to ask my parents or other people.   Did I start slowly?   Did I get distracted?   How far behind was I?

Practice Time Planning for Longer-Term Assignments

Directions to parents: When you are holding a Time-Planning Conference, consider the homework that needs to be completed that day. Also, decide whether any longer-term assignments or tests need to be worked on that day as well. If your child does not have any longer-term assignments, use one of these as practice for your discussion (you and your child can choose which one to use). This will help your child become more aware of time demands and help keep the Time Bandit under control.

Spelling: For this week, there are 15 new words to learn. In order to study for the spelling test on Friday, please copy each word three times and write each one in a sentence.

Math: The class has to learn the squares of numbers from 1 to 15. You have to write out a definition of a square, and memorize the squares of 1 to 15. A test on squares will be held in 5 days.

Social Studies: In 5 days, you will need to present a short report for the class about the states that surround your home state. You need to find out the capital cities, the population of each state, and the nickname of each state, and create a labeled map of each state.

OTMP Checklist: Things to Remember for Session 14

Please bring with you:

- ☐ Your OTMP parent's folder with:
    - ☐ Handout 19, Home Behavior Record
- ☐ The accordion binder with:
    - ☐ The child's DAR folder with completed DARs and Assignment and Test Calendars
    - ☐ All school papers
    - ☐ The child's OTMP folder with completed copies of:
        - ☐ Handout 34, Time-Planning Conference (with Handout 32, Time Tracker for Homework [including longer-term assignments] attached)
        - ☐ Handout 37, Time-Planning Conference for Problem Situations
        - ☐ Teacher Form 9, Skills Check-Up
- ☐ The child's school bag with backpack checklist and luggage tag attached
- ☐ Any questions or ideas that you want to discuss

Ideas for Battling the Time Bandit

What strategies can I use to battle the Time Bandit when working on my **homework**?	1. 2. 3. 4. 5.
What strategies can I use to battle the Time Bandit in the **problem situation**?	1. 2. 3. 4. 5.
What can I do to battle the Time Bandit in one of my **regular routines**?	1. 2. 3. 4. 5.
What can I do to battle the Time Bandit in another **regular routine**?	1. 2. 3. 4. 5.

Time-Planning Conference for Regular Routines

Describe a regular routine (such as getting ready for bed)				
How long should it take to complete?				
What time does it have to be completed?				
When should I fit this in?				
How long did it take you to do it? (Look at clock as you start and after you are finished.)				
Were you done on time?				
What Time Bandit tactics interfered?				

Time Planning Conference, Including Review of the Problem Situation

Step 1: Get out the Daily Assignment Record (DAR) and Assignment and Test Calendar.

Step 2: Discuss assignments (short-term and long-term) that must be worked on today.

Step 3: Look at the Personal Calendar. What other activities are occurring tonight?

Step 4: Discuss what you want to do for leisure time today.

Step 5: Don't forget eating and getting ready for bed.

Step 6: Discuss how long each part of homework will take and how long all of homework will take.

Step 7: Decide when you will complete homework today.

Step 8: Fill in the Time Tracker for Homework as you complete each assignment.

Time-Planning Steps	Mon.	Tues.	Wed.	Thurs.	Fri.
Check the DAR for assignments.					
Check the Assignment and Test Calendar for other things to work on.					
Decide what schoolwork has to be worked on today.					
Check the Personal Calendar. Do you have any other activities?					
What do you want to do for leisure time today, and for how long?					
How long will your homework take?					

(continued)

Subject 1:					
Subject 2:					
Subject 3:					
Total time:					
When should you fit in this homework?					
Do I have to fit in the Problem Situation today? If so, how can I get this done on time?					

OTMP Checklist: Things to Remember for Session 15

Please bring with you:

- ☐ Your OTMP parent's folder with:

  - ☐ Handout 19, Home Behavior Record

- ☐ The accordion binder with:

  - ☐ The child's DAR folder with completed DARs and Assignment and Test Calendars

  - ☐ All school papers

  - ☐ The child's OTMP folder with completed copies of:

    - ☐ Handout 42, Time-Planning Conference, Including Review of the Problem Situation with (Handout 32, Time Tracker for Homework, attached)

    - ☐ Handout 41, Time Planning Conference Sheet for Regular Routines

- ☐ The child's school bag with backpack checklist and luggage tag attached

- ☐ Any questions or ideas that you want to discuss

Steps in Task Planning

Let's Control the Go-Ahead-Don't-Plan Glitch

1. **Think About the Goal**: Describe your goal in a short sentence.

2. **Get Ready to Go:**

    a. **Break it down:** What steps do you need to take to reach your goal?

    b. **Stuff you need:** What materials do you need to complete the steps?

3. **Manage your time:**

    a. **Arrange the steps:** In what order will you complete the steps?

    b. **Plan your time:** How much time will you need for each step?

    c. **Fit it in:** How will you fit the steps into your schedule?

4. **Check It Out:** Did you get everything done—neatly and completely?

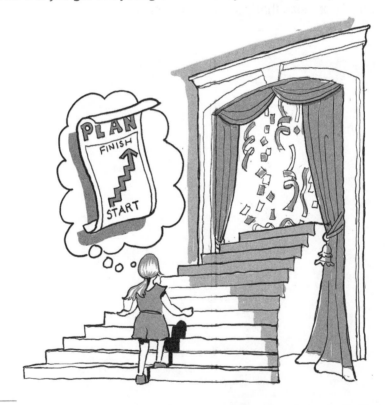

Task-Planning Conference: First Steps

List the activity used to practice task planning (e.g., bike ride).
1. **Think about the goal:** Describe your goal in a short sentence (e.g., "I want to ride my bike to the park").

2a. **Break it down: What steps do you have to take to reach your goal?** (e.g., pack a water bottle, check tires, put on helmet and knee pads)

Home Exercise Ideas: Task Planning

Directions to parents: Select an activity from this list (or think of your own), and ask your child to complete a Task-Planning Conference for this activity, using Handout 45 (Task-Planning Conference: First Steps).

1. Getting ready for bed
2. Practicing a musical instrument
3. Doing the dishes
4. Clearing your desk
5. Cleaning your room
6. Doing the laundry
7. Going for a walk
8. Riding your bike
9. Making and packing your lunch for school
10. Completing some math problems for homework
11. Studying for a test
12. Doing a book report
13. Completing a report for social studies
14. Preparing for a science fair
15. Writing an essay about your favorite game or movie, describing what you enjoy and why
16. Making a diorama about a state in the United States
17. Making a homemade card for someone's birthday
18. Going to purchase a pack of gum
19. Building a plastic model of a car or airplane
20. Getting ready for soccer practice
21. Inviting two friends over to watch a movie and have snacks
22. Cleaning out a closet
23. Bathing the dog
24. Borrowing a book from the library
25. Going on a hike
26. Going camping overnight

OTMP Checklist: Things to Remember for Session 16

Please bring with you:

☐ Your OTMP parent's folder with:

☐ Handout 19, Home Behavior Record

☐ The accordion binder with:

☐ The child's DAR folder with completed DARs and Assignment and Test Calendars

☐ All school papers

☐ The child's OTMP folder with completed copies of:

☐ Handout 42, Time-Planning Conference, Including Review of the Problem Situation (with Handout 32, Time Tracker for Homework, attached)

☐ Handout 45, Task-Planning Conference: First Steps

☐ The child's school bag with backpack checklist and luggage tag attached

☐ Any questions or ideas that you want to discuss

Task-Planning Conference

| 1. The Goal | 2. Getting Ready to Go | | 3. Time Management | | | 4. Checking It Out |
	a. Breaking it down into steps	b. What stuff is needed?	a. Ordering the steps	b. How long?	c. When to fit it in?	(All done—neat and complete)

OTMP Checklist: Things to Remember for Session 17

Please bring with you:

- ☐ Your OTMP parent's folder with:

    - ☐ Handout 19, Home Behavior Record

- ☐ The accordion binder with:

    - ☐ The child's DAR folder with completed DARs and Assignment and Test Calendars

    - ☐ All school papers

    - ☐ The child's OTMP folder with completed copies of Handout 48, Task-Planning Conference (for school, homework, and other activities)

- ☐ The child's school bag with backpack checklist and luggage tag attached

- ☐ Any questions or ideas that you want to discuss

OTMP Checklist: Things to Remember for Session 18

Please bring with you:

- ☐ Your OTMP parent's folder with:

    - ☐ Handout 19, Home Behavior Record

    - ☐ A note regarding an upcoming family activity/project/event that will require planning

- ☐ The accordion binder with:

    - ☐ The child's DAR folder with completed DARs and Assignment and Test Calendars

    - ☐ All school papers

    - ☐ The child's OTMP folder with completed copies of Handout 48, Task-Planning Conference

- ☐ The child's school bag with backpack checklist and luggage tag attached

- ☐ Any questions or ideas that you want to discuss

OTMP Checklist: Things to Remember for Session 19

Please bring with you:

- ☐ Your OTMP parent's folder with:

    - ☐ Handout 19, Home Behavior Record

- ☐ The accordion binder with:

    - ☐ The child's DAR folder with completed DARs and Assignment and Test Calendars

    - ☐ All school papers

    - ☐ The child's OTMP folder with completed copies of Handout 48, Task-Planning Conference

- ☐ The child's school bag with backpack checklist and luggage tag attached

- ☐ Any questions or ideas that you want to discuss

Personalized Commercial Script Outline

Why did you get involved in OST?
What Glitches used to get you?
What did you do in the program? What skills did you learn?
Was it helpful? What was the most helpful part?
Was it fun?
Did the program work for you?

Helping Your Child Maintain Good Organizational Skills

Your child has learned a number of important organizational, time management, and planning (OTMP) skills during the organizational skills training (OST) program. You have been taught how to prompt your child to use these skills (e.g., "Remember to put your completed homework in your backpack," "Don't forget to clear your desk before you start working") and how to reward your child for doing so. Now that the program is ending, it is important for your child to continue to use the OTMP skills without becoming overly dependent on prompts and rewards. The procedures described below, known as "fading" and "thinning," have been developed for just this purpose. "Fading" means reducing how often you prompt. "Thinning" means reducing how often you reward. Here are useful guidelines and suggestions on how to use fading and thinning with your child.

Fading: Reducing How Often You Prompt

The ideal goal is for your child to use the OTMP tools and skills learned in this program without always having to be reminded to do so. Reducing how often you prompt gives your child opportunities to become self-reliant and to use these skills when needed. This will also help your child to better recognize situations that call for OTMP skills, and to use them even when you are not present.

There is no "one right" fading schedule. What works best for one child does not work best for another. Also, a child may do fine in some situations without being prompted, but may need prompts in other situations. Therefore, deciding how to fade prompting with your child will depend in part on three factors: (1) how often you currently remind your child to use the OTMP skills, (2) how well your child does when these prompts are not given, and (3) whether there are situations that require more or fewer prompts. With these factors in mind, you can begin the process of reducing (fading) the number of prompts you give your child.

First, let your child know that you will be reducing how often you provide reminders to be organized, and explain why you are doing this. Second, discuss with your child how visual or written cues can be useful reminders to use skills and stay organized instead of relying on your prompts. For example, point out how your child can use the tag on the backpack that asks, "Is everything in my bag?" as a prompt to make sure that all materials have been packed. Third, keep track of what happens when you do not give prompts. Does your child carry out or fail to carry out the required skills? Make notes about this. Fourth, whenever your child independently uses an OTMP skill, praise your child for having done so without being reminded. Finally, use the information you have tracked to make any necessary adjustments to the fading schedule. For example, if you notice that materials have been left out of the backpack, you might have to increase how often you prompt your child to check that everything needed for school the next day has been packed. If you notice that your child is playing with items on the desk during homework time, you might have to increase how often you prompt your child to check that the desk is Ready to Go.

Thinning: Reducing How Often You Reward

Throughout the treatment, you have been rewarding your child regularly and frequently for using the skills taught in OST. Now that treatment is ending, it is important to reduce how often you give "concrete" rewards to your child, such as extra video game time, choosing the dessert for dinner, or playing a word game with Mom or Dad. There are different ways to reduce concrete rewards, and these are briefly described below. However, it is essential to continue regularly praising your child and giving

(continued)

"social" rewards for OTMP behaviors. That is, when you are praising your child for being organized, also give a hug, a smile, or some other expression of affection and approval. This kind of positive feedback is as important to your child as concrete rewards.

The easiest and most effective ways to "thin" rewards are (1) *increasing the length of time* before your child is rewarded for being well organized, or (2) *increasing the number of times* your child has to show good OTMP skills before being rewarded. Often these two criteria are related. Here are some examples:

1. Instead of giving your child a "concrete" reward every day that the Daily Assignment Record (DAR) is completed, signed by the teacher, and brought home, reward your child at the end of the week if the DAR was completed and signed on at least 4 days, and give a "bonus" if the DAR was completed and signed every day. *Remember to praise your child* each day for having brought home a completed and signed DAR.

2. Instead of giving a "concrete" reward each day that your child shows good time management for homework, wait to give the reward until your child has shown this on three occasions. For example, you would reward your child after three instances of accurately estimating the amount of time it took to complete homework. Remember to praise, hug, or give a "high-five" to your child each day good management of homework time happens. To keep track of when to give a reward, you can continue to record your child's behavior on a simple chart, like the Rewards Menu or Home Behavior Record (copies follow). Such a chart can also remind you to praise your child for using organizational tools and routines.

REWARD MENU
Daily Rewards

If I get 60% of my daily points, I can choose from:

If I get more than 60% of my daily points, I can choose from:

Weekly Rewards

If I get 60% of my daily points, I can choose from:

If I get more than 60% of my daily points, I can choose from:

(continued)

HOME BEHAVIOR RECORD

Directions: Give your child 1 point for each behavior that is performed on a given day. There are 5 possible points to be earned each day.

Behaviors	Day 1	Day 2	Day 3	Day 4	Day 5	Day 6	Day 7
School Behavior 1 _____ _____							
School Behavior 2 _____ _____							
Home Behavior 1 _____ _____							
Home Behavior 2 _____ _____							
Home Behavior 3 _____ _____							
Total points (out of 5)							
Points for the week							

OTMP Checklist: Things to Remember for Session 20

Please bring with you:

- ☐ Your OTMP parent's folder with:

    - ☐ Handout 19, Home Behavior Record

- ☐ The accordion binder with:

    - ☐ The child's DAR folder with completed DARs and Assignment and Test Calendars

    - ☐ All school papers

    - ☐ The child's OTMP folder with completed copies of:

        - ☐ Handout 48, Task-Planning Conference

        - ☐ Hnadout 52, Personalized Commercial Script Outline

        - ☐ Personalized commercial script

- ☐ The child's school bag with backpack checklist and luggage tag attached

- ☐ Any questions or ideas that you want to discuss

Owner's Manual for Organizational Skills

Table of Contents

Appendix: Helpful Handouts

1. KEEPING THE GLITCHES UNDER CONTROL

In organizational skills training (OST), you learned about the "Glitches," little creatures that live inside our brains and get in the way when we least expect it. They trick us by making us forget to use important skills. They make us get in trouble, in school and at home, by making us less organized. Glitches can bother anyone, but Glitches get to some people—such as people with attention/deficit/hyperactivity disorder (ADHD)—more often. These people have to work hard to help their "Mastermind" get control of the Glitches. Kids and adults can take action and use special tools to keep the Glitches under control. It is important to keep using those tools to keep the Mastermind in charge.

You learned that you probably have to work harder than other kids to control the Glitches. This means using the same routines over and over again. In OST, you learned routines for keeping track of assignments, managing your materials (like books and papers), managing your time, and planning for important tasks. Your parents and teachers helped you remember what to do at home and in school by prompting, praising, and rewarding you. Together, we kept the Glitches under control. If you want to keep control of the Glitches, you have to keep using these routines at home and in school.

Remember: the Glitches are tricky. It can be fun to let the Glitches come out and play. We all need a vacation when we don't have to worry about planning ahead or getting things done on time. But when

(continued)

we forget to manage the Glitches after a vacation, it can be hard to get back on track. As you know, the Glitches can cause major problems during the school year. So keep using your skills all the time when school is in session. And whenever a vacation ends, it is important to get the Mastermind back in shape. You've come a long way in being more organized since you started this program, but you won't magically *stay* organized. If you want to keep on top of the Glitches, you have to keep using the new tools you've learned. Your parents will also have to help, by providing reminders and lots of praise when you use the OST steps.

If you follow the suggestions in this manual, you should have a better school year. You can keep your Mastermind in charge. In this manual, we give ideas for managing each one of the Glitches. You will probably think of some extra ideas on your own. Go ahead! Be creative! You know what works best for you. This manual also spells out steps that you can take to stay organized from the beginning to the end of each day. These ideas may help set up a routine that will keep the Glitches under control.

2. TIPS FOR CONTROLLING THE GO-AHEAD-FORGET-IT GLITCH

Keeping Track of Homework, Tests, and Assignments

1. Use a Daily Assignment Record (DAR) every day. You can copy and use the blank DAR at the end of this manual. Or you and your parents can use the instructions (also at the end of this manual) to create your own DAR on the computer.
2. Make a quick checklist of the items you need for each assignment.
3. Write down due dates for assignments and tests on your Assignment and Test Calendar.
4. Copy due dates for tests and assignments to a calendar. Keep the calendar at the front or back of your DAR folder or planner. You can copy and use the blank Assignment and Test Calendar at the end of this manual. You can also use a calendar that shows the month in a planner.

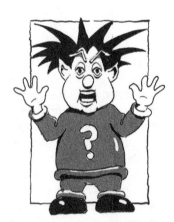

The Go-Ahead-Forget-It Glitch.

Managing Your Books, Supplies, and Papers

1. Make yourself a reminder checklist for your backpack, so you will remember to pack your books, notebooks, papers, and other important materials.
2. Look at your reminder checklist when you pack up at school.
3. Look at your reminder checklist when you pack up at home.
4. Include important items on your checklist that must go back and forth between home and school (lunch money, a musical instrument, gym clothes, etc.).

(continued)

368

3. TIPS FOR CONTROLLING THE GO-AHEAD-LOSE-IT GLITCH

Managing Your Papers

1. Use a binder with pockets to hold your papers. An accordion binder is an excellent choice.
2. Label a section for each subject.
3. Whenever you get papers, put them in the binder. Don't wait until later to do it. Don't cram the papers into your backpack and say that you're going to file them later. Put them in the binder right away.
4. If you take out papers and use them, make sure you return them to the binder immediately after you are done.
5. If you need to use a three-ring binder for school, get folders with pockets for your papers—but also make sure the folders have closing flaps, so nothing can fall out.
6. If you have to transfer papers to another folder or binder, do it carefully so you don't lose the papers.

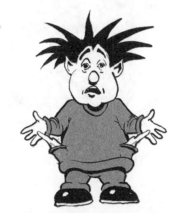

The Go-Ahead-Lose-It Glitch.

Managing Other Stuff

1. For really important items (like special toys, a calculator, or a cell phone), try to pick one place where you will keep those items all the time. Return the items to this place after you have used them. That way, you will not have to remember where you put something. You can just go back to the special place. For example, if you have a cell phone, keep it in one special spot in your room.
2. If you have several items that you want to keep track of at home, consider getting a basket or a box where you put them all together.
3. Try to use a similar plan for your items at school. You may have lost clothing, gloves or other belongings at school before. Try to make sure that you have one place where you keep things.
4. If you need to take something to school that you usually don't have with you, put the item on your checklist, so you remember that it has to be taken to school or brought back home.

4. TIPS FOR CONTROLLING THE TIME BANDIT

Managing Your Time at School

1. When you are given an assignment to do at school, estimate how long each step should take.
2. Use a watch or clock to help you stay close to those time estimates. For example, if you think it will take 10 minutes to do one step, look at the clock when you begin and when you end. See if you were

(continued)

right. Adjust your plans if you were wrong. Try to remember how closely you kept to your predictions. This will help you plan your time in the future.

3. Don't use up work time getting distracted. If you do, you may not complete your work, and your teacher will be disappointed. You will probably have to finish your work later or at home. You may even have to miss out on recess time, to complete the work that you were supposed to do during the class period.

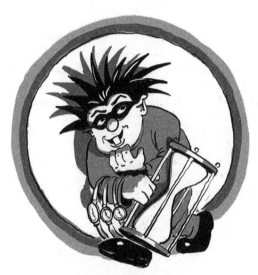

The Time Bandit.

Managing Your Time at Home

1. Hold Time-Planning Conferences with one of your parents or someone else before you begin your homework. Set up your schedule for the evening so you can get all of your assignments done, while taking reasonable breaks. Make sure to review your Assignment and Test Calendar so you can include projects and studying in your schedule.

2. Clear your work area of distractions; they steal your time. Although it may be fun to play with things on your desk, it is probably not as much fun as playing your favorite game, watching a good TV show, or reading a good book after your work has been completed. So save your time for really fun activities.

3. When you have activities and chores, try to estimate how much time they will take to complete. Try to stay close to your estimates, so you don't waste time that could be spent doing other fun things.

4. Don't forget to think about the steps it takes to prepare for activities. For example, if you have a karate class that lasts 1 hour, don't forget that it takes time to travel to and from the class. Travel time is part of the time required to do that activity. Cleaning up and storing your stuff after you have played sports or games also takes time, but it is an important step. It may be faster to leave the equipment all over the place, but doing that will slow you down the next time you play, because you will have to go look for the equipment.

5. TIPS FOR CONTROLLING THE GO-AHEAD-DON'T-PLAN GLITCH

1. Remember that everything you do can be broken down into steps. Think about the steps you need to take to complete assignments, projects, and fun activities.

2. For important tasks, use your task-planning skills: Think about the steps, write them down, consider
(continued)

what materials you will need to complete each step, put them in the right order, decide how long they will take, and check them off as you complete them.

3. Use task planning steps as often as you can. If you practice these skills on smaller tasks (e.g., preparing a snack), you will be better prepared for bigger tasks (e.g., completing a book report).

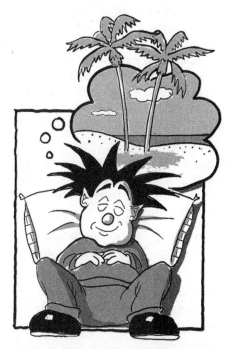

The Go-Ahead-Don't-Plan Glitch.

6. PLANNING A DAILY ROUTINE TO CONTROL THE GLITCHES

Let's put all of the tips together into one plan for how to stay organized and control the Glitches every day. If you follow the basic steps below every day, staying organized will be part of your routine, and it will be easier for you to keep the Mastermind in control all day. You know these steps—you've practiced them in sessions, at home, and at school for the past few months. Now your job is to make sure that you use these steps every day. If you do, it will be a lot harder for the Glitches to cause trouble for you.

Basic Steps to Follow for a School Day

Step 1: Handle the Go-Ahead-Forget-It Glitch from the start of the day, by making a backpack checklist, and checking it every morning before you go to school. Use it as a reminder to pack your books; your binder (or other folder) with papers; special papers like permission slips; your lunch or lunch money; and anything else you always need (e.g., pencils, pens, bus or subway card, money, gym clothes, or portable video games for the bus ride). This will help you leave home with everything you need.

Step 2: Keep controlling the Go-Ahead-Forget-It Glitch. Make sure you keep track of your assignments and the items you need to complete those assignments. Make yourself an assignment record that has a place to write down what books and materials you need for each assignment. If your school uses a planner, make sure you add a place to list the items you need for each assignment. Then get yourself a calendar or make one, so you can write down information about long-term assignments on it. This will

(continued)

help you keep track of long-term assignments, which can be forgotten when you turn the page on a planner or assignment record.

Make sure you pick a time each day to write down your assignments on your assignment record. There might be a set time in your class when you are supposed to write down the assignments; if so, use this time to check that you have written down all of the important information. If you feel rushed during this time and often don't have a chance to write down all of the assignments, talk to your teacher about this problem, and ask if you can work out another time to complete your DAR or fill in your planner. No matter what, make sure you write down Avall of your assignments—even the ones you think you'll definitely remember. You might think that you will remember everything, but don't believe it. That's just another one of the Go-Ahead-Forget-It Glitch's tricks. At the beginning of the school year, ask your teacher to check your list each day, to make sure you wrote everything down correctly.

If you have several teachers, make sure to fill in your assignment record before the end of each class period. Give yourself enough time to do this carefully, so the Go-Ahead-Forget-It Glitch does not sneak up on you.

Step 3: To help the Mastermind control the Go-Ahead-Forget-It Glitch and the Go-Ahead-Lose-It Glitch, set up a special place to store your papers, like an accordion binder. When you get a paper, immediately put it in the right place in your binder. You may get papers throughout the day, so make sure your binder or special storage place is with you all the time.

Step 4: At the end of the day, use your backpack checklist to pack up your stuff. The checklist will help you figure out what you should put in your backpack. It will remind you to check to make sure that you have everything.

Step 5: When you get home and are ready to start your homework, take your backpack to the place where you do homework, and show your parent (or other adult) your assignment record. Show this person that you know what your assignments are, and that you have all the materials you need to complete those assignments.

Step 6: Next, manage the Time Bandit. Briefly, hold a Time-Planning Conference for the evening with your parent or other adult. Look at your Assignment and Test Record to see what's for homework, and check your Personal Calendar to see which long-term assignments and tests are coming up. Figure out what work you need to do that evening. Decide when you will do your homework, so you leave enough time to do something fun afterward. Decide on the order in which you will do your assignments. Be a Time Detective and decide how long each assignment or part of an assignment should take. Plan brief breaks, if you need them, and be realistic about how much time you will need to get everything done.

Step 7: Get your homework area Ready to Go. Make sure that you have everything you need to complete assignments. Consider everything, including the kitchen sink! Then put away anything that will distract you. Leave yourself enough space to work free of clutter.

Step 8: Carry out your plan.

Step 9: When you're finished, check your work for neatness and completeness. This will help you control the Go-Ahead-Don't-Plan Glitch.

Step 10: Congratulate yourself! You have put your Mastermind in charge, and you are working hard to control the Glitches. Keep up the good work!

Good luck, and don't let the Glitches get you!

(continued)

APPENDIX

Helpful Handouts

(continued)

DAILY ASSIGNMENT RECORD

Date: _____

Subject	What Is for Homework?	What Do I Need to Take?	Other Assignments and Due Dates	Teacher: Check for School Points—Did the child use the skill? If yes, provide a point.
Language Arts		___ Workbook ___ Handouts ___ Textbook ___ Other		**Target Skills:** 1.
Social Studies		___ Workbook ___ Handouts ___ Textbook ___ Other		
Science		___ Workbook ___ Handouts ___ Textbook ___ Other		
Math		___ Workbook ___ Handouts ___ Textbook ___ Other		**Check/Initials** _____
Spelling		___ Workbook ___ Handouts ___ Textbook ___ Other		**Target Skills:** 2.
Second Language		___ Workbook ___ Handouts ___ Textbook ___ Other		
Announcements or Special Papers		___ Handouts ___ Other ___ Permission slip		
Anything Else?				**Check/Initials** _____

(continued)

374

HOW TO CREATE YOUR OWN DAILY ASSIGNMENT RECORD

You may need to create a new DAR for the next school year, if your subjects change. The following directions will help you and your parents create your own DAR on your computer.

- Using Microsoft Word, open a new document.
- Click on the "Page Layout" tab at the top of the screen. Then click on "Orientation" and set the orientation to "Landscape."
- Click on the "Insert" drop-down menu at the top of the screen.
- Click on "Table," then "Insert Table."
- A small screen will pop up. For the number of columns, type in the number 5; for the number of rows, type in the number of subjects you have in school (this will generally be about 4—for example, math, science, social studies, and English).
- A table with the correct number of rows and column will appear on the computer screen. Using the "Enter" button, increase the length of each column. Use your mouse to adjust the width of each column, by dragging the vertical lines that separate the columns to the right or left.
- The five rows should have the following titles:

Subject	What Is for Homework?	What Do I Need to Take?	Other Assignments and Due Dates	Teacher: Check for School Points—Did the child use the skill? If yes, provide a point.

- Use one sheet per day. You can staple a number of sheets into a manila folder to create a notepad for each week. Be creative; if you feel that your DAR should include other headings, feel free to adjust it so it suits your needs.

(continued)

ASSIGNMENT AND TEST CALENDAR

Month _____

What Is Due?:
Look at Your Daily Assignment Record

Monday	Tuesday	Wednesday	Thursday	Friday

(continued)

376

TIME-PLANNING CONFERENCE

Step 1: Get out the Daily Assignment Record (DAR) and Assignment and Test Calendar.

Step 2: Discuss assignments (short-term and long-term) that must be worked on today.

Step 3: Look at the Personal Calendar. What other activities are occurring tonight?

Step 4: Discuss what you want to do for leisure time today.

Step 5: Don't forget eating and getting ready for bed.

Step 6: Discuss how long each part of homework will take and how long all of homework will take.

Step 7: Decide when you will complete homework today.

Step 8: Fill in the Time Tracker for Homework as you complete each assignment.

Time-Planning Steps	Mon.	Tues.	Wed.	Thurs.	Fri.
Check the DAR for assignments.					
Check the Assignment and Test Calendar for other things to work on.					
Decide what schoolwork has to be worked on today.					
Check the Personal Calendar. Do you have any other activities?					
What do you want to do for leisure time today, and for how long?					
How long will your homework take?					
Subject 1:					
Subject 2:					
Subject 3:					
Total time:					
When should you fit in this homework?					

(continued)

377

TIME TRACKER FOR HOMEWORK

Step 1: Think about the amount of homework that you have.

Step 2: Think about how much time you think each assignment will take.

Step 3: Write down the time that you think you will start, and then the time that you think you will finish.

Step 4: When you start each assignment, write down the time.

Step 5: When you finish each assignment, write down the time.

DAY 1

	Subject 1	Subject 2	Subject 3
I plan to start at:			
I plan to finish at:			
I actually started at:			
I actually finished at:			
Is my work complete?			
How much more time did I spend to complete it?			

DAY 2

	Subject 1	Subject 2	Subject 3
I plan to start at:			
I plan to finish at:			
I actually started at:			
I actually finished at:			
Is my work complete?			
How much more time did I spend to complete it?			

(continued)

TIME TRACKER FOR HOMEWORK *(continued)*

DAY 3

	Subject 1	Subject 2	Subject 3
I plan to start at:			
I plan to finish at:			
I actually started at:			
I actually finished at:			
Is my work complete?			
How much more time did I spend to complete it?			

DAY 4

	Subject 1	Subject 2	Subject 3
I plan to start at:			
I plan to finish at:			
I actually started at:			
I actually finished at:			
Is my work complete?			
How much more time did I spend to complete it?			

DAY 5

	Subject 1	Subject 2	Subject 3
I plan to start at:			
I plan to finish at:			
I actually started at:			
I actually finished at:			
Is my work complete?			
How much more time did I spend to complete it?			

(continued)

PERSONAL CALENDAR

Fill in your schedule for the week:

1. When do I get home?

2. What time do I have to go to bed?

3. Do I have any special activities after school? If so, what are they, and what times are they scheduled?

	Su	M	Tu	W	Th	F	Sa
Get home							
Go to bed							
Any special activities							

(continued)

TASK-PLANNING CONFERENCE

1. The Goal	2. Getting Ready to Go			3. Time Management			4. Checking It Out
	a. Breaking it down into steps	b. What stuff is needed?	a. Ordering the steps	b. How long?	c. When to fit it in?		(All done—neat and complete)

OST Graduation Certificate

Congratulations!

_____

has completed a full course of organizational skills training (OST).

The Mastermind is in control!

_____   _____
Name   Date

TEACHER FORMS

Teacher's Guide to Organizational Skills Training

WHAT IS ORGANIZATIONAL SKILLS TRAINING?

- Organizational skills training (OST) is a comprehensive treatment program that helps children to improve their organization, time management, and planning (OTMP) skills.
- Your student will meet with an OST therapist twice a week for 10 weeks, and will be taught new organizational skills and routines, one at a time. Skills will be taught in four broad areas that are critical for the child's functioning at home and in school:
  - Tracking Assignments (e.g., writing down homework assignments and due dates for long-term projects or tests)
  - Managing Materials (e.g., storing and transferring papers and books between school and home; setting up a workspace with appropriate items)
  - Time Management (e.g., completing assignments on time; creating and following a schedule)
  - Task Planning (e.g., breaking larger projects down into steps, developing a reasonable plan for completing long-term projects)
- The student will practice each new skill in session, and will be given "homework" to practice that skill at home and in school, as part of the regular routines.
- The Detailed OST Schedule (Teacher Form 2) lists the skills that the student will probably learn and need to use in class each week. However, each student is treated as an individual; the therapist will only move on to a new skill when the child has improved and become more competent in using the previous skill.

HOW ARE TEACHERS INVOLVED IN OST?

- Teachers play a crucial role in the OST program, as they can support students' use of new organizational skills in the classroom setting.
- For each new skill that a student must use in the classroom, a teacher is asked to:
  - Prompt the student to use the skill/routine.
  - Monitor the student's use of the skill/routine.
  - Praise the student for following the prompt and using the skill/routine.
  - Provide a point on the child's Daily Assignment Record (see Teacher Form 4) after the child has used the skill/routine.
- The whole process of prompting, monitoring, praising, and providing points should take **no more than 2–4 minutes daily** to complete . . . because the OST program's developers know how precious a teacher's time is.
- In OST, teachers and therapists work together to help students learn new organizational skills that can give them a better chance of success in school. Your student's therapist will schedule five in-person or phone meetings over the course of treatment to help keep you informed about which skills the student should use in school and how you can best support the student in using those skills. In addition, you can always feel free to contact the therapist via phone or email, to discuss any questions or concerns you may have.

Detailed OST Schedule

Week	Session	Topic	Target behavior: Teacher will prompt, monitor, praise, and provide a school point if the child performed the behavior
1	1	Orientation meeting for parent and child	No target behavior Therapist and teacher meet to discuss: 1. The child's OTMP difficulties in school 2. The DAR and the prompt–monitor–praise–point system
	2	Behavior management training for parents	No target behavior
2	3	Introduction of method for keeping track of assignments, the Daily Assignment Record (DAR); controlling the Go-Ahead-Forget-It Glitch	Completed the DAR
	4	Review of school assignments and papers	Completed the DAR
3	5	Introduction of method for storing and transferring papers, the accordion binder; controlling the Go-Ahead-Lose-It Glitch	1. Completed the DAR accurately 2. Put papers in the binder
	6	Review of routines for tracking assignments and managing papers	1. Completed the DAR accurately 2. Put papers in the binder
4	7	Introduction of the backpack checklist	1. Completed the DAR accurately 2. Used the binder and turned in all papers
	8	Continued use of backpack checklist	1. Used the binder and turned in all papers 2. Used the backpack checklist
5	9	Getting work area Ready to Go	1. Used the binder and backpack checklist, and turned in all papers 2. Got the desk Ready to Go
	10	Understanding time and calendars; controlling the Time Bandit	1. Turned in all assignments 2. Got the desk Ready to Go
6	11	Time management for homework	1. Got the desk Ready to Go 2. Completed the Time Tracker for In-Class Work for an in-class assignment

(continued)

	12	Holding onto free time	1. Got the desk Ready to Go 2. Completed the Time Tracker for In-Class Work for an in-class assignment
7	13	Time planning for longer-term assignments; managing the Time Bandit	1. Got the desk Ready to Go 2. Completed the Time Tracker for In-Class Work for an in-class assignment
	14	Time management for regular routines	1. Completed all in-class assignments on time 2. Completed the Time Tracker for In-Class Work for an in-class assignment
8	15	Introduction to task planning and first steps in planning; controlling the Go-Ahead-Don't-Plan Glitch	Same as Session 14
	16	Next steps in task planning: Managing materials and time	1. Completed all in-class assignments on time 2. Completed the Time Tracker for In-Class Work for an in-class assignment, *or* Completed a Task-Planning Conference for an in-class assignment
9	17	Coordinating planning and time management	Same as Session 16
	18	Planning for long-term projects	Same as Session 16
10	19	Task planning: Checking It Out	1. Completed all in-class assignments on time 2. Checked all assignments for neatness and completeness
	20	Program summary	Discussed with the therapist ways to encourage and praise continued effective organization

Guide to the Daily Assignment Record

Your student has been taught and practiced a new method for writing down school assignments: using a Daily Assignment Record, or DAR. The DAR is designed to help students keep track of their assignments and the materials they need to complete those assignments. A sample DAR is provided as Teacher Form 4, so you can see its basic features:

1. A space to write down homework assignments for each subject
2. A space to check what items need to go home (e.g., textbooks, notebooks, worksheets)
3. A space to write down any other assignments or tests that are due in the future.
4. A space called "Teacher: Check for School Points . . ." where you can give the child school points for completing the target behavior for the day

For the next week, the target behavior will be completing the DAR. Please check your student's DAR each day, and give the student a point for any attempt to complete the DAR (even if you have to correct mistakes in filling it out).

After this week, you will give the child a point for completing the DAR only if it is completed accurately. You will see this change noted under the "Teacher; Checking for School Points . . ." column.

Please remember the prompt–monitor–praise–point procedure:

1. *Prompt* your student to use the behavior.
2. *Monitor* the student's use of the behavior.
3. *Praise* the student for using the behavior.
4. *Provide a point* if the student showed the behavior.

Sample Daily Assignment Record

Date: _____

Subject	What Is for Homework?	What Do I Need to Take?	Other Assignments and Due Dates	Teacher: Check for School Points—Did the child use the skill? If yes, provide a point.
Language Arts		___ Workbook ___ Handouts ___ Textbook ___ Other		**Target Skills:** 1.
Social Studies		___ Workbook ___ Handouts ___ Textbook ___ Other		
Science		___ Workbook ___ Handouts ___ Textbook ___ Other		
Math		___ Workbook ___ Handouts ___ Textbook ___ Other		**Check/Initials** _____
Spelling		___ Workbook ___ Handouts ___ Textbook ___ Other		**Target Skills:** 2.
Second Language		___ Workbook ___ Handouts ___ Textbook ___ Other		
Announcements or Special Papers		___ Handouts ___ Other ___ Permission slip		
Anything Else?				**Check/Initials** _____

Guide to the Accordion Binder

The child should follow the following steps:

1. Fill in the Daily Assignment Record (DAR).
2. Put all papers in the accordion binder (including the DAR).
3. Check that papers are in the right spot in the binder.

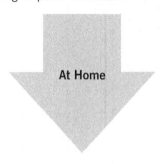

At Home

4. Fill in Assignment and Test Calendars
5. Work with papers
6. Put back in binder

REMINDER . . .

The target behaviors for this week are these:

1. Complete the DAR accurately. Please prompt use of the DAR, and encourage accurate completion.
2. Put papers in the binder. Please prompt the child to put all of the papers given during the day into the binder. *If the child responds to your prompt, please give the child a school point.* You do not need to worry about accuracy of placement.

Please remember:

1. *Prompt* your student to use the behavior.
2. *Monitor* the student's use of the behavior.
3. *Praise* the student for using the behavior.
4. Give a *point* if the student showed the behavior.

Ready to Go: Teacher Guidelines

Before starting an in-class assignment, prompt the student to consider these questions:

1. Do you have everything you need? (Consider everything including the kitchen sink!)
2. What should you put away?
3. Is your work area clear?
4. Are there any things that could distract you?

Then tell the student: "You are now Ready to Go!"

Introduction to Time Management

LET'S REVIEW . . .

So far, in OST, the child has learned skills for:

- Keeping track of assignments
- Keeping track of materials needed to complete assignments
- Filing, storing, and transferring school papers
- Packing bags with necessary items
- Getting workspaces ready for work

NEW FOCUS: TIME MANAGEMENT

OST will now be focusing on "time management," which includes:

- Learning how behavior is connected to time
- Using a calendar to keep track of assignments and activities
- Estimating how long specific tasks will take to complete
- Keeping track of how long specific tasks actually take to complete
- Planning a schedule so that important tasks get done

HOW CAN YOU HELP THE CHILD WORK ON TIME MANAGEMENT IN SCHOOL?

The child will be learning how to use a special form, the Time Tracker for In-Class Work (see Teacher Form 8), to keep track of how time is spent for an in-class assignment. Using the form, the child will be asked before beginning one in-class assignment each day (a sheet of math word problems, a reading response, etc.) to estimate how long the assignment will take. The child will then write down when work is started on the assignment and when the work period ends, and will note whether the assignment is complete. You may choose which assignment to use for this practice with the Time Tracker.

The child should be able to complete the Time Tracker for In-Class Work independently, after some practice. However, especially when the child is first starting to use this form, please make sure to prompt the child to fill in the appropriate spaces, and to provide any support the child might need in writing in the times. Finally, help the child determine whether the assignment is complete or not. When the child is done using the Time Tracker, the form should be filed in the binder, in the section designated for OTMP papers.

You will give the child a school point for completing the Time Tracker for In-Class Work, regardless of whether or not the work has been completed on time. The important skill to reinforce, at this point, is the awareness of how time is being used when an assignment must be completed.

Time Tracker for In-Class Work

Please complete this form once a day, when your teacher asks you to.

Step 1: Think about the in-class assignment that you have to do.

Step 2: Decide how much time you think the assignment will take.

Step 3: Write down the time that you think you will start and the time you think you will finish.

Step 4: When you start the assignment, write down the time.

Step 5: When you are all finished, write down the time.

	Monday	Tuesday	Wednesday	Thursday	Friday
How long will this assignment take?					
What time is it at the start of the assignment?					
What time is it at the end of the assignment?					
Is the assignment complete?					
Did I need more time or less time?					
Did anything slow me down?					
Teacher initials					

Skills Check-Up

Child's Name: _____

Date of Day 1: _____

	Day 1	Day 2	Day 3	Day 4
Is the child completing in-class activities on time?				
Is the child handing in homework on time?				
Does the child have the books, supplies, and materials needed for class?				

Teacher's Name: _____

Introduction to Task Planning

The final few sessions of OST will focus on helping the child learn skills to control the Go-Ahead-Don't-Plan Glitch. This Glitch sometimes tells the child to engage in tasks willy-nilly, without much planning. As you can imagine, this lack of planning can result in problems for the child. The child is learning to use a Task-Planning Conference to plan for important tasks and/or projects, and will practice the steps listed below in sessions and at home. If there are opportunities in your classroom to use task planning, the therapist will discuss with you how to help the child use a Task-Planning Conference for in-class work or projects. A sample Task-Planning Conference is provided as Teacher Form 11, so you can see its basic features.

STEPS IN TASK PLANNING

1. **Think about the goal:** Describe your goal in a short sentence.

2. **Get Ready to Go**
   a. **Break it down:** What steps do you need to take to reach your goal?
   b. **Stuff you need:** What materials do you need to complete the steps?

3. **Manage your time:**
   a. **Arrange the steps:** In what order will you complete the steps?
   b. **Plan your time:** How much time will you need for each step?
   c. **Fit it in:** How will you fit the steps into your schedule?

4. **Check It Out:** Did you meet your goal completely and accurately?

Sample Task Planning Conference Worksheet

| 1. The Goal | 2. Getting Ready to Go | | 3. Time Management | | | 4. Checking It Out |
	a. Breaking it down into steps	b. What stuff is needed?	a. Ordering the steps	b. How long?	c. When to fit it in?	(All done—neat and complete)

References

Abikoff, H. (1985). Efficacy of cognitive training interventions in hyperactive children: A critical review. *Clinical Psychology Review, 5*, 479–512.

Abikoff, H., & Gallagher, R. (2003, October). Assessment and treatment of organizational skills deficits in ADHD children. In T. Wilens (Chair), *Clinical issues of executive functioning disturbances (EF) in ADHD*. Symposium conducted at the annual meeting of the American Academy of Child and Adolescent Psychiatry, Miami Beach, FL.

Abikoff, H., & Gallagher, R. (2008). Assessment and remediation of organizational skills deficits in children with ADHD. In K. McBurnett & L. Pfiffner (Eds.), *Attention deficit hyperactivity disorder: Concepts, controversies, new directions* (pp. 137–152). New York: Information Healthcare USA.

Abikoff, H., & Gallagher, R. (2009). *The Children's Organizational Skills Scales: Technical manual*. North Tonawanda, NY: Multi-Health Systems.

Abikoff, H., Gallagher, R., & Alvir, J. (2003, June). *A teacher rating scale of children's organizational, time management and planning skills: The COSS-T*. Poster presented at the annual meeting of the International Society for Research in Child and Adolescent Psychopathology, Sydney, Australia.

Abikoff, H., Gallagher, R., Wells, K. C., Murray, D. W., Huang, L., Lu, F., et al. (2013). Remediating organizational functioning in children with ADHD: Immediate and long-term effects from a randomized controlled trial. *Journal of Consulting and Clinical Psychology, 81*(1), 113–128.

Abikoff, H., Jensen, P. S., Arnold, L. L., Hoza, B., Hechtman, L., Pollack, S., et al. (2002). Observed classroom behavior of children with ADHD: Relationship to comorbidity and gender. *Journal of Abnormal Child Psychology, 30*, 349–359.

Abikoff, H., Nissley-Tsiopinis, J., Gallagher, R., Zambenedetti, M., Seyffert, M., Boorady, R., et al. (2009). Effects of MPH-OROS on the organizational, time management, and planning behaviors of children with ADHD. *Journal of the American Academy of Child and Adolescent Psychiatry, 48*, 166–175.

American Psychiatric Association. (1994). *Diagnostic and statistical manual of mental disorders* (4th ed.). Washington, DC: Author.

Assouline, S. G., & Whiteman, C. S. (2011). Twice-exceptionality: Implications for school psychologists in the post-IDEA 2004 era. *Journal of Applied School Psychology, 27*(4), 380–402.

Axelrod, M. I., Zhe, E. J., Haugen, K. A., & Klein, J. A. (2009). Self-management of on-task homework behavior: A promising strategy for adolescents with attention and behavior problems. *School Psychology Review, 38*(3), 325–333.

Baker, J. A., Bridger, R., & Evans, K. (1998). Models of underachievement among gifted preadolescents: The role of personal, family, and school factors. *Gifted Child Quarterly, 42*(1), 5–15.

Barkley, R. A. (2006). *Attention deficit hyperactivity disorder: A handbook for diagnosis and treatment* (3rd ed.). New York: Guilford Press.

Barkley, R. A. (2012). *Executive functions: What they are, how they work, and why they evolved*. New York: Guilford Press.

Barkley, R. A., & Fischer, M. (2011). Predicting impairment in major life activities and occupational functioning in hyperactive children as adults: Self-reported executive function (EF) deficits versus EF tests. *Developmental Neuropsychology, 36*, 137–161.

Barkley, R. A., Fischer, M., Smallish, L., & Fletcher, K. (2006). Young adult outcome of hyperactive children: Adaptive functioning in major life activities. *Journal of the American Academy of Child and Adolescent Psychiatry, 45*(2), 192–202.

Barkley, R. A., & Murphy, K. R. (2011). The nature of executive function (EF) deficits in daily life activities in adults with ADHD and their relationship to performance on EF tests. *Journal of Psychopathology and Behavioral Assessment, 33*, 137–158.

Bernardi, S., Faraone, S. V., Cortese, S., Kerridge, B. T., Pallanti, S., Wang, S., et al. (2012). The lifetime impact of attention deficit hyperactivity disorder: Results from the National Epidemiologic Survey on Alcohol and Related Conditions (NESARC). *Psychological Medicine, 47*, 875–884.

Biederman, J. (2005). Attention-deficit/hyperactivity disorder: A selective overview. *Biological Psychiatry, 57*(11), 1215–1220.

Castellanos, F. X., Sonuga-Barke, E. J. S., Milham, M. P., & Tannock, R. (2006). Characterising cognition in ADHD: Beyond executive dysfunction. *Trends in Cognitive Science, 10*, 117–123.

Clemons, T. L. (2008). *Underachieving gifted students: A social cognitive model*. Storrs, CT: National Research Center on the Gifted and Talented.

Conners, C. K. (2008). *Conners 3rd Edition: Technical manual*. North Tonawanda, NY: Multi-Health Systems.

Connor, D. F., Steeber, J., & McBurnett, K. (2010). A review of attention-deficit/hyperactivity disorder complicated by symptoms of oppositional defiant disorder and conduct disorder. *Journal of Developmental and Behavioral Pediatrics, 31*(5), 427–440.

Currie, D., Lee, D. L., & Scheeler, M. C. (2005). Using PDAs to increase the homework completion of students with ADHD. *Journal of Evidence-Based Practices for Schools, 6*(2), 151–162.

Diamantopoulou, S., Rydell, A., Thorell, L. B., & Bohlin, G. (2007). Impact of executive functioning and symptoms of attention deficit hyperactivity disorder on children's peer relations and school performance. *Developmental Neuropsychology, 32*(1), 521–542.

Dorminy, K. P., Luscre, D., & Gast, D. L. (2009). Teaching organizational skills to children with high functioning autism and Asperger's syndrome. *Education and Training in Developmental Disabilities, 44*(4), 538–550.

Doshi, J. A., Hodgkins, P., Kahle, J., Sikirica, V., Cangelosi, M. J., Setyawan, J., et al. (2012). Economic impact of childhood and adult attention-deficit/hyperactivity disorder in the United States. *Journal of the American Academy of Child and Adolescent Psychiatry, 51*, 990–1002.

DuPaul, G. J. (2006). Academic achievement in children with ADHD. *Journal of the American Academy of Child and Adolescent Psychiatry, 45*(7), 766.

DuPaul, G. J., & Stoner, G. (2003). *ADHD in the schools: Assessment and intervention strategies* (2nd ed.). New York: Guilford Press.

Eisenberg, D., & Schneider, H. (2007). Perceptions of academic skills of children diagnosed with ADHD. *Journal of Attention Disorders, 10*, 390–397.

Faraone, S. V., & Doyle, A. E. (2001). The nature and heritability of attention-deficit/hyperactivity disorder. *Child and Adolescent Psychiatric Clinics of North America, 10*(2), 299–316.

Gallagher, R., Fleary, S., & Abikoff, H. (2007, November). *The Children's Organizational Skills Scales (COSS): Parent and teacher ratings in children with ADHD and typical development on organization, time management, and planning behaviors*. Poster presented at the annual meeting of the Association for Behavioral and Cognitive Therapies, Philadelphia.

Germano, E., Gagliano, A., & Curatolo, P. (2010). Comorbidity of ADHD and dyslexia. *Developmental Neuropsychology, 35*(5),475–493.

Gioia, G. A., Isquith, P. K., Guy, S. C., & Kenworthy, L. (2000). *Behavior Rating Inventory of Executive Function*. Odessa, FL: Psychological Assessment Resources.

Gureasko-Moore, S., DuPaul, G. J., & White, G. P. (2006). The effects of self-management in general education classrooms on the organizational skills of adolescents with ADHD. *Behavior Modification, 30*(2), 159–183.

Gureasko-Moore, S., DuPaul, G. J., & White, G. P. (2007). Self-management of classroom preparedness and homework: Effects on school functioning of adolescents with attention deficit hyperactivity disorder. *School Psychology Review, 36*(4), 647–664.

Hinshaw, S. P. (1992). Academic underachievement, attention deficits, and aggression: Comorbidity and implications for intervention. *Journal of Consulting and Clinical Psychology, 60,* 893–903.

Hinshaw, S. P., Klein, R. G., & Abikoff, H. (2007). Childhood attention-deficit/hyperactivity disorder: Nonpharmacologic treatments and their combination with medication. In P. E. Nathan & J. M. Gorman (Eds.), *A guide to treatments that work* (3rd ed., pp. 3–27). New York: Oxford University Press.

Kaufman, J., Birmaher, B., Brent, D., Rao, U., Flynn, C., Moreci, P., et al. (1997). Schedule for Affective Disorders and Schizophrenia for School-Age Children—Present and Lifetime Version (K-SADS-PL): Initial reliability and validity data. *Journal of the American Academy of Child and Adolescent Psychiatry, 36*(7), 980–988.

Kos, J. M., Richdale, A. L., & Hay, D. A. (2006). Children with attention deficit hyperactivity disorder and their teachers: A review of the literature. *International Journal of Disability, Development and Education, 53*(2), 147–160.

Langberg, J. M., Epstein, J. N., Becker, S. P., Girio-Herrera, E., & Vaughn, A. J. (2012). Evaluation of the Homework, Organization, and Planning Skills (HOPS) intervention for middle school students with attention deficit hyperactivity disorder as implemented by school mental health providers. *School Psychology Review, 41,* 342–364.

Langberg, J. M., Molina, B. S. G., Arnold, L. E., Epstein, J. N., Altaye, M., Hinshaw, S. P., et al. (2011). Patterns and predictors of adolescent academic achievement and performance in a sample of children with attention/deficit hyperactivity disorder (ADHD). *Journal of Clinical Child and Adolescent Psychology, 40,* 519–531.

Leroux, J. A., & Levitt-Perlman, M. (2000). The gifted child with attention deficit disorder: An identification and intervention challenge. *Roeper Review, 22*(3), 171–176.

Martinussen, R., Hayden, J., Hogg-Johnson, S., & Tannock, R. (2005). A meta-analysis of working memory impairments in children with attention-deficit hyperactivity disorder. *Journal of the American Academy of Child and Adolescent Psychiatry, 44,* 377–384.

Mikami, A. M. (2010). The importance of friendship for youth with attention-deficit/hyperactivity disorder. *Clinical Child and Family Psychology Review, 13,* 181–198.

Minde, K., Eakin, L., Hechtman, L., Ochs, E., Bouffard, R., Greenfield, B., et al. (2003). The psychosocial functioning of children and spouses of adults with ADHD. *Journal of Child Psychology and Psychiatry, 44*(4), 637–646.

MTA Cooperative Group. (1999). A 14-month randomized clinical trial of treatment strategies for attention-deficit/hyperactivity disorder. *Archives of General Psychiatry, 56,* 1073–1086.

Naglieri, J. A., & Goldstein, S. (2012). *comprehensive Executive Function Inventory.* North Tonawanda, NY: Multi-Health Systems.

Pennington, B. F., & Ozonoff, S. (1996). Executive functions and developmental psychopathology. *Journal of Child Psychology and Psychiatry, 37,* 51–87.

Pliszka, S., & Workgroup on Quality Issues. (2007). Practice parameters for the assessment and treatment of children and adolescents with attention-deficit/hyperactivity disorder. *Journal of the American Academy of Child and Adolescent Psychiatry, 46*(7), 894–921.

Power, T. J., Karustis, J. L., & Habboushe, D. F. (2001). *Homework success for children with ADHD: A family-school intervention program.* New York: Guilford Press.

Power, T. J., Mautone, J. A., Soffer, S. L., Clarke, A. T., Marshall, S. A., Sharman, J., et al. (2012). A family–school intervention for children with ADHD: Results of a randomized clinical trial. *Journal of Consulting and Clinical Psychology, 80*(4), 611–623.

Power, T. J., Werba, B. E., Watkins, M. W., Angelucci, J. G., & Eiraldi, R. B. (2006). Patterns of parent-reported homework problems among ADHD-referred and non-referred children. *School Psychology Quarterly, 21,* 13–33.

Raggi, V. L., & Chronis, A. M. (2006). Interventions to address the academic impairment of children and adolescents with ADHD. *Clinical Child and Family Psychology Review, 9*(2), 85–111.

Reck, S. G., Hund, A. M., & Landau, S. (2010). Memory for object locations in boys with and without ADHD. *Journal of Attention Disorders, 13,* 505–515.

Ronk, M. J., Hund, A. M., & Landau, S. (2011). Assessment of social competence of boys with attention-deficit/hyperactivity disorder: Problematic peer entry, host responses, and evaluations. *Journal of Abnormal Child Psychology, 39*, 829–840.

Rutledge, K. J., van den Bos, W., McClure, S. M., & Schweitzer, J. B. (2012). Training cognition in ADHD: Current findings, borrowed concepts, and future directions. *Neurotherapeutics, 9*, 542–558.

Schaffer, D., Fisher, P., Lucas, C. P., Dulcan, M. K., & Schwab-Stone, M. E. (2000). NIMH Diagnostic Interview Schedule for Children Version IV (NIMH DISC-IV): Description, differences from previous versions, and reliability of some common diagnoses. *Journal of the American Academy of Child and Adolescent Psychiatry, 39*(1), 28–38.

Sexton, C. C., Gelhorn, H., Bell, J., & Classi, P. (2012). The co-occurrence of reading disorder and ADHD: Epidemiology, treatment, psychosocial impact, and economic burden. *Journal of Learning Disabilities, 45*(6), 538–564.

Solanto, M. V., Marks, D. J., Wasserstein, J., Mitchell, K., Abikoff, H., Alvir, J. M. J., et al. (2010). Efficacy of meta-cognitive therapy for adult ADHD. *American Journal of Psychiatry, 167*(8), 958–968.

Sonuga-Barke, E., Bitsakou, P., & Thompson, M. (2010). Beyond the dual pathway model: Evidence for the dissociation of timing, inhibitory, and delay-related impairments in attention-deficit/hyperactivity disorder. *Journal of the American Academy of Child and Adolescent Psychiatry, 49*, 345–355.

Subcommittee on Attention-Deficit/Hyperactivity Disorder, Steering Committee on Quality Improvement and Management. (2011). ADHD: Clinical practice guidelines for the diagnosis, evaluation, and treatment of attention-deficit/hyperactivity disorder in children and adolescents. *Pediatrics, 128*(5), 1007–1022.

Swanson, J. M. (1992). *School-based assessments and interventions for ADD students.* Irvine, CA: K. C. Publications.

Tallal, P. (2000). Experimental studies of language learning impairments: From research to remediation. In D. V. M. Bishop & L. B. Leonard (Eds.), *Speech and language impairments in children: Causes, characteristics, intervention, and outcomes* (pp. 131–155). Philadelphia: Taylor & Francis Group.

Tannock, R., Martinussen, R., & Frijters, J. (2000). Naming speed performance and stimulant effects indicate effortful, semantic processing deficits in attention-deficit/hyperactivity disorder. *Journal of Abnormal Child Psychology, 28*(3), 237–252.

Thorell, L. B. (2007). Do delay aversion and executive function deficits make distinct contributions to the functional impact of ADHD symptoms?: A study of early academic skill deficits. *Journal of Child Psychology and Psychiatry, 48*, 1061–1070.

Torralva, T., Gleichgerrcht, E., Lischinsky, A., Roca, M., & Manes, F. (2013). "Ecological" and highly demanding executive tasks detect real-life deficits in high-functioning adult ADHD patients. *Journal of Attention Disorders, 17*(1), 11–19.

Volkow, N. D., Wang, G. J., Kollins, S. H., Wigal, T. L., Newcorn, J. H., Telang, F., et al. (2009). Evaluating dopamine reward pathway in ADHD: Clinical implications. *Journal of the American Medical Association, 302*, 1084–1091.

Wells, K., Murray, D., Gallagher, R., & Abikoff, H. (2007). *PATHKO (Parents and Teachers Helping Kids Organize) manual.* Unpublished manual. Durham, NC: Duke University Medical Center.

Willcutt, E. G., Doyle, A. E., Nigg, J. T., Faraone, S. V., & Pennington, B. F. (2005). Validity of the executive function theory of attention-deficit/hyperactivity disorder: A meta-analytic review. *Biological Psychiatry, 57*, 1336–1346.

Woodward, L., Taylor, E., & Dowdney, L. (1998). The parenting and family functioning of children with hyperactivity. *Journal of Child Psychology and Psychiatry, 39*, 161–169.

Index

Accordion Binder Instructions (Handout 20), 97, 101, 102, 323
Accordion binders
  alternative procedures, 103–104
  explaining the use of to the teacher, 41
  in-session practice
    in using, 101–102
    in weeding out the binder, 110
  introducing to the child, 99–100
  reviewing use of, 42, 108, 116
  setting up the child's personal binder, 100–101
Analog clocks, 157–158
Anxiety disorders, 27, 28
Assessment
  child assessments
    for ADHD, 24
    for common comorbidities and their impact on providing OST, 27–29
    for OTMP difficulties, 25–27, 55–58
  of parent participation, 29–30
  of teacher participation, 30–31
Assignment and Test Calendar (Handout 11)
  conducting in-session practice, 89–90
  handout, 313
  reviewing, 98–99, 109, 116
  support the child in discussing, 93
  teaching the child to use, 89
  use in tracking assignments, 21, 71, 80, 83, 84
Attention-deficit/hyperactivity disorder (ADHD)
  assessment for, 24
  impact of parental ADHD on parent participation, 29–30
  providing information about ADHD to parents, 61–62

symptoms/functional difficulties during childhood, 4
  See also Children with ADHD
Autism spectrum disorder (ASD), 29

Backpack/Activity bag
  creating a new backpack checklist, 125, 127
  determining a routine for packing at home, 128
  discussing backpack organization, 125–126
  discussing items that must be packed in, 124
  discussing "other stuff" the child must pack for school, 124–125, 127
  in-session practice with packing, 126–127
Backpack checklist
  conducting a child interview on school materials, 116–117
  creating a new list with "other stuff," 125, 127
  creating a personalized checklist, 118
  demonstrating how to use, 117–118
  explaining the rationale for using, 117
  explaining to the teacher, 41
  in-session practice, 119
  reviewing for student use of, 42
Behavior management. *See* Implementing Behavior Management Procedures session
Behavior monitoring. *See* Monitoring
Behavior Rating Inventory of Executive Function (BRIEF), 25, 26

Calendars
  discussing with the child, 140–141
  helping the child develop a personal calendar, 141
  See also Assignment and Test Calendar; Personal Calendar; Understanding Time and Calendars session

401